Multidisciplinary Approach to Neurofibromatosis Type 1

Gianluca Tadini • Eric Legius • Hilde Brems
Editors

Multidisciplinary Approach to Neurofibromatosis Type 1

Springer

Editors
Gianluca Tadini
Center for Inherited Cutaneous Diseases
University of Milan
Milan
Milano
Italy

Hilde Brems
Department of Human Genetics
KU Leuven
Leuven
Belgium

Eric Legius
Center for Human Genetics
Universitaire Ziekenhuizen Leuven Center for Human Genetics
Leuven
Oost-Vlaanderen
Belgium

ISBN 978-3-319-92449-6 ISBN 978-3-319-92450-2 (eBook)
https://doi.org/10.1007/978-3-319-92450-2

This Springer imprint is published by the registered company Springer Nature Switzerland AG
The registered company address is: Gewerbestrasse 11, 6330 Cham, Switzerland

Foreword

This textbook represents a highly up-to-date resource for clinicians on the clinical aspects of neurofibromatosis type 1 (NF1). Virtually every clinician in any field of practice will at some time in his/her career be faced with the challenge of a patient with NF1. Many in certain specialties such as paediatrics and paediatric oncology will see many often as the first person to diagnose the condition in a given individual. For those for whom diagnosis and recommendations for management is their "bread and butter" such as clinical geneticists, this is a really useful handbook. As one of the more frequent rare disorders with a birth incidence reaching the very top end of the definition of "rare" (1 in 2000), a comprehensive book like this one is a great resource. It is written for clinicians by clinical and laboratory experts and contains an up-to-date review of the new revised diagnostic criteria as well as covering the manifestations across protean organ systems. Chapters range from specific chapters on ocular, bone and cancer manifestations to recommendations for management and surveillance. For those who want to delve further into the molecular mechanism of the disease, there are chapters on molecular diagnostics, the genomics of tumours and involvement of the RAS-MAPK pathway and genotype–phenotype correlations. Importantly, this book contains the rationale and process behind the recent changes to the diagnostic criteria. For a condition that until recently had no effective medical treatments, this book contains important up-to-date information on treatment with MEK inhibitors. An insight into the problems with learning and behaviour including the recently described autistic spectrum disorder within NF1 is well covered. Overall I would strongly recommend this book for those who have even slightly more than a passing acquaintance with NF1.

Manchester, UK — D. Gareth Evans, MD FRCP

Preface

Few textbooks are devoted to a single rare disease. This textbook is an example of a comprehensive compilation of clinical aspects of neurofibromatosis type 1 (NF1), one of the more frequent rare disorders. It is written for clinicians by clinical experts. Several other textbooks deal with the larger group of "neurofibromatoses", including neurofibromatosis type 1, neurofibromatosis type 2 (NF2) and schwannomatosis. It is obvious now that NF1 is very different from NF2 and schwannomatosis. NF1 can be easily distinguished clinically from NF2 and schwannomatosis. The two latter conditions are characterized by schwannomas and not by neurofibromas. This distinction will be reflected in an adaptation of the diagnostic criteria for this group of disorders. Conversely, a clear distinction between (mosaic) NF2 and schwannomatosis is frequently not possible without an extensive molecular diagnostic investigation, including molecular analysis of tumour tissue. Clinical examination in children without a family history of NF1 does not always allow to differentiate NF1 from other syndromes characterized by multiple café-au-lait spots such as Legius syndrome and constitutive mismatch repair syndrome. In this book, specific attention is given to the diagnostic algorithm in children with multiple café-au-lait macules, the limitations of the NIH diagnostic criteria and the importance of a correct molecular diagnosis.

NF1 is a genetic disorder that can affect many different organ systems both in children and adults, also influencing learning and behaviour. Scientific progress in many different disciplines has changed the care for individuals with NF1 substantially over the past years. Virtually every clinician will be confronted with patients (suspected of) having neurofibromatosis type 1. The book is quite unique in its kind because it covers clinical aspects of the different organ and body systems potentially affected in children and adults with NF1. It is illustrated with beautiful images of most clinical presentations and complications of the disease. NF1 is an autosomal dominant disease and the genetic, molecular diagnostic and reproductive aspects relevant for the clinician are well covered. The chapter on molecular diagnosis is also dealing with specific NF1 mutations that are associated with a higher risk for certain complications. This emerging genotype–phenotype correlation can be of value for the personalized medical follow-up in an increasing number of NF1 individuals. Molecular diagnosis of mosaic NF1 poses specific challenges for the diagnostic lab because it is not straightforward to obtain affected cells from biopsies for a proper molecular diagnosis. Nevertheless, it might be important to provide a patient with a mosaic presentation of NF1 with the proper reproductive options. The diagnosis and treatment of nervous system and non-nervous system tumours are reported for both benign and malignant tumours. The book integrates the monitoring, diagnosis and potential treatments of NF1-related phenotypes. The *NF1* gene is a tumour suppressor gene but many non-tumoral phenotypes can be present in NF1 individuals and these are covered in specific chapters dealing with potential skeletal, pigmentation, learning and behavioural problems.

Recent literature has shed light on the natural history of NF1 in children and adults. Research on tissues from NF1 patients and in animal model systems has unravelled many of the biological mechanisms underlying complications of the disease. We are better in recognizing individuals at high risk for specific complications. We have learned how to monitor for a specific complication and when to treat or not to treat. The increased knowledge on the importance of aberrant RAS-MAPK pathway signalling for neurofibroma development resulted for the first time in significant "targeted treatments" for plexiform neurofibromas using MEK inhibitors, some of which are being introduced in clinical practice at the moment. There is no doubt that we will witness an increasing number of new therapeutic approaches in the near future. A specific chapter on therapeutic approaches in NF1 was a high priority.

NF1 belongs to a group of genetic diseases resulting from a constitutive deranged RAS-MAPK pathway signalling. This group of diseases is referred to as "the RASopathies". A specific chapter deals with the clinical overlap with NF1 and the increased risk for specific tumours and leukaemias in the group of RASopathies. The book ends with specific suggestions to update the current NIH diagnostic criteria.

We wish to thank Springer Nature for facilitating the publication of "Multidisciplinary Approach to Neurofibromatosis type 1", and all the expert authors who spent their valuable time contributing to this book.

Milan, Italy Gianluca Tadini
Leuven, Belgium Eric Legius
Leuven, Belgium Hilde Brems

Acknowledgements

We would like to dedicate this book to the patients, their families and patient support groups.

We also acknowledge colleagues from all over the world who have provided us with their deep knowledge, summarized in this volume, a job lasting over 2 years.

Contents

Epidemiology of Neurofibromatosis Type 1

1

Lidia Pezzani and Donatella Milani

Content

Neurofibromatosis type 1 (NF1, OMIM #162200) is one of the most frequent Mendelian diseases, and the majority of the epidemiological studies report a prevalence that range from 1/3000 to 1/6000, while incidence varies between 1/2558 and 1/3333 live births [1–4]. No significant difference in prevalence is reported due to ethnicity [5–9]. NF1 is characterized by an autosomal dominant transmission and by a complete penetrance, but the clinical expression of the disease may be extremely variable, and a very mild presentation is possible, leading to hypothetical underdiagnosis. Furthermore, its diagnosis is currently still based on the very specific clinical criteria encoded by National Institute of Health Consensus Conference statement in 1988 [10], that are however not so sensitive because the onset of many features is age dependent, and some of them are not present in early infancy, thus leading to a delayed or missed diagnosis [11]. It has been anyhow observed that about 95% of NF1 patients meet the current diagnostic criteria by the age of 8 years, while all do so by the age of 20 years [12]. Some more recent studies hypothesized that the real incidence rate of the disease is higher; the enhanced efficacy to make a diagnosis of the last decades thanks to the diagnostic criteria and to genetic tests seems indeed to shift the rate closer to 1/2000 live births [13].

L. Pezzani · D. Milani (✉)
Department of Pathophysiology and Transplantation, Fondazione IRCCS Ca' Granda Ospedale Maggiore Policlinico di Milano, Pediatric Highly Intensive Care Unit, Milan, Italy
e-mail: lidiapezzani@yahoo.it; donatella.milani@policlinico.mi.it

G. Tadini et al. (eds.), *Multidisciplinary Approach to Neurofibromatosis Type 1*,
https://doi.org/10.1007/978-3-319-92450-2_1

In half of the cases, NF1 is inherited, while in the other half, it arises from a de novo mutation with a prevalence of *NF1* mutations of paternal origin [14]. Moreover, in some studies higher paternal age has been found in NF1 de novo cases [15–18].

Several studies have shown excess of mortality of NF1 patients compared with the general population and a high proportion of deaths caused by NF1 serious complications which could affect diverse body systems, in particular vasculopathy and malignant tumors (frequently malignancy of peripheral and central nerve tissue [19–22]). However, given that NF1 has a variety of clinical manifestations and complications of varying degrees of severity, it may not be recorded as the official cause of death, so information on NF1-associated mortality is limited [23].

Mortality in NF1 patients seems anyway to dramatically increase from adolescence to 40 years of age, with one third of the deaths occurring before 40 years; after 40 years, the mortality decreases until 50 years of age and then shows a constant increase in older ages, with the highest absolute number of deaths among 70–74 years old [23]. So, most of the mortality excess in NF1 is noticed before 50 years of age and NF1 contributes only for a small minority of deaths after that age. Therefore individuals living beyond 50 years without a serious NF1 complication could expect to live a near normal life expectancy [22].

Moreover, the gender difference in age at death was smaller among persons with NF1 compared to the general population, suggesting this life-threatening disease is more deleterious to women than to men or that NF1 is more likely to be reported on the death certificates of young women. Some studies have shown that women with NF1 have a higher risk of malignancies than males, and the difference was accounted for, almost entirely, by the newly identified association between NF1 and breast cancer [24, 25].

In conclusion, NF1 incidence rate seems to be higher than previously expected. It is worth noting that in the next years the widespread availability and the easier access to genetic tests of new generation (NGS) [26] maybe will cause further rise of this rate due to the decrease of delayed or missed diagnosis, thanks to a more precocious diagnosis in patients with paucisymptomatic forms (early infancy, segmental forms) and to an easier differential diagnosis with other Rasopathies [27] or other similar conditions.

References

1. Huson SM, Compston DA, Clark P, Harper PS. A genetic study of von Recklinghausen neurofibromatosis in south East Wales. I. Prevalence, fitness, mutation rate, and effect of parental transmission on severity. J Med Genet. 1989;26(11):704–11.
2. Poyhonen M, Kytölä S, Leisti J. Epidemiology of neurofibromatosis type 1 (NF1) in northern Finland. J Med Genet. 2000;37:632–6.
3. Lammert M, Friedman JM, Kluwe L, Mautner VF. Prevalence of neurofibromatosis 1 in German children at elementary school enrollment. Arch Dermatol. 2005;141(1):71–4.
4. Evans DG, Howard E, Giblin C, Clancy T, Spencer H, Huson SM, Lalloo F. Birth incidence and prevalence of tumor-prone syndromes: estimates from a UK family genetic register service. Am J Med Genet A. 2010;152A:327–32.

5. Niimura M. Neurofibromatosis in Japan. In: Ishibashi Y, Hori Y, editors. Tuberous sclerosis and neurofibromatosis: epidemiology, pathophysiology, biology, and management. Amsterdam: Elsevier; 1990. p. 23–31.
6. Wong VC. Clinical manifestations of neurofibromatosis-1 in Chinese children. Pediatr Neurol. 1994;11:301–7.
7. Friedman JM, Birch PH. Type 1 neurofibromatosis: a descriptive analysis of the disorder in 1,728 patients. Am J Med Genet. 1997;70:138–43.
8. Poyhonen M, Niemela S, Herva R. Risk of malignancy and death in neurofibromatosis. Arch Pathol Lab Med. 1997;121:139–43.
9. Cnossen MH, de Goede-Bolder A, van den Broek KM, Waasdorp CM, Oranje AP, Stroink H, Simonsz HJ, van den Ouweland AM, Halley DJ, Niermeijer MF. A prospective 10 year follow up study of patients with neurofibromatosis type 1. Arch Dis Child. 1998;78(5):408–12.
10. National Institutes of Health Consensus Development Conference Statement: neurofibromatosis. Bethesda, Md., USA, July 13–15, 1987. Neurofibromatosis. 1988;1(3):172–8.
11. Tadini G, Milani D, Menni F, Pezzani L, Sabatini C, Esposito S. Is it time to change the neurofibromatosis 1 diagnostic criteria? Eur J Intern Med. 2014;25(6):506–10.
12. DeBella K, Szudek J, Friedman JM. Use of the national institutes of health criteria for diagnosis of neurofibromatosis 1 in children. Pediatrics. 2000;105:608–14.
13. Uusitalo E, Leppävirta J, Koffert A, Suominen S, Vahtera J, Vahlberg T, Pöyhönen M, Peltonen J, Peltonen S. Incidence and mortality of neurofibromatosis: a total population study in Finland. J Invest Dermatol. 2015;135(3):904–6.
14. Kong A, Frigge ML, Masson G, Besenbacher S, Sulem P, Magnusson G, Gudjonsson SA, Sigurdsson A, Jonasdottir A, Jonasdottir A, Wong WS, Sigurdsson G, Walters GB, Steinberg S, Helgason H, Thorleifsson G, Gudbjartsson DF, Helgason A, Magnusson OT, Thorsteinsdottir U, Stefansson K. Rate of de novo mutations and the importance of father's age to disease risk. Nature. 2012;488(7412):471–5.
15. Takano T, Kawashima T, Yamanouchi Y, Kitayama K, Baba T, Ueno K, Hamaguchi H. Genetics of neurofibromatosis 1 in Japan: mutation rate and paternal age effect. Hum Genet. 1992;89(3):281–6.
16. Bunin GR, Needle M, Riccardi VM. Paternal age and sporadic neurofibromatosis 1: a case-control study and consideration of the methodologic issues. Genet Epidemiol. 1997;14(5):507–16.
17. Liu Q, Zoellner N, Gutmann DH, Johnson KJ. Parental age and Neurofibromatosis type 1: a report from the NF1 patient registry initiative. Familial Cancer. 2015 Jun;14(2):317–24.
18. Dubov T, Toledano-Alhadef H, Bokstein F, Constantini S, Ben-Shachar S. The effect of parental age on the presence of de novo mutations - lessons from neurofibromatosis type I. Mol Genet Genomic Med. 2016;4(4):480–6.
19. Friedman JM, Arbiser J, Epstein JA, Gutmann DH, Huot SJ, Lin AE, McManus B, Korf BR. Cardiovascular disease in neurofibromatosis 1: report of the NF1 Cardiovascular Task Force. Genet Med. 2002;4(3):105–11.
20. Evans DGR, Baser ME, McGaughran J, Sharif S, Howard E, Moran A. Malignant peripheral nerve sheath tumours in neurofibromatosis 1. J Med Genet. 2002 May;39(5):311–4.
21. Duong TA, Sbidian E, Valeyrie-Allanore L, Vialette C, Ferkal S, Hadj-Rabia S, Glorion C, Lyonnet S, Zerah M, Kemlin I, Rodriguez D, Bastuji-Garin S, Wolkenstein P. Mortality associated with neurofibromatosis 1: a cohort study of 1895 patients in 1980-2006 in France. Orphanet J Rare Dis. 2011;6:18.
22. Evans DG, O'Hara C, Wilding A, Ingham SL, Howard E, Dawson J, Moran A, Scott-Kitching V, Holt F, Huson SM. Mortality in neurofibromatosis 1: in north West England: an assessment of actuarial survival in a region of the UK since 1989. Eur J Hum Genet. 2011;19(11):1187–91.
23. Masocco M, Kodra Y, Vichi M, Conti S, Kanieff M, Pace M, Frova L, Taruscio D. Mortality associated with neurofibromatosis type 1: a study based on Italian death certificates (1995-2006). Orphanet J Rare Dis. 2011;6:11.
24. Walker L, Thompson D, Easton D, Ponder B, Ponder M, Frayling I, Baralle D. A prospective study of neurofibromatosis type 1 cancer incidence in the UK. Br J Cancer. 2006;95(2):233–8.

25. Sharif S, Moran A, Huson SM, Iddenden R, Shenton A, Howard E, Evans DG. Women with neurofibromatosis 1 are at a moderately increased risk of developing breast cancer and should be considered for early screening. J Med Genet. 2007;44(8):481–4.
26. Pasmant E, Parfait B, Luscan A, Goussard P, Briand-Suleau A, Laurendeau I, Fouveaut C, Leroy C, Montadert A, Wolkenstein P, Vidaud M, Vidaud D. Neurofibromatosis type 1 molecular diagnosis: what can NGS do for you when you have a large gene with loss of function mutations? Eur J Hum Genet. 2015 May;23(5):596–601.
27. Santoro C, Giugliano T, Melone MAB, Cirillo M, Schettino C, Bernardo P, Cirillo G, Perrotta S, Piluso G. Multiple spinal nerve enlargement and SOS1 mutation: further evidence of overlap between neurofibromatosis type 1 and Noonan phenotype. Clin Genet. 2017;93:138. [Epub ahead of print].

Genetics and Pathway in Neurofibromatosis Type 1

2

Ellen Denayer, Eric Legius, and Hilde Brems

Contents

Neurofibromatosis type 1 (NF1) is an autosomal dominant inherited disorder, characterized by typical clinical manifestations including multiple café-au-lait spots (CALs), skin fold freckling, Lisch nodules in the iris, optic pathway gliomas, and neurofibromas. The condition is caused by heterozygous inactivating germline mutations in the *NF1* gene located on chromosome band 17q11.2. In this chapter we will focus on the knowledge about the *NF1* gene, its encoded protein neurofibromin and the cellular pathways in which it is involved.

E. Denayer
Clinical Department of Human Genetics, KU Leuven-University of Leuven, University Hospitals Leuven, Leuven, Belgium
e-mail: ellen.denayer@uzleuven.be

E. Legius · H. Brems (✉)
Clinical Department of Human Genetics, KU Leuven-University of Leuven, University Hospitals Leuven, Leuven, Belgium

Department of Human Genetics, KU Leuven-University of Leuven, Leuven, Belgium
e-mail: eric.legius@uzleuven.be; hilde.brems@kuleuven.be

G. Tadini et al. (eds.), *Multidisciplinary Approach to Neurofibromatosis Type 1*,
https://doi.org/10.1007/978-3-319-92450-2_2

2.1 The NF1 Gene

The *NF1* gene was identified by positional cloning in 1990 showing mutations in individuals affected with NF1 [1–3]. *NF1* is located on chromosome band 17q11.2 and is composed of 61 exons. The *NF1* gene is a large gene spanning 350 kb of genomic DNA [4]. The processed full-length NF1 mRNA transcript is expressed in nearly all adult tissues and is about 11–13 kb in length [5]. The *NF1* gene contains at least 4 alternatively spliced exons which are expressed in a developmental and tissue-specific pattern: exons 9a, 10a-2, 23a, and 48a. These exons do not alter the reading frame [6–9].

The *NF1* gene has been recognized as a tumor suppressor gene by the finding of biallelic inactivation of *NF1* in the tumors like MPNSTs associated with NF1 [10]. This implies that apart from the germline *NF1* mutation, an additional somatic inactivation (mutation or loss) of the remaining wild-type *NF1* allele is needed to initiate tumor formation, following the Knudson two-hit hypothesis of tumor formation. In neurofibromas a second hit is found in the Schwann cells, the glial cells of the peripheral nervous system [11, 12]. Biallelic inactivation of the *NF1* gene was also shown in the tumor cells of pheochromocytomas [13], gastro-intestinal stromal tumors (GIST), a rare mesenchymal tumor of the gastro-intestinal tract, that occurs more often in patients with NF1 [14] as well as in glomus cells from glomus tumors. These are small, benign but painful tumors that originate from the glomus body, a thermoregulatory shunt in the fingers and toes [15]. Double inactivation of *NF1* is also present in other non-tumoral manifestations of NF1, e.g. in tibial pseudarthrosis [16] and in melanocytes of the CALs [17].

Different *NF1*-related sequences (pseudogenes) are distributed throughout the human genome. These *NF1* pseudogenes are believed to have arisen by duplication and transposition of the NF1 locus and are non-processed and non-functional [18, 19]. Three genes, *OMGP*, *EVI2A*, and *EVI2B* are embedded in *NF1* intron 27b and are transcribed in the opposite orientation [20, 21]. *OMGP* (oligodendrocyte-myelin glycoprotein) is a membrane glycoprotein expressed in the human central nervous system during myelinization and seems to operate as a cell adhesion molecule. It is an important inhibitor of fibroblast and neuron proliferation *in vitro*. The other two genes, *EVI2A* and *EVI2B* (ecotropic viral integration site), are human homologues of the murine *Evi-2A* and *Evi-2B*, which are involved in the development of leukemia in those animals.

2.2 Neurofibromin

The protein encoded by the *NF1* gene is neurofibromin. The *NF1* gene has a coding sequence of 8454 bp and the resulting neurofibromin contains 2818 amino acids. It has a molecular mass of 250–280 kDa [22, 23]. The protein is localized in the cytoplasm, but also nuclear localization has been reported [22–24]. Neurofibromin is ubiquitously expressed but has highest expression in neurons, Schwann cells, oligodendrocytes, and leukocytes [25].

The alternatively spliced exons are responsible for the production of different neurofibromin isoforms. Normal neurofibromin type I does not contain any of the insertions and is predominantly expressed in brain. Neurofibromin type II is the result of the insertion of exon 23a in the NF1-GRD, is expressed in Schwann cells, and has a reduced GAP activity [26]. Costa et al. showed that mice lacking this alternatively spliced exon 23a are viable and physically normal, and do not have an increased tumor predisposition, but show specific learning impairments. These findings implicated that the GAP domain of NF1 modulates learning and memory [27]. Neurofibromin type III contains exon 48a and neurofibromin type IV contains both exons 23a and exon 48a. These isoforms are mainly expressed in cardiac and muscle tissue. Neurofibromin IXa results from the inclusion of exon 9a and has limited neuronal expression. Neurofibromin Xa-2 with inclusion of exon 10a-2 is observed in the majority of human tissues.

Several animal models have been developed for studying the functions of neurofibromin. *Nf1* knockout (−/−) mice are embryonically lethal dying at 12–14 days of gestation due to cardiac defects [28]. *Nf1* heterozygous mice are viable. They have an increased predisposition for developing malignancies, but not neurofibromas, and they show learning difficulties. Using Cre-lox technology a mouse model was created in which the *Nf1* gene inactivated only in the stem cells that give rise to Schwann cells. A floxed *Nf1* allele was deleted by a Cre transgene under the control of the Schwann cell-specific promoter, Krox 20. These mice develop neurofibromas if heterozygous surrounding cells are present. This supports the idea that a micro-environment with *Nf1* heterozygous cells is important for neurofibroma formation [29]. Conditional knockout models with complete deletion of *Nf1* in neurons (Nf1Syn1) and glia (Nf1GFP) were used to study the contribution of these cell types to learning difficulties and tumor development, respectively [30, 31]. Multiple other animal models have been created depending on the research questions being asked and recently a minipig NF1 model mimicking the human NF1 condition.

The neurofibromin protein is highly conserved among species and is composed of different domains. The SEC14 domain is located at amino acids 1545–1816 [32]. Sec14 is found in secretory proteins and in lipid-regulated proteins, such as RhoGAPs and RhoGEFs. The RAS-GTPase (Guanosine TriPhosphatase) activating protein(GAP)-related domain (NF1-GRD) is the best studied functional domain of the *NF1* gene and corresponds to a small region located in the central region of the protein. This domain was recognized as showing significant similarity to the catalytic domain of yeast IRA1, IRA2 proteins, and the mammalian GTPase-Activating Proteins (GAPs). GAPs accelerate the hydrolysis of RAS-GTP to RAS-GDP, converting it from the active to the inactive form. The NF1-GRD spans approximately 60 amino acids and corresponds to exons 20–27a (residues 1125–1537) [33–35]. Its crystallographic structure (NF1–333, residues 1198–1530) was reported by Scheffzek et al. [36]. This NF1-GRD interacts with active RAS through binding of

RAS-GTP in a groove of this domain by residues including the switch regions I and II on RAS and an arginine finger on NF1. This interaction results in GAP-stimulated hydrolysis of GTP [37].

Sites flanking the GRD of neurofibromin bind to the EVH1 domain of SPRED1 and neurofibromin is recruited to the membrane by SPRED1. SPRED1 is attached to the membrane by its sprouty related domain (SPR). Once neurofibromin is recruited to the membrane it can bind and downregulated RAS-GTP [38–40]. *SPRED1* heterozygous inactivating mutations are known to be the cause of the autosomal dominant Legius syndrome which is also characterized by multiple café-au-lait spots (discussed in the chapter on Legius syndrome).

2.3 The RAS-MAPK Pathway

RAS proteins are small molecular weight proteins (21 kDa) that exist in three major isoforms: HRAS, KRAS, and NRAS. These three RAS-family members share 85% amino acid sequence identity. They are widely expressed, with *KRAS* being expressed in almost all cell types. *RAS* genes were first identified as homologues of rodent sarcoma virus genes. In 1982 human DNA sequences homologous to the transforming oncogenes of the v-Harvey (*HRAS)* and Kirsten (*KRAS*) rat sarcoma virus were identified in DNA sequences derived from a human bladder and a human lung cancer cell line, respectively [41]. RAS proteins control signaling pathways that are involved in cell proliferation, differentiation, and apoptosis. These proteins are covalently anchored to the plasma membrane by a farnesyl group and a palmitoyl group (except KRAS4b isoform) [42] and link cell surface receptors to intracellular effector pathways. RAS proteins are guanosine nucleotide-bound proteins which cycle between an inactive GDP-bound conformation and an active GTP- conformation that interacts with effector proteins in different downstream pathways. RAS proteins have a low intrinsic GTPase activity that is increased 10^5 times by GTP activating proteins (GAPs) such as p120–GAP and neurofibromin. Neurofibromin, by means of its NF1-GRD domain, increases the GTP hydrolysis rate and functions as a tumor suppressor by reducing the activity of RAS. On the other hand, the guanine nucleotide exchange factors (GEFs), such as SOS, perform the reverse path, reactivating RAS by promoting the exchange of GDP for GTP.

RAS can be activated through binding of a growth factor to a receptor tyrosine kinase such as the epidermal-growth-factor receptor (EGFR) or through other receptor types, such as the G-protein-coupled receptors. Binding of a growth factor to a receptor tyrosine kinase results in dimerization and autophosphorylation on tyrosine residues of the receptor, which then recruits and activates enzymes (e.g., the phosphatase SHP2), adaptors (e.g., GRB2), and docking proteins (e.g., GAB). Binding of the receptor to the SH2 domain of the adaptor protein GRB2 results in binding of GRB2 to SOS, through its SH3 domain, which is then recruited to the plasma membrane. SOS1 works as a GEF by displacing the Switch I and distorting the Switch II region of RAS leading to enhanced GDP release and rebinding of GTP and thus increased levels of active RAS-GTP. There are however variations on the

GRB2-SOS-RAS signaling mechanism with GRB2 recognizing other adaptor proteins (e.g., GAB2), and linking with yet other receptor tyrosine kinases.

Different downstream effector pathways of RAS exist such as the MAPK, PI3kinase/AKT, and Rho GTPase pathways and others [42]. The RAS-MAPK pathway is the best studied among these. In its active GTP-bound form RAS interacts with the RAF serine/threonine kinase (MAPKKK = MAPkinasekinasekinase). RAF proteins (ARAF, BRAF and CRAF or RAF1) are located in the cytosol in an autoinhibited inactive conformation, stabilized by a protein called 14-3-3. Membrane recruitment of RAF via RAS-GTP induces the release of 14-3-3 from the N-terminal binding site. Activated RAF phosphorylates and activates a second kinase named MAP kinase/ERK kinase (MEK or MAPKK = MAPkinasekinase). Active MEK (MEK1 or MEK2) phosphorylates a threonine and tyrosine residue on its substrate ERK (Extracellular signal-Regulated kinase or MAPK = MAPkinase). Active ERK phosphorylates a variety of targets, including other kinases, such as RSK (ribosomal S6 kinase), and transcription factors, such as ETS1, ETS2, JUN, FOS, ELK1, and cyclic adenosine monophosphate (cAMP) response element-binding protein (CREB), resulting in a change in the pattern of expression of genes involved in cell cycle, apoptosis, cell differentiation, or migration. Signaling through this pathway is terminated when RAS-GTP is hydrolyzed to RAS-GDP either by the intrinsic GTPase activity of RAS (slow), or by GTPase activating proteins, GAPs, such as neurofibromin or p120GAP, the protein product of *RASA1*. While it is now well-appreciated that this single linear pathway is an oversimplification of the complex RAS signaling network, this representation helps to understand the basis of the mechanisms of maintaining cellular RAS-signaling. For example different feedback mechanisms and different ERK scaffolding proteins and signaling modulators have been demonstrated to play critical roles in determining the strength and duration of RTK-mediated signaling. Moreover activation of RAS-MAPK signaling can occur at various intracellular compartments and not merely at the cell membrane [43].

Another effector of active RAS is PI3Kinase (PI3K), which phosphorylates the protein kinase B (Akt or PKB). Akt then phosphorylates and inactivates the TSC1-TSC2 complex. Mutations in *TSC1* or *TSC2* are found in tuberous sclerosis complex, an autosomal dominant condition characterized by intellectual disability, seizures, cardiac rhabdomyomas, specific skin lesions, benign hamartomas, and increased risk for malignancies. The inhibition of the TSC1-TSC2 complex by Akt leads to the activation of the GAP Rheb (RAS homology enriched in brain), which in turn activates mTOR (mechanistic Target OF Rapamycin). mTOR is an evolutionary conserved protein regulating cell proliferation and many cellular processes [44].

The RAS-MAPK pathway has been studied extensively in oncology, since somatic mutations in different components of the RAS-MAPK pathway are found in human tumors. Some (20–30%) human tumors have activating point mutations in *RAS*, the prevalence being the highest in adenocarcinoma of the pancreas (90%), colon (50%), thyroid (50%), lung (30%), and melanoma (25%) [45]. Mutations are found most frequently in *KRAS* (about 85% of total), less in *NRAS* (about 15%), and rarely in *HRAS* (less than 1%).

Somatic mutation hotspots in *RAS* genes are located in amino acids G12, G13, and Q61. The key biochemical defect of mutant RAS proteins is GAP insensitivity, resulting in impaired intrinsic GTP hydrolysis of RAS as well as impaired GAP-stimulated GTP hydrolysis. This results in persistent accumulation of constitutive active GTP-bound RAS and constitutive activation of downstream effectors such as the MAPK pathway [46], leading to deregulation of cell growth, programmed cell death and invasiveness, and the ability for neo-angiogenesis. RAS signaling pathways are also active in tumors in which growth-factor-receptor tyrosine kinases have been overexpressed, such as *EGFR* and *ERBB2* (also known as *HER2/neu*) in breast, ovarian, and stomach carcinomas [47].

A statistical evaluation of the combined prevalence of somatic mutations and copy number alterations in human cancers confirmed RTK signaling and the RAS/MAPK pathway to be one of the most significantly altered pathways, across all cancer types, except for prostate [48]. This study also identified the *NF1* gene as one of the genes mutated frequently in different human cancer types.

Following the extensive amount of research on the importance in tumor formation of somatic mutations in genes of the RAS-MAPK pathway, and on the *NF1* gene as a cause of NF1, germline mutations in different other genes of this pathway were found in patients with partly overlapping phenotypes including variable degrees of developmental delay/intellectual disability, cardiac involvement, facial dysmorphism, cutaneous manifestations, and increased risk for malignancies. Costello syndrome is a rare sporadic occurring disorder presenting with high birth weight followed by feeding problems and subsequent failure to thrive, coarse facial features, cardiac abnormalities, intellectual disability, and predisposition for malignancy. The tumor risk in patients with Costello syndrome is about 15% by age 20 years, with the most frequently found tumor type being rhabdomyosarcoma, followed by neuroblastoma and bladder cancer [49]. Costello syndrome is caused by germline mutations in *HRAS*. Germline mutations in *PTPN11*, encoding SHP2, a regulator of RAS signaling, as well as in *KRAS*, *NRAS*, *SOS1*, *BRAF*, *RAF1* and in *SHOC2*, *RIT1*, *CBL*, and *LZTR1* are found in Noonan syndrome, with a lower incidence of malignancy, estimated about 4% by age 20. Interestingly the mutational hotspots for somatic mutations in *KRAS* do not coincide with germline mutations in Noonan syndrome. This probably reflects the important role of KRAS during embryogenesis, as it is believed that the strongly activating mutations that are found in cancer would not be tolerated in the germline and would result in embryonic lethality. A comprehensive review of this group of disorders that is now referred to as the RASopathies will be given in chapter on RASopathies.

RAS and its downstream effectors have also been extensively studied for their involvement in neuronal processes such as learning, memory, and synaptic plasticity. Dasgupta et al. demonstrated that reduced (Nf1+/−) and absent (Nf1−/−) expression in neural stem/progenitor cells results in a substantially increased cell proliferation in vitro in a dose-dependent manner and Nf1−/− cells harbor abnormalities in cell differentiation and survival advantage over wild-type cells. This effect reflected impaired RAS regulation. These findings supported the hypothesis that alterations in neurofibromin expression in the developing brain have significant consequences for astrocyte growth and differentiation relevant to normal brain development and astrocytoma formation in children [50]. Learning difficulties are recognized in patients with NF1 and are present in *Nf1* deficient (Nf1+/−) mice. The learning difficulties in *Nf1*+/− mice have been explained by an increased GABA-mediated inhibition. GABA (gamma-aminobutyric acid) acts as an inhibitory transmitter in the hippocampus, a region in the brain that is implicated in memory formation. Costa et al. and Li et al. showed that learning deficits in *Nf*1+/− mice can be reversed by genetic or pharmacologic manipulation of RAS activity or by GABA antagonist receptors, pointing to the fact that correct modulation of RAS is essential for learning and memory [51, 52].

2.4 Other Pathways in Which Neurofibromin Is Involved

Another pathway in which neurofibromin involved is the cAMP pathway by regulation of adenylyl cyclase (AC) activity, which has been studied in Drosophila [53, 54]. In this cAMP pathway activation of the Gα subunit of G-protein coupled receptors stimulates, upon ligand binding, the enzyme AC that synthesizes cyclic AMP (cAMP) from ATP. cAMP then activates protein kinase A (PKA), which in turn phosphorylates target proteins involved in a wide range of biological processes. The NF1-regulated AC/cAMP pathway has been shown to be involved in controlling body size [54], the regulation of the cellular response to the neuropeptide PACAP38 (pituitary adenylyl cyclase-activating polypeptide) at the neuromuscular junction [53] and learning and short-term memory [55]. Also in mice *Nf1*-dependent regulation of AC activity has been shown [56]. Hannan et al. demonstrated that sequences in the C-terminal region of NF1 are sufficient for *Nf1* AC activity, and for rescue of body size defects in *Nf1* mutant flies [57].

Defective cAMP generation was shown to underly the sensitivity of CNS neurons in *Nf1* heterozygous mice [58]. However neurofibromin regulation of cAMP requires RAS activation in human and mouse neurons through the activation of atypical protein kinase C ζ, leading to GRK2-driven $G\alpha_s$ inactivation. These findings reveal a novel mechanism by which RAS can regulate cAMP levels in the mammalian brain [59].

Neurofibromin has also been associated with microtubules and specific *NF1* mutations interrupt the association of neurofibromin with the microtubules [60].

References

1. Cawthon RM, Weiss R, Xu GF, Viskochil D, Culver M, Stevens J, Robertson M, Dunn D, Gesteland R, O'Connell P, White R. A major segment of the neurofibromatosis type 1 gene: cDNA sequence, genomic structure, and point mutations. Cell. 1990;62(1): 193–201.
2. Viskochil D, Buchberg AM, Xu G, Cawthon RM, Stevens J, Wolff RK, Culver M, Carey JC, Copeland NG, Jenkins NA, et al. Deletions and a translocation interrupt a cloned gene at the neurofibromatosis type 1 locus. Cell. 1990;62(1):187–92.

3. Wallace MR, Marchuk DA, Andersen LB, Letcher R, Odeh HM, Saulino AM, Fountain JW, Brereton A, Nicholson J, Mitchell AL, et al. Type 1 neurofibromatosis gene: identification of a large transcript disrupted in three NF1 patients. Science. 1990;249(4965):181–6.
4. Li Y, O'Connell P, Breidenbach HH, Cawthon R, Stevens J, Xu G, Neil S, Robertson M, White R, Viskochil D. Genomic organization of the neurofibromatosis 1 gene (NF1). Genomics. 1995;25(1):9–18.
5. Marchuk DA, Saulino AM, Tavakkol R, Swaroop M, Wallace MR, Andersen LB, Mitchell AL, Gutmann DH, Boguski M, Collins FS. cDNA cloning of the type 1 neurofibromatosis gene: complete sequence of the NF1 gene product. Genomics. 1991;11(4):931–40.
6. Gutmann DH, Geist RT, Rose K, Wright DE. Expression of two new protein isoforms of the neurofibromatosis type 1 gene product, neurofibromin, in muscle tissues. Dev Dyn. 1995;202(3):302–11.
7. Gutmann DH, Geist RT, Wright DE, Snider WD. Expression of the neurofibromatosis 1 (NF1) isoforms in developing and adult rat tissues. Cell Growth Differ. 1995;6(3):315–23.
8. Nishi T, Lee PS, Oka K, Levin VA, Tanase S, Morino Y, Saya H. Differential expression of two types of the neurofibromatosis type 1 (NF1) gene transcripts related to neuronal differentiation. Oncogene. 1991;6(9):1555–9.
9. Vandenbroucke I, Vandesompele J, De Paepe A, Messiaen L. Quantification of NF1 transcripts reveals novel highly expressed splice variants. FEBS Lett. 2002;522(1–3):71–6.
10. Legius E, Marchuk DA, Collins FS, Glover TW. Somatic deletion of the neurofibromatosis type 1 gene in a neurofibrosarcoma supports a tumour suppressor gene hypothesis. Nat Genet. 1993;3:122–6.
11. Kluwe L, Friedrich R, Mautner VF. Loss of NF1 allele in Schwann cells but not in fibroblasts derived from an NF1-associated neurofibroma. Genes Chromosomes Cancer. 1999;24(3):283–5.
12. Serra E, Rosenbaum T, Winner U, Aledo R, Ars E, Estivill X, Lenard HG, Lázaro C. Mutations affecting mRNA splicing are the most common molecular defects in patients with neurofibromatosis type 1. Hum Mol Genet. 2000;9(20):3055–64.
13. Xu W, Mulligan LM, Ponder MA, Liu L, Smith BA, Mathew CG, Ponder BA. Loss of NF1 alleles in phaeochromocytomas from patients with type I neurofibromatosis. Genes Chromosomes Cancer. 1992;4(4):337–42.
14. Maertens O, Prenen H, Debiec-Rychter M, Wozniak A, Sciot R, Pauwels P, De Wever I, Vermeesch JR, de Raedt T, De Paepe A, Speleman F, van Oosterom A, Messiaen L, Legius E. Molecular pathogenesis of multiple gastrointestinal stromal tumors in NF1 patients. Hum Mol Genet. 2006;15(6):1015–23.
15. Brems H, Park C, Maertens O, Pemov A, Messiaen L, Upadhyaya M, Claes K, Beert E, Peeters K, Mautner V, Sloan JL, Yao L, Lee CC, Sciot R, De Smet L, Legius E, Stewart DR. Glomus tumors in neurofibromatosis type 1: genetic, functional, and clinical evidence of a novel association. Cancer Res. 2009;69(18):7393–401.
16. Stevenson DA, Zhou H, Ashrafi S, Messiaen LM, Carey JC, D'Astous JL, Santora SD, Viskochil DH. Double inactivation of NF1 in tibial pseudarthrosis. Am J Hum Genet. 2006;79(1):143–8.
17. De Schepper S, Maertens O, Callens T, Naeyaert JM, Lambert J, Messiaen L. Somatic mutation analysis in NF1 café au lait spots reveals two NF1 hits in the melanocytes. J Invest Dermatol. 2008;128(4):1050–3.
18. Luijten M, Wang Y, Smith BT, Westerveld A, Smink LJ, Dunham I, Roe BA, Hulsebos TJ. Mechanism of spreading of the highly related neurofibromatosis type 1 (NF1) pseudogenes on chromosomes 2, 14 and 22. Eur J Hum Genet. 2000;8(3):209–14.
19. Luijten M, Redeker S, Minoshima S, Shimizu N, Westerveld A, Hulsebos TJ. Duplication and transposition of the NF1 pseudogene regions on chromosomes 2, 14, and 22. Hum Genet. 2001;109(1):109–16.
20. Cawthon RM, Andersen LB, Buchberg AM, Xu GF, O'Connell P, Viskochil D, Weiss RB, Wallace MR, Marchuk DA, Culver M, et al. cDNA sequence and genomic structure of EV12B, a gene lying within an intron of the neurofibromatosis type 1 gene. Genomics. 1991;9(3):446–60.

21. Viskochil D, Cawthon R, O'Connell P, Xu GF, Stevens J, Culver M, Carey J, White R. The gene encoding the oligodendrocyte-myelin glycoprotein is embedded within the neurofibromatosis type 1 gene. Mol Cell Biol. 1991;11(2):906–12.
22. DeClue JE, Cohen BD, Lowy DR. Identification and characterization of the neurofibromatosis type 1 protein product. Proc Natl Acad Sci U S A. 1991;88(22):9914–8.
23. Gutmann DH, Wood DL, Collins FS. Identification of the neurofibromatosis type 1 gene product. Proc Natl Acad Sci U S A. 1991;88(21):9658–62.
24. Vandenbroucke I, Van Oostveldt P, Coene E, De Paepe A, Messiaen L. Neurofibromin is actively transported to the nucleus. FEBS Lett. 2004;560(1–3):98–102.
25. Daston MM, Scrable H, Nordlund M, Sturbaum AK, Nissen LM, Ratner N. The protein product of the neurofibromatosis type 1 gene is expressed at highest abundance in neurons, Schwann cells, and oligodendrocytes. Neuron. 1992;8(3):415–28.
26. Andersen LB, Ballester R, Marchuk DA, Chang E, Gutmann DH, Saulino AM, Camonis J, Wigler M, Collins FS. A conserved alternative splice in the von Recklinghausen neurofibromatosis (NF1) gene produces two neurofibromin isoforms, both of which have GTPase-activating protein activity. Mol Cell Biol. 1993;13(1):487–95.
27. Costa RM, Yang T, Huynh DP, Pulst SM, Viskochil DH, Silva AJ, Brannan CI. Learning deficits, but normal development and tumor predisposition, in mice lacking exon 23a of Nf1. Nat Genet. 2001;27(4):399–405.
28. Brannan CI, Perkins AS, Vogel KS, Ratner N, Nordlund ML, Reid SW, Buchberg AM, Jenkins NA, Parada LF, Copeland NG. Targeted disruption of the neurofibromatosis type-1 gene leads to developmental abnormalities in heart and various neural crest-derived tissues. Genes Dev. 1994;8(9):1019–29.
29. Zhu Y, Ghosh P, Charnay P, Burns DK, Parada LF. Neurofibromas in NF1: Schwann cell origin and role of tumor environment. Science. 2002;296(5569):920–2.
30. Bajenaru ML, Zhu Y, Hedrick NM, Donahoe J, Parada LF, Gutmann DH. Astrocyte-specific inactivation of the neurofibromatosis 1 gene (NF1) is insufficient for astrocytoma formation. Mol Cell Biol. 2002;22(14):5100–13.
31. Zhu Y, Romero MI, Ghosh P, Ye Z, Charnay P, Rushing EJ, Marth JD, Parada LF. Ablation of NF1 function in neurons induces abnormal development of cerebral cortex and reactive gliosis in the brain. Genes Dev. 2001;15(7):859–76.
32. Bonneau F, D'Angelo I, Welti S, Stier G, Ylänne J, Scheffzek K. Expression, purification and preliminary crystallographic characterization of a novel segment from the neurofibromatosis type 1 protein. Acta Crystallogr D Biol Crystallogr. 2004;60(Pt 12 Pt 2):2364–7.
33. Ballester R, Marchuk D, Boguski M, Saulino A, Letcher R, Wigler M, Collins F. The NF1 locus encodes a protein functionally related to mammalian GAP and yeast IRA proteins. Cell. 1990;63(4):851–9.
34. Martin GA, Viskochil D, Bollag G, McCabe PC, Crosier WJ, Haubruck H, Conroy L, Clark R, O'Connell P, Cawthon RM, et al. The GAP-related domain of the neurofibromatosis type 1 gene product interacts with ras p21. Cell. 1990;63(4):843–9.
35. Xu GF, Lin B, Tanaka K, Dunn D, Wood D, Gesteland R, White R, Weiss R, Tamanoi F. The catalytic domain of the neurofibromatosis type 1 gene product stimulates ras GTPase and complements ira mutants of S. cerevisiae. Cell. 1990;63(4):835–41.
36. Scheffzek K, Ahmadian MR, Wiesmüller L, Kabsch W, Stege P, Schmitz F, Wittinghofer A. Structural analysis of the GAP-related domain from neurofibromin and its implications. EMBO J. 1998;17(15):4313–27.
37. Ahmadian MR, Kiel C, Stege P, Scheffzek K. Structural fingerprints of the Ras-GTPase activating proteins neurofibromin and p120GAP. J Mol Biol. 2003;329(4):699–710.
38. Dunzendorfer-Matt T, Mercado EL, Maly K, McCormick F, Scheffzek K. The neurofibromin recruitment factor Spred1 binds to the GAP related domain without affecting Ras inactivation. Proc Natl Acad Sci U S A. 2016;113(27):7497–502.
39. Hirata Y, Brems H, Suzuki M, Kanamori M, Okada M, Morita R, Llano-Rivas I, Ose T, Messiaen L, Legius E, Yoshimura A. Interaction between a domain of the negative regulator of the Ras-ERK pathway, SPRED1 protein, and the GTPase-activating protein-related domain of

neurofibromin is implicated in Legius syndrome and neurofibromatosis type 1. J Biol Chem. 2016;291(7):3124–34.
40. Stowe IB, Mercado EL, Stowe TR, Bell EL, Oses-Prieto JA, Hernández H, Burlingame AL, McCormick F. A shared molecular mechanism underlies the human rasopathies Legius syndrome and Neurofibromatosis-1. Genes Dev. 2012;26(13):1421–6.
41. Der CJ, Krontiris TG, Cooper GM. Transforming genes of human bladder and lung carcinoma cell lines are homologous to the ras genes of Harvey and Kirsten sarcoma viruses. Proc Natl Acad Sci U S A. 1982;79(11):3637–40.
42. Simanshu DK, Nissley DV, McCormick F. RAS proteins and their regulators in human disease. Cell. 2017;170(1):17–33.
43. McKay MM, Morrison DK. Integrating signals from RTKs to ERK/MAPK. Oncogene. 2007;26(22):3113–21.
44. Johannessen CM, Reczek EE, James MF, Brems H, Legius E, Cichowski K. The NF1 tumor suppressor critically regulates TSC2 and mTOR. Proc Natl Acad Sci U S A. 2005;102(24):8573–8.
45. Malumbres M, Barbacid M. RAS oncogenes: the first 30 years. Nat Rev Cancer. 2003;3(6):459–65.
46. Bos JL. Ras oncogenes in human cancer: a review. Cancer Res. 1989;49(17):4682–9.
47. Mendelsohn J, Baselga J. The EGF receptor family as targets for cancer therapy. Oncogene. 2000;19(56):6550–65.
48. Kan Z, Jaiswal BS, Stinson J, Janakiraman V, Bhatt D, Stern HM, Yue P, Haverty PM, Bourgon R, Zheng J, Moorhead M, Chaudhuri S, Tomsho LP, Peters BA, Pujara K, Cordes S, Davis DP, Carlton VE, Yuan W, Li L, Wang W, Eigenbrot C, Kaminker JS, Eberhard DA, Waring P, Schuster SC, Modrusan Z, Zhang Z, Stokoe D, de Sauvage FJ, Faham M, Seshagiri S. Diverse somatic mutation patterns and pathway alterations in human cancers. Nature. 2010;466(7308):869–73.
49. Kratz CP, Rapisuwon S, Reed H, Hasle H, Rosenberg PS. Cancer in Noonan, Costello, cardiofaciocutaneous and LEOPARD syndromes. Am J Med Genet C Semin Med Genet. 2011;157C(2):83–9.
50. Dasgupta B, Gutmann DH. Neurofibromin regulates neural stem cell proliferation, survival, and astroglial differentiation in vitro and in vivo. J Neurosci. 2005;25(23):5584–94.
51. Costa RM, Federov NB, Kogan JH, Murphy GG, Stern J, Ohno M, Kucherlapati R, Jacks T, Silva AJ. Mechanism for the learning deficits in a mouse model of neurofibromatosis type 1. Nature. 2002;415(6871):526–30.
52. Li W, Cui Y, Kushner SA, Brown RA, Jentsch JD, Frankland PW, Cannon TD, Silva AJ. The HMG-CoA reductase inhibitor lovastatin reverses the learning and attention deficits in a mouse model of neurofibromatosis type 1. Curr Biol. 2005;15(21):1961–7.
53. Guo HF, The I, Hannan F, Bernards A, Zhong Y. Requirement of Drosophila NF1 for activation of adenylyl cyclase by PACAP38-like neuropeptides. Science. 1997;276(5313):795–8.
54. The I, Hannigan GE, Cowley GS, Reginald S, Zhong Y, Gusella JF, Hariharan IK, Bernards A. Rescue of a Drosophila NF1 mutant phenotype by protein kinase A. Science. 1997;276(5313):791–4.
55. Guo HF, Tong J, Hannan F, Luo L, Zhong Y. A neurofibromatosis-1-regulated pathway is required for learning in Drosophila. Nature. 2000;403(6772):895–8.
56. Tong J, Hannan F, Zhu Y, Bernards A, Zhong Y. Neurofibromin regulates G protein-stimulated adenylyl cyclase activity. Nat Neurosci. 2002;5(2):95–6.
57. Hannan F, Ho I, Tong JJ, Zhu Y, Nurnberg P, Zhong Y. Effect of neurofibromatosis type I mutations on a novel pathway for adenylyl cyclase activation requiring neurofibromin and Ras. Hum Mol Genet. 2006;15(7):1087–98.
58. Brown JA, Gianino SM, Gutmann DH. Defective cAMP generation underlies the sensitivity of CNS neurons to neurofibromatosis-1 heterozygosity. J Neurosci. 2010;30(16):5579–89.
59. Anastasaki C, Gutmann DH. Neuronal NF1/RAS regulation of cyclic AMP requires atypical PKC activation. Hum Mol Genet. 2014;23(25):6712–21.
60. Xu H, Gutmann DH. Mutations in the GAP-related domain impair the ability of neurofibromin to associate with microtubules. Brain Res. 1997;759(1):149–52.

Molecular Diagnosis for NF1

3

Ludwine M. Messiaen

Contents

3.1 Introduction

The *NF1* gene, a large and complex gene spread over 280 kb of genomic DNA on chromosome 17q11.2, was identified independently by 2 groups using standard techniques of positional cloning [1, 2]. It comprises 57 constitutive and at least 3 alternatively spliced exons and is ubiquitously expressed. In addition, 3 two-exon genes, located on the opposite strand and transcribed in the opposite direction compared to *NF1,* are embedded in the 60 kb *NF1* intron 36[27b]: *EVI2B*, *EVI2A,* and *OMGP*.

After full cloning of the gene, an initial exon numbering system and genomic organization of all *NF1* exons, exon boundaries, and flanking intronic sequences was reported in 1995 [3] and the exon numbering published therein, referred to as the "legacy" or "historical" numbering, has been widely used for many years.

As a transition from this legacy numbering towards a nomenclature compliant with the recommendations of the Human Genome Variation Society (HGVS; http://www.hgvs.org/) and National Center for Biotechnology Information (NCBI) was highly desirable, and as discussed at an *NF1* Best Practice meeting organized by

L. M. Messiaen (✉)
Department of Genetics at UAB, Medical Genomics Laboratory, Birmingham, AL, USA
e-mail: lmessiaen@uabmc.edu

G. Tadini et al. (eds.), *Multidisciplinary Approach to Neurofibromatosis Type 1*,
https://doi.org/10.1007/978-3-319-92450-2_3

Prof. M. Upadhyaya in Cardiff, UK, in 2010, an *NF1* Locus Reference Genetic record (LRG) was requested and subsequently created (http://ftp.ebi.ac.uk/pub/databases/lrgex/LRG_214.xml) [4, 5]. LRGs are created, compiled, and maintained by the NCBI and the European Bioinformatics Institute (EBI).

The *NF1* LRG_214 has hereafter become the preferred reference sequence, and has been implemented in the largest public locus specific *NF1* database (NF1 LOVD: https://databases.lovd.nl/shared/genes/NF1, 2620 unique public variants reported as of May 15, 2019), by diagnostic laboratories following the recommendations of the HGVS, and papers reporting on the *NF1* mutational spectrum and genotype-phenotype correlations.

The transcript NM_000267.3, i.e. the transcript including the 57 constitutive exons but excluding the alternatively spliced exon 31[23a], has an open reading frame of 8457 nucleotides, encoding a 2818 amino acid protein. This transcript is most widely used in variant analyses, as no clear pathogenic variants have been reported in the alternatively spliced exon 31[23a]. Exon numbering, start and end position of all *NF1* exons using transcript reference NM_000267.3 and genomic reference record LRG_214 is provided in Table 3.1. In this chapter, exon numbering is used according to the HGVS recommendations, with the legacy numbering provided between square brackets.

Table 3.1 Exon numbering, start and end position of all exons using transcript reference NM_000267.3 and genomic reference record LRG_214

Exon	Exon legacy	c.start Exon	c.end Exon	g.start Exon	g.end Exon	Length Exon	Length Intron
1	1	−383	60	5001	5443	443	60,613
2	2	61	204	66,057	66,200	144	2883
3	3	205	288	69,084	69,167	84	4092
4	4a	289	479	73,260	73,450	191	6514
5	4b	480	586	79,965	80,071	107	11,424
6	4c	587	654	91,496	91,563	68	220
7	5	655	730	91,784	91,859	76	722
8	6	731	888	92,582	92,739	158	17,756
9	7	889	1062	110,496	110,669	174	441
10	8	1063	1185	111,111	111,233	123	251
11	9	1186	1260	111,485	111,559	75	4754
12	10a	1261	1392	116,314	116,445	132	8079
13	10b	1393	1527	124,525	124,659	135	4419
14	10c	1528	1641	129,079	129,192	114	2731
15	11	1642	1721	131,924	132,003	80	1514
16	12a	1722	1845	133,518	133,641	124	1527
17	12b	1846	2001	135,169	135,324	156	1184
18	13	2002	2251	136,509	136,758	250	533
19	14	2252	2325	137,292	137,365	74	231
20	15	2326	2409	137,597	137,680	84	1418
21	16	2410	2850	139,099	139,539	441	369
22	17	2851	2990	139,909	140,048	140	285
23	18	2991	3113	140,334	140,456	123	459

Table 3.1 (continued)

Exon	Exon legacy	c.start Exon	c.end Exon	g.start Exon	g.end Exon	Length Exon	Length Intron
24	19a	3114	3197	140,916	140,999	84	1147
25	19b	3198	3314	142,147	142,263	117	510
26	20	3315	3496	142,774	142,955	182	120
27	21	3497	3708	143,076	143,287	212	2397
28	22	3709	3870	145,685	145,846	162	145
29	23-1	3871	3974	145,992	146,095	104	12,962
30	23-2	3975	4110	159,058	159,193	136	9224
32	24	4111	4269	168,418	168,576	159	529
33	25	4270	4367	169,106	169,203	98	1239
34	26	4368	4514	170,443	170,589	147	1195
35	27a	4515	4661	171,785	171,931	147	3371
36	27b	4662	4772	175,303	175,413	111	60,480
37	28	4773	5205	235,894	236,326	433	1246
38	29	5206	5546	237,573	237,913	341	2456
39	30	5547	5749	240,370	240,572	203	4339
40	31	5750	5943	244,912	245,105	194	1301
41	32	5944	6084	246,407	246,547	141	161
42	33	6085	6364	246,709	246,988	280	453
43	34	6365	6579	247,442	247,656	215	236
44	35	6580	6641	247,893	247,954	62	144
45	36	6642	6756	248,099	248,213	115	564
46	37	6757	6858	248,778	248,879	102	1699
47	38	6859	6999	250,579	250,719	141	2363
48	39	7000	7126	253,083	253,209	127	5984
49	40	7127	7258	259,194	259,325	132	931
50	41	7259	7394	260,257	260,392	136	1938
51	42	7395	7552	262,331	262,488	158	4045
52	43	7553	7675	266,534	266,656	123	377
53	44	7676	7806	267,034	267,164	131	178
54	45	7807	7907	267,343	267,443	101	1110
55	46	7908	8050	268,554	268,696	143	346
56	47	8051	8097	269,043	269,089	47	1471
57	48	8098	8314	270,561	270,777	217	13,309
58	49	8315	*3522	284,087	287,751	3665	

3.2 Molecular Analysis and the *NF1* Mutational Spectrum

Pathogenic variants in the large and complex *NF1* gene can be located across the entire coding region as well as across non-coding regions and include a wide variety of types of variants such as *NF1* microdeletions comprising the *NF1* gene and multiple flanking genes (recently reviewed by [6]), smaller intragenic copy number changes, i.e. deletions/duplications involving 1 to several exons [7], frameshift, nonsense, and missense variants [8–10], splice site, exonic as well as deep intronic variants affecting normal splicing (25–30% of all variants, with ~1/3 of these *not* detected, misclassified, or classified as a variant of uncertain significance by gDNA sequencing [8, 9, 11–16]), in-frame deletions or duplications involving 1 to several codons, substitutions altering the methionine translational start codon, complex insertion/deletion variants, (balanced) translocations and Alu/LiNE insertions [17].

In a cohort of 8080 unrelated *NF1*-variant positive individuals analyzed at the Medical Genomics Laboratory using comprehensive variant analysis using a previously described RNA-based core assay supplemented with methods to identify *NF1* microdeletions as well as smaller copy number changes affecting one-to-multiple exons [8, 9, 18], we identified >3200 different (likely) pathogenic variants. Approximately 4.4% of the probands carry one of 4 different sized *NF1* microdeletions (i.e., either type I, II, III or atypical, all deletions extending beyond the entire *NF1* gene and including an array of additional flanking genes [6]), therefore *NF1* microdeletions are the most recurrent type of pathogenic *NF1* variant. Besides the microdeletion, another 28 different pathogenic variants were identified with a frequency of ≥0.5% (i.e., found in ≥40 unrelated probands out of the 8080 individuals; Table 3.2) and together account for ~21.3% of pathogenic variants. Another 2700 different variants were identified only once or twice in 3310 unrelated probands. Frequency of the different types of variants is provided in Fig. 3.1. Types of pathogenic variants, ordered in decreasing frequency, include splice (27.6%), frameshift (24%), nonsense (21%), missense and/or 1-to-8 amino acid deletions/duplications (19.5%), microdeletions, type I–IV (4.4%), intragenic one-to-multiple exon deletions/duplications (3.2%), and complex other (indels, balanced translocation, methionine start codon; <1%).

Given the wide variety of types of variants, no *single* molecular technique can identify all possible pathogenic types of *NF1* variants in individuals in whom NF1 is suspected.

Comprehensive *NF1* variant analysis using an RNA-based core assay supplemented with methods to identify *NF1* microdeletions as well as smaller copy number changes identifies a pathogenic variant in >95% of non-founder NF1 patients fulfilling NIH criteria [8]. The sensitivity of a comprehensive RNA-based approach was confirmed in multiple independent studies that included well characterized patients [9, 14–16, 19]. The efficiency and reliability of this approach are based on the application of a set of complementary techniques that not only allow the detection of different variant types, but also of unusual splicing defects occurring outside the evolutionarily conserved canonical AG/GT splice site sequences of the *NF1* gene.

gDNA-*only* variant detection approaches involve the sequencing of the entire *NF1* coding region and flanking splice sites from the genomic DNA either by Sanger sequencing or Next Generation Sequencing (NGS), complemented by copy number analyses to detect entire *NF1* gene or one-to-multiple exon deletions/duplications.

Table 3.2 Recurrent pathogenic variants identified in ≥0.5% of the unrelated individuals in this cohort

Pathogenic variant	Exon	Type/effect	# of patients	% of pathogenic variants in 8080 cohort
c.4537C>T; p.R1513X	E35[27a]	Nonsense	100	1.24
c.1466A>G; p.Y489∗	E13[10b]	Splice, skipping last 62 nucleotides of E13[10b]	99	1.23
c.1756_1759delACTA	E16[12a]	Frameshift	80	0.99
c.5425C>T; p.R1809C	E38[29]	Missense	78	0.97
c.3826C>T; p.R1276X	E28[22]	Nonsense	74	0.92
c.2033dupC	E18[13]	Frameshift	72	0.89
c.2970_2972delAAT; p.991delM	E22[17]	1 AA deletion	72	0.89
c.6792C>A	E46[37]	Splice, in-frame skipping E46[37]	69	0.85
c.499_502delTGTT	E5[4b]	Frameshift	68	0.84
c.4084C>T; p.R1362X	E30[23]-2	Nonsense	67	0.83
c.574C>T; p.R192X	E5[4b]	Nonsense	64	0.79
c.6709C>T; p.R2237X	E45[36]	Nonsense	63	0.78
c.5839C>T; p.R1947X	E40[31]	Nonsense	62	0.77
c.1541_1542delAG	E14[10]c	Frameshift	58	0.72
c.910C>T; p.R304X	E9[7]	Nonsense/splice (low proportion of transcripts with in-frame skipping E9[7])	57	0.71
c.1246C>T; R416X	E11[9]	Nonsense	55	0.68
c.5242C>T; p.R1748X	E38[29]	Nonsense	55	0.68
c.7846C>T; p.R2616X	E54[45]	Nonsense	55	0.68
c.2041C>T; p.R681X	E18[13]	Nonsense	54	0.67
c.7486C>T; p.R2496X	E51[42]	Nonsense	54	0.67
c.1318C>T; p.R440X	E12[10]a	Nonsense	50	0.62
c.4267A>G; p.K1423E	E32[24]	Missense	49	0.61
c.3827G>A; p.R1276Q	E28[22]	Missense	48	0.59
c.2446C>T; p.R816X	E20[15]	Nonsense	47	0.58
c.5546G>A; "p.R1849Q"	E38[29]	Splice, out-of-frame skipping of E38 [29] and E38+39[29+30]	47	0.58
c.1381C>T; p.R461X	E12[10a]	Nonsense	44	0.54
c.7285C>T; p.R2429X	E50[41]	Nonsense	42	0.52
c.1885G>A	E17[12b]	Splice, out-of-frame skipping first 41 nucleotides of E17[12b]	40	0.50
28 different pathogenic variants	E5[4b]–E54[45]		1723	21.32%

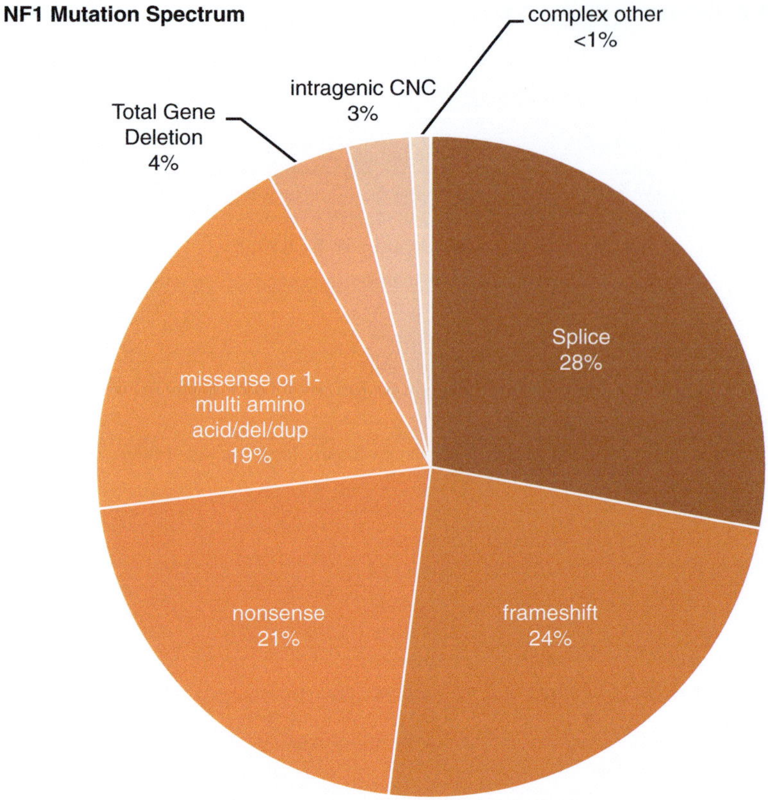

Fig. 3.1 Spectrum of variants identified in cohort of 8080 unrelated individuals identified by RNA-based comprehensive molecular analysis complemented by dosage analysis using MLPA

These approaches have a lower diagnostic sensitivity and specificity (Table 3.3) [10, 20–23]. The lower sensitivity and specificity of gDNA-only variant detection approaches compared to comprehensive RNA-based approaches are largely explained by the frequent occurrence of unusual splicing defects in the *NF1* gene that either completely escape detection by gDNA-*only* approaches as they can reside deep into the large *NF1* introns and cause missplicing (e.g., Fig. 3.2a) or that, although technically identifiable by gDNA-only approaches, remain classified as a variant of uncertain significance if located outside the 100% evolutionarily conserved AG/GT splice sites (e.g., Fig. 3.2b), or are *mis*classified as a nonsense, missense, or silent variant although RNA-based functional evaluation shows they disable the normal *NF1* splicing of the variant allele (e.g., Fig. 3.2c). Comprehensive RNA-based approaches intrinsically provide a functional evaluation of the effect any coding and non-coding intragenic *NF1* variant has on splicing. Therefore, laboratories offering clinical gDNA-based-only *NF1* testing (including copy number analysis) should be aware of the shortcomings of this approach compared to the comprehensive RNA-based approach with sensitivity reduced by ~5% (no detection of deep intronic variants and

Table 3.3 Molecular genetic testing approaches used in neurofibromatosis 1

Gene	Test method	Proportion of non-founder probands with a pathogenic variant detectable by this method
NF1	Multistep approach based on cDNA and gDNA sequence analysis complemented with copy number analysis using, e.g. multiplex ligation-dependent probe analysis	>95%
	Genomic DNA sequence analysis[a] (Sanger or NGS) of all exons and flanking intronic sequence	~80 to 85%
	Gene-targeted copy number analysis by MLPA (includes the microdeletions as well as single-to-multiple exon deletions/duplications)	~7%
	Chromosomal microarray	~5%
	Cytogenetic analysis	<1%

[a]gDNA sequence analysis, either by Sanger sequencing or next generation sequencing, detects variants that are benign, likely benign, of uncertain significance, likely pathogenic, or pathogenic. Deep intronic pathogenic splice variants typically are *not* detected by a gDNA-based sequencing analysis, unless those variants were previously reported and these intronic regions were included in the gDNA-based sequencing analysis. Typically, both Sanger and NGS-based sequencing assays restrict the region of analysis/reporting to 10–15 nt of intronic sequence flanking each exon. Pathogenic variants may include small intragenic deletions/insertions and missense, nonsense, and splice site variants within 10–15 nt of the exon borders; typically, exon or whole-gene deletions/duplications are not detected

splice site variants beyond the intronic sequence closely flanking the exons) and specificity reduced by ~10% (of those variants that will be detected, ~10% will be classified as VUS or misclassified due to unknown effect on splicing).

However, as even the most comprehensive RNA-based approaches complemented with copy number analysis fail to detect a pathogenic variant in ~<5% of non-founder individuals with classic features of NF1, there is a need to further improve *NF1* detection strategies, with special emphasis on the 5′ and 3′ untranslated regions (UTR), routinely not included in clinical testing. A few candidate nucleotides within the 5'UTR have recently been reported, i.e. c.-272 and c.-273 [16], but as these variants were still associated with bi-allelic RNA expression in vitro, it is unclear if they affect normal *NF1* transcription/translation of the variant allele. Furthermore, complex rearrangements such as inversions typically are refractory to the currently used molecular approaches and efforts should be made to develop the necessary technologies to facilitate detection of such variants. Lastly, balanced translocations, found in <1% of unrelated NF1 individuals, will not be identified by RNA- or gDNA-based Sanger or NGS sequencing approaches nor by MLPA or chromosomal microarray copy number analyses. A cytogenetic analysis is needed to detect this type of pathogenic variant.

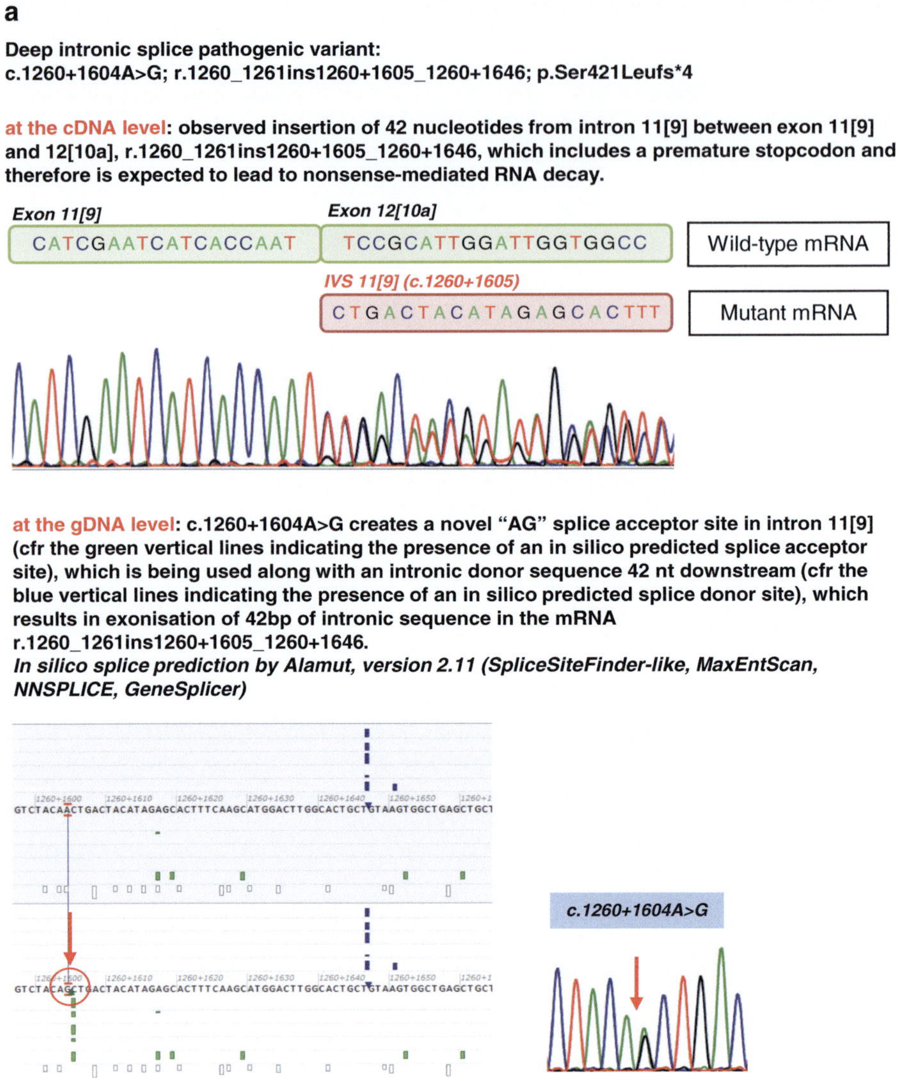

Fig. 3.2 Comprehensive RNA-based approaches intrinsically provide a functional evaluation of the effect any coding and non-coding intragenic *NF1* variant has on splicing. (**a**) Effect of deep intronic c.1260+1604A>G at the cDNA and gDNA level

b

Intronic Splice site variant, located outside the +/- 15 nucleotides flanking every exon and therefore outside the area ordinarily covered by DNA based Sanger sequencing, NGS panel or whole exome sequencing:
c.6579+18A>G; r. 6579_6580ins6579+1_6579+17; p.Ala2194Valfs*2

at the cDNA level: observed insertion of the first 17 nt of intron 43[34] between exon 43[34] and exon 44[35], r. 6579_6580ins6579+1_6579+17, which includes a premature stopcodon and therefore is expected to lead to nonsense-mediated RNA decay.

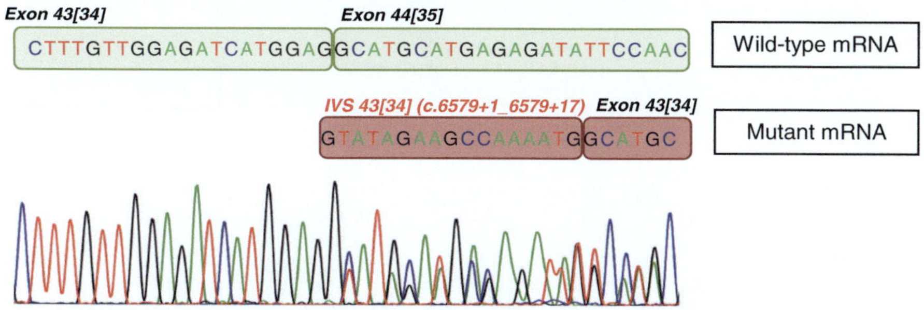

at the gDNA level: : c.6579+18A>G creates a strong novel intronic splice donor site in intron 43[34], which is used by the splice machinery and results in intron retention of the first 17 nt intron 43[34] in the mRNA: r. 6579_6580ins6579+1_6579+17 l.
In silico splice prediction by Alamut, version 2.11 (SpliceSiteFinder-like, MaxEntScan, NNSPLICE, GeneSplicer)

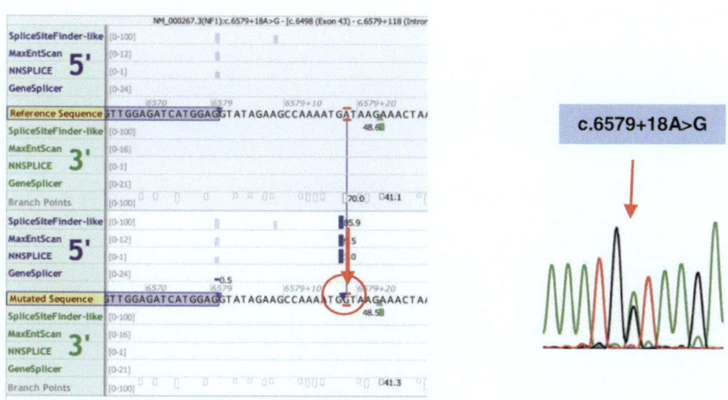

Fig. 3.2 (continued) Comprehensive RNA-based approaches intrinsically provide a functional evaluation of the effect any coding and non-coding intragenic NF1 variant has on splicing. (**b**) effect of intronic c.6579+18A>G at the cDNA and gDNA level

c

Exonic "synonymous" variant affecting correct splicing
c.2709G>A; r.2707_2850del; p.Cys904_Leu951del (and not p.Val903=)

at the cDNA level: observed in-frame skipping of the last 144 nucleotides of exon 21[16]; at the DNA level this variant mimics a synonymous variant p.Val903=

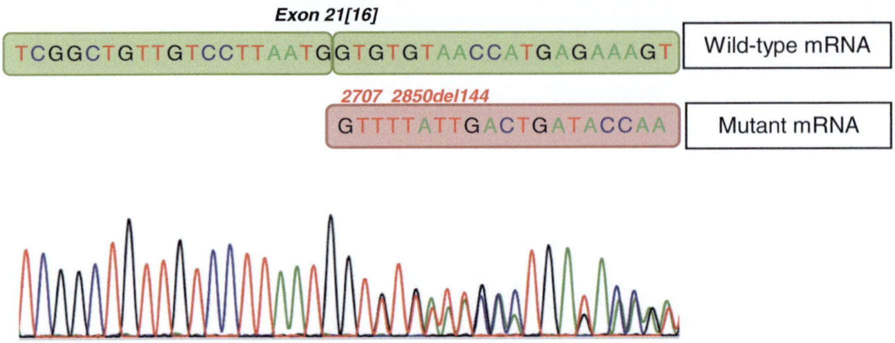

at the gDNA level: c.2709G>A increases the strength of a cryptic exonic splice donor site in exon 21[16], which is being used and results in in-frame skipping of the last 144 nt of exon 21[16] in the mRNA: r.2707_2850del. *In silico splice prediction by Alamut, version 2.11 (SpliceSiteFinder-like, MaxEntScan, NNSPLICE, GeneSplicer)*

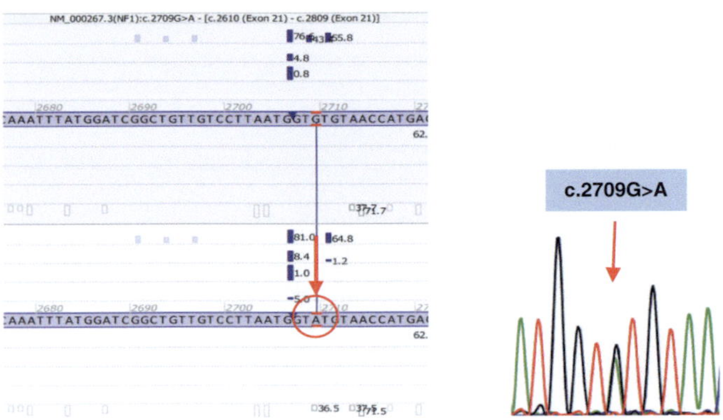

Fig. 3.2 (continued) Comprehensive RNA-based approaches intrinsically provide a functional evaluation of the effect any coding and non-coding intragenic NF1 variant has on splicing. (**c**) effect of synonymous exonic c.2709G>A at the cDNA and gDNA level

3.3 Molecular Analysis and Mosaic/Segmental NF1

As many as 30–50% of NF1 patients have no affected parent from whom the disorder was inherited, therefore are "sporadic" or "founder" patients. A proportion of these "founder" patients have the disorder due to acquiring a *somatic NF1* pathogenic variant in a specific cell *after* fertilization; during embryonic development this cell further clonally expands and this "founder" or sporadic NF1 patient will therefore carry this *NF1* pathogenic "first hit" variant only in a subpopulation of the body, as opposed to in all body cells if the *NF1* pathogenic variant would be present at fertilization, i.e. in the germ cell (egg or sperm). In addition, in accordance with the "two-hit Knudson hypothesis" of tumor-suppressor genes, somatic "second hit" pathogenic *NF1* variants are well documented in *NF1*-associated tumors including cutaneous and plexiform neurofibromas, gastrointestinal stromal tumors, glomus tumors, pheochromocytomas, juvenile myelomonocytic leukemia, astrocytomas (reviewed by [24]) as well as in tissues from some distinctive non-tumor lesions such as tibial pseudarthrosis [25, 26] and café-au-lait macules (CALMs) [27], thereby resulting in bi-allelic *NF1* activation.

Mosaic patients often present with a milder presentation (often referred to as *generalized* mosaic NF1), or with NF1-associated features limited to one or more segments of the body, typically not crossing the midline (often referred to as mosaic *localized* or segmental NF1). It is thought that the somatic pathogenic variant in patients with *generalized* NF1 occurred in an earlier stage of embryonic development compared to patients with *segmental* NF1. Importantly, however, as NF1 is a progressive disorder, the mosaic phenotypic presentation may/will evolve with time and more features still may appear as the patient ages (exemplified, e.g. in [28]). Depending on the *timing* and *types of progenitor cells* affected by the first hit somatic *NF1* pathogenic variant, the externally visible phenotype observed in a mosaic NF1 patient may include pigmentary features only, cutaneous neurofibromas-only, plexiform neurofibroma-only or a combination of pigmentary lesions and (cutaneous or plexiform) neurofibromas (reviewed by [28]). Pure *gonadal* mosaicism, with the somatic pathogenic *NF1* variant present only in the gonads in an individual with no clinical features of NF1 at all, is rare given that presence of at least two siblings carrying the same pathogenic *NF1* variant, absent in the blood in both unaffected parents has been reported only in 4 families so far, with ¾ and ¼ proven to be of paternal, respectively, maternal original [29–32].

Detection of the causal pathogenic variants in patients with a mosaic/segmental phenotype requires special attention to (1) the sensitivity of the technology used to detect variants with very low allele frequency, as well as (2) the type of cells to be analyzed. In patients with generalized mosaic NF1, the pathogenic *NF1* variant may still be detectable in blood, depending on the type of pathogenic variant, its allele frequency and the molecular diagnostic approaches used. As an example, gonosomal mosaicism was proven in an adult male with 4 typical CALMs on the midline of his back as the only known manifestation but with multiple affected offspring [33]. An intragenic deletion of the exons 15–29[11–23.1], present in <10% of the alleles, was detectable due to the preferential amplification of the shorter pathogenic transcript by reverse-transcriptase PCR (RT-PCR) as part of the comprehensive RNA-based testing approach, but remained undetectable by Multiplex Ligation-dependent Probe Amplification (MLPA) copy number analysis and array Comparative Genomics Hybridization (aCGH). Low-level mosaic variants with variant allele frequency (VAF) <10% frequently escape detection by Sanger sequencing, aCGH or MLPA. As part of an overall comprehensive screen to pick up any type of low-level *NF1* variants in DNA extracted from blood, RT-PCR has a high sensitivity to detect low-level mosaic intragenic copy number changes, whereas FISH, digital droplet PCR or quantitative PCR will pick up low-level microdeletions and deep coverage (>1500×) NGS, customized and targeted to the *NF1* coding and intronic regions, will detect all types of missense, nonsense, frameshift, indel, and splice site variants even if present in only 2–3% of the alleles (Messiaen, unpublished). Although there is no sharp phenotypic demarcation between *generalized* mosaic and *segmental* NF1, in general, a pathogenic *NF1* variant usually remains undetected in DNA extracted from blood in patients with a clear segmental presentation as the percentage of cells carrying the *NF1* first hit is either too low or even completely absent [34, 35], Messiaen, unpublished]. In such patients, comprehensive analysis specifically of neural crest-derived cells from the affected body lesions is required, i.e. specifically the melanocytes (but not keratinocytes or fibroblasts) from the CALMs [27, 35] or Schwann cells from the cutaneous neurofibromas [36, 37]. Such clinical testing from neural crest-derived cells is currently only available in a few specialized genetic laboratories in the world.

Identification of a *common "first hit"* pathogenic *NF1* hit in the Schwann cells and/or melanocytes from neurofibromas and/or CALMs, but not in unaffected tissues/cells (such as blood), from a patient clinically presenting with possible mosaic/segmental NF1, confirms the diagnosis of mosaic/segmental NF1 and this *"first hit"* pathogenic variant *may* be at risk to be transmitted to the next generation, if gonads were involved. This is important information for counseling related to recurrence risk for parents and offspring. Besides a *common NF1* first hit, a *different NF1* second hit is typically identified in *every* neurofibroma or CALM. As the second hit in every CALM or neurofibroma is different, each patient carries an entirely unique set of *NF1* mutations. An example of such analysis is discussed in Fig. 3.3.

a

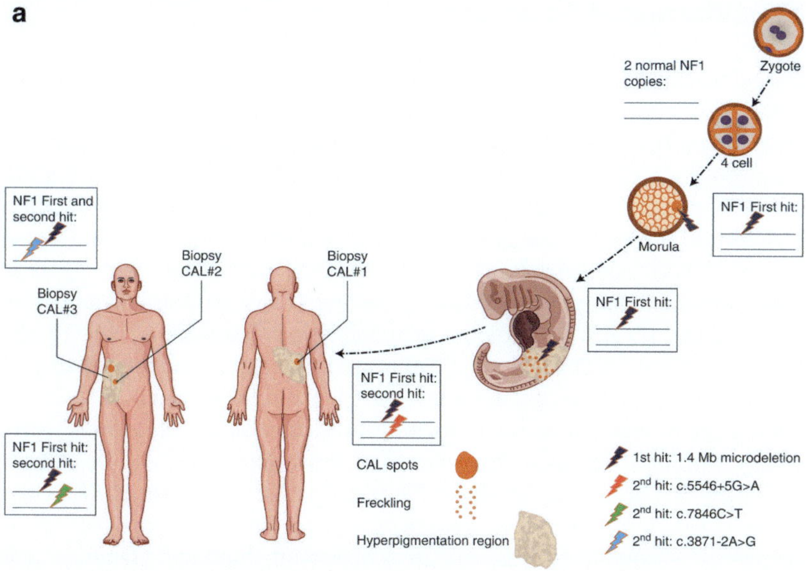

b

tissue	*NF1* pathogenic variant first hit	*NF1* pathogenic variant second hit	mRNA/protein effect second hit
Blood	none	none	NA
CALM 1	1.4 Mb microdeletion	c.5546+5G>A	Out of frame missplicing: r.[5206_5546del,5206_5749del]; p.[Gly1737Serfs*4,Gly1737Leufs*3]
CALM 2	1.4 Mb microdeletion	c.7846C>T	Nonsense: r.7846c>u; p.Arg2616Ter
CALM 3	1.4 Mb microdeletion	c.3871-2A>G	Out of frame missplicing: r.3871_3974del; p.Tyr1292Argfs*7

Fig. 3.3 Segmental or localized mosaic NF1 is caused by somatic *NF1* pathogenic variants. (**a**) Example of genetic testing for a segmental/localized mosaic patient with pigmentary lesions-only and referred for genetic testing to the UAB Medical Genomics Laboratory with biopsies taken by Dr. John G. Pappas, NYU Langone Medical center, New York City, US. The biopsies were submitted in a sterile shipping medium with the location of the biopsies (3-mm punch biopsies) indicated on the body diagram of the Medical Genomics Laboratory's phenotypic checklist (see Fig. S1 in reference Koczkowska et al., 2018). Upon receipt in the laboratory, in vitro selective culture of melanocytes was initiated. Melanocyte cultures were harvested at passage 4 and subjected to comprehensive RNA-based *NF1/SPRED1* genetic testing. If a somatic "first hit" pathogenic variant, resulting from a replication error, occurs in a neural crest precursor cell after fertilization in early embryonic development, further cell divisions from the initial cell will result in an affected body segment. CALMs then originate from melanocyte precursor cells that acquire an additional somatic *NF1* second hit during further cell divisions. In the patient here discussed, genetic testing from blood and melanocytes, cultured from the CALMs, showed a common somatic *NF1* first hit in all 3 biopsied CALMs (here a 1.4 Mb microdeletion), which was absent in the blood. In addition, a different somatic *NF1* "second hit" pathogenic variant was found in the melanocytes from every *CALM* confirming the diagnosis of segmental/mosaic localized NF1. (**b**) The somatic second hit pathogenic variants identified in cultured melanocytes from 3 different CALMs, and their effect at the RNA/protein level

3.3.1 Classification of Variants

Early papers describing *NF1* variants did not always provide the rationale leading to their classification and the interpretation was rather simplistic (for a discussion, see [38, 39]). Over the years, the exponential increase of sequencing efforts led to the identification of a myriad of genetic variants found in normal control populations [and submitted in databases such as the genome Aggregation Database (gnomAD), the Exome Aggregation Consortium (ExAC), the Exome Variant Server (EVS), and other] and/or in cohorts of individuals with specific genetic disorders or phenotypic features [including ClinVar, Online Mendelian Inheritance in Man (OMIM), Leiden Open Variation Database (LOVD), the Human Genome Mutation Database (HGMD), and other]. Our understanding of the clinical significance of any given variant ranges from those in which the variant is certainly pathogenic for a given disorder to those that are almost certainly benign. Many variants fall somewhere between those extremes. As the importance and utility of clinical molecular *NF1* testing has increased, so does the importance to create and implement standards and guidelines for the classification of sequence variants. The American College of Medical Genetics and Genomics (ACMGG), the Association for Molecular pathology (AMP), and the College of American Pathologists (CAP) have developed standards and guidelines for the interpretation of sequence variants [40], which have now been widely used and implemented in laboratories offering clinical molecular genetic testing. Variants identified in genes that cause Mendelian disease are classified using standard terminology as being "pathogenic," "likely pathogenic," "uncertain significance," "likely benign," or "benign." The guidelines describe a process for classifying such variants into one of these five categories, based on evidence derived from several types of data, such as population data, in silico computational predictive data, functional data, genetic data (segregation of the variant with disorder in the family versus the variant proven *de novo* in sporadic cases with unaffected parents), allelic data, data from the literature or public databases, and other data. These guidelines provide an evidence framework to objectively classify variants, improving inter-laboratory consistency of classification, and offer a set of criteria that, if fulfilled, can result in the reclassification of a variant of uncertain significance to likely pathogenic or pathogenic. An example of how such reclassification for a missense or intronic variant can be obtained is provided in Fig. 3.4a, b. These examples illustrate the importance of *additional* genetic, clinical (detailed phenotyping), or functional work-up after the initial identification of an "uncertain significance" or "likely pathogenic" variant and the importance of a close collaboration between the clinical laboratory, the health care provider and families to improve variant classification. Sometimes, however, a final classification will necessarily need to await availability of additional data from other patients carrying the same variant, which is challenging given the complex *NF1* mutational spectrum with many families carrying a "private" variant, only observed once so far.

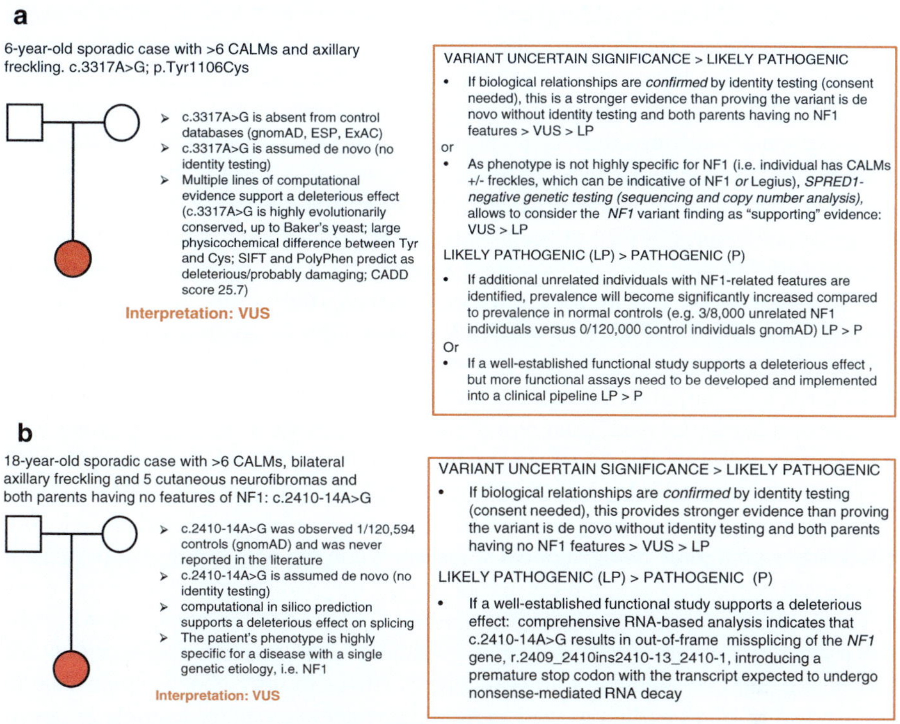

Fig. 3.4 (**a**, **b**) Example of the interpretation and reclassification of a missense variant (c.3317A>G; p.Tyr1106Cys) and an intronic variant (c.2410-14A>G), illustrating this is often a multistep process requiring a close collaboration between the clinical laboratory, the health care provider, and families to improve the interpretation

3.3.2 Molecular Diagnosis and Genotype-Phenotype Correlations

NF1 is a frequent neurocutaneous disorder with a birth frequency of approximately 1 in 2000 [41]. Criteria to make a clinical diagnosis of NF1 were originally established at the NIH Consensus Conference in 1987 [42] and are currently being revised and updated to include results from molecular and clinical studies reported since that time, one such novel criterion being the presence of a pathogenic *NF1* variant.

There is a need for a *reliable, specific,* and *sensitive NF1* variant detection approach: *first,* to assist with family planning including prenatal or preimplantation diagnosis, if desired; *second,* to establish an immediate diagnosis of NF1 in a young child with a serious tumor (e.g., a high-grade optic glioma, rhabdomyosarcoma, …) that may be associated with NF1 or with a different cancer predisposition syndrome, autosomal recessive constitutional mismatch repair deficiency syndrome (CMMRD), with CMMRD patients frequently also presenting with non-malignant features of NF1 (especially CALMs and freckling) and differentiation between both disorders being of ultimate importance for therapy, cancer surveillance in the patient and relatives, and recurrence risk in siblings [43, 44]; and third, to resolve diagnostic dilemmas in individuals not fulfilling the NIH diagnostic criteria, especially young children presenting with pigmentary features *only* or atypical patients, such as individuals with spinal neurofibromatosis, NF-Noonan syndrome or segmental NF. Only about half of sporadic NF1 patients (i.e., founder patients) fulfill the NIH diagnostic criteria by 1 year of age. More features of NF1 develop with age but *still* ~5% of founder NF1 patients will not fulfill these criteria by the age of 8 years [45]. CAL-spots are almost always the first signs of NF1, with their number increasing during the first years of life. Waiting for more symptoms to appear with time in order to ascertain the diagnosis of NF1 on clinical grounds can be very stressful for families. Moreover, the diagnosis for individuals with multiple CAL-spots with (or without) freckling-*only*, but no neurofibromas or other tumor manifestations of Neurofibromatosis type 1, can be either NF1 *or* Legius syndrome, the latter caused by *SPRED1* pathogenic variants [46, 47]. Approximately 2% of individuals fulfilling the NIH diagnostic criteria for NF1, based on pigmentary features, carry a *SPRED1* but no *NF1* pathogenic variant [47, 48]. Given the overall more benign course of Legius syndrome with absence of peripheral and central nervous system tumors, establishing a diagnosis with *certainty* and *early* in these patients through molecular diagnosis, as opposed to not being able to establish a diagnosis of either NF1 or Legius syndrome with confidence, is important for counseling and management. Earlier diagnosis allows to offer genetic counseling to parents and relatives earlier, as well as to initiate interventions for learning or developmental problems sooner. Earlier diagnosis will become even more important once more therapeutic options become available.

Furthermore, an increasing number of *clinically relevant* genotype-phenotype correlations have been reported. First, individuals with a constitutional *NF1* microdeletion, i.e. deletion of the *NF1* gene and flanking regions/genes, usually show a more severe phenotype compared to the general NF1 population. Patients carrying an *NF1* microdeletion (MIM: 613675) typically present with a larger number of neurofibromas at a younger age, may have dysmorphic facial features including downslanted palpebral fissures, hypertelorism, low set ears, broad nasal bridge, micrognathia, facial asymmetry, an increased lifetime risk for malignant peripheral nerve sheath tumors (MPNSTs) and may have a more severe developmental delay and/or intellectual disability. In the UAB cohort, ~5% of all NF1 patients carry such microdeletion. Genotype-phenotype correlations associated with the *NF1* microdeletions have recently been reviewed by [6].

We recently described another *NF1* region associated with a more severe phenotype: individuals carrying constitutional missense variants affecting one of 5 neighboring *NF1* codons Leu844, Cys845, Ala846, Leu847, and Gly848, located outside of the central GAP-Related Domain known to downregulate Ras-GTP to Ras-GDP, have a high prevalence of a severe phenotype, including plexiform and symptomatic spinal neurofibromas, symptomatic optic pathway gliomas, malignant neoplasms as well as bone abnormalities [39]. A pathogenic variant in one of the amino acids in this cluster was identified in ~0.8% of unrelated NF1 individuals in the UAB cohort (67/8400).

There also has been significant progress in the identification of *NF1* genotypes associated with a *milder* presentation, similar to Legius syndrome, i.e. presence of multiple CALMs with or without skinfold freckling but without neurofibromas or other tumor manifestations of NF1. Legius syndrome accounts for ~2% of individuals fulfilling NIH criteria based on pigmentary features [47, 48]. In the UAB cohort, ~0.9% (74/8400) of all unrelated *NF1*-positive individuals carry the Methionine codon 992 deletion (c.2970_2972del; p.Met992del): these individuals, as well as their affected relatives and individuals from the independently assessed European cohort, all present with this milder phenotype [49, 50], except, however, for benign brain tumors being observed in the p.Met992del-positive cohort (4.8%), but not in Legius syndrome [50]. *NF1* missense mutations affecting the Arginine codon at position 1809, found in ~1.2% of unrelated NF1 individuals in the UAB cohort, are equally associated with a presentation without tumor manifestations of NF1, however, pulmonic stenosis and Noonan-like features are significantly more prevalent in this group as compared to the general NF1 population [51, 52]. Cognitive impairment and/or learning disabilities remain part of the clinical phenotype associated with both the p.Met992del or p.Arg1809 pathogenic missense variants. Two other missense pathogenic variants, i.e. p.Leu1390Phe and p.Arg1038Gly, have been reported with all affected having pigmentary features but none showing any cutaneous neurofibromas (six p.Leu1390Phe-positive adults, aged 19–63 years, from a 5-generation family and five p.Arg1038Gly-positive adults, aged 30–72 years, from 2 families) [53, 54]. Certainly, additional recurrent variants associated with a clinically relevant genotype-phenotype correlation exist and wait to be reported, however, large cohorts of individuals with accurate standardized phenotypic information and carrying the identical pathogenic *NF1* variant are needed to provide statistically significant evidence.

Although each of the so far reported *NF1* variants associated with a clinically relevant genotype-phenotype correlation affects only a small percentage of NF1 individuals, *together*, they already affect counseling and management of almost 10% of the NF1 population.

While the clinical course will remain unpredictable for the majority of patients, especially those carrying truncating pathogenic variants, there clearly exist specific pathogenic *NF1* variants that, if present in an individual, allow a more precise forecasting of the expected course of NF1 and of the symptoms more likely to occur, or not to occur. As more genotype-phenotype correlations are unveiled, sensitive and specific *NF1* genetic testing will be essential to personalized medicine by improving an early definite diagnosis, facilitating disease surveillance and stratification of NF1-affected individuals.

References

1. Wallace MR, Andersen LB, Saulino AM, Gregory PE, Glover TW, Collins FS. A de novo Alu insertion results in neurofibromatosis type 1. Nature. 1991;353(6347):864–6.
2. Viskochil D, Buchberg AM, Xu G, Cawthon RM, Stevens J, Wolff RK, et al. Deletions and a translocation interrupt a cloned gene at the neurofibromatosis type 1 locus. Cell. 1990;62(1):187–92.

3. Li Y, O'Connell P, Breidenbach HH, Cawthon R, Stevens J, Xu G, Neil S, et al. Genomic organization of the neurofibromatosis 1 gene (*NF1*). Genomics. 1995;25(1):9–18.
4. MacArthur JA, Morales J, Tully RE, Astashyn A, Gil L, Bruford EA, et al. Locus reference genomic: reference sequences for the reporting of clinically relevant sequence variants. Nucleic Acids Res. 2014;42(Database issue):D873–8.
5. Dalgleish R, Flicek P, Cunningham F, Astashyn A, Tully RE, Proctor G, et al. Locus reference genomic sequences: an improved basis for describing human DNA variants. Genome Med. 2010;2(4):24.
6. Kehrer-Sawatzki H, Mautner VF, Cooper DN. Emerging genotype-phenotype correlations in patients with large *NF1* deletions. Hum Genet. 2017;136(4):349–76.
7. Hsiao MC, Piotrowski A, Callens T, Fu C, Wimmer K, Claes KB, et al. Decoding *NF1* intragenic copy-number variations. Am J Hum Genet. 2015;97(2):238–49.
8. Messiaen LM, Callens T, Mortier G, Beysen D, Vandenbroucke I, Van Roy N, et al. Exhaustive mutation analysis of the *NF1* gene allows identification of 95% of mutations and reveals a high frequency of unusual splicing defects. Hum Mutat. 2000;15(6):541–55.
9. Messiaen LM, Wimmer K. *NF1* mutational spectrum. In: Kaufmann D, editor. Neurofibromatoses. Monographs in Human Genetics, vol. 16. Basel: Karger; 2008. p. 63–77.
10. van Minkelen R, van Bever Y, Kromosoeto JN, Withagen-Hermans CJ, Nieuwlaat A, Halley DJ, et al. A clinical and genetic overview of 18 years neurofibromatosis type 1 molecular diagnostics in the Netherlands. Clin Genet. 2014;85(4):318–27.
11. Ars E, Serra E, García J, Kruyer H, Gaona A, Lázaro C, et al. Mutations affecting mRNA splicing are the most common molecular defects in patients with neurofibromatosis type 1. Hum Mol Genet. 2000;9(2):237–47. Erratum in: Hum Mol Genet 2000;9(4):659.
12. Zatkova A, Messiaen L, Vandenbroucke I, Wieser R, Fonatsch C, Krainer AR, Wimmer K. Disruption of exonic splicing enhancer elements is the principal cause of exon skipping associated with seven nonsense or missense alleles of *NF1*. Hum Mutat. 2004;24(6):491–501.
13. Pros E, Gómez C, Martín T, Fábregas P, Serra E, Lázaro C. Nature and mRNA effect of 282 different *NF1* point mutations: focus on splicing alterations. Hum Mutat. 2008;29(9):E173–93.
14. Valero MC, Martín Y, Hernández-Imaz E, Marina Hernández A, Meleán G, Valero AM, et al. A highly sensitive genetic protocol to detect *NF1* mutations. J Mol Diagn. 2011;13(2):113–22.
15. Sabbagh A, Pasmant E, Imbard A, Luscan A, Soares M, Blanché H, et al. *NF1* molecular characterization and neurofibromatosis type I genotype-phenotype correlation: the French experience. Hum Mutat. 2013;34(11):1510–8.
16. Evans DG, Bowers N, Burkitt-Wright E, Miles E, Garg S, Scott-Kitching V, Penman-Splitt M, et al. Comprehensive RNA analysis of the *NF1* gene in classically affected *NF1* affected individuals meeting NIH criteria has high sensitivity and mutation negative testing is reassuring in isolated cases with pigmentary features only. EBioMedicine. 2016;7:212–20.
17. Wimmer K, Callens T, Wernstedt A, Messiaen L. The *NF1* gene contains hotspots for L1 endonuclease-dependent de novo insertion. PLoS Genet. 2011;7(11):e1002371.
18. Messiaen L, Wimmer K. Mutation analysis of the *NF1* gene by cDNA-based sequencing of the coding region. In: KSG C, Geller M, editors. Advances in neurofibromatosis research. New York: Nova Science Publishers; 2012. p. 89–108.
19. Wimmer K, Roca X, Beiglböck H, Callens T, Etzler J, Rao AR, et al. Extensive in silico analysis of *NF1* splicing defects uncovers determinants for splicing outcome upon 5′ splice-site disruption. Hum Mutat. 2007;28(6):599–612.
20. Maruoka R, Takenouchi T, Torii C, Shimizu A, Misu K, Higasa K, et al. The use of next-generation sequencing in molecular diagnosis of neurofibromatosis type 1: a validation study. Genet Test Mol Biomarkers. 2014;18(11):722–35.
21. Pasmant E, Parfait B, Luscan A, Goussard P, Briand-Suleau A, Laurendeau I, et al. Neurofibromatosis type 1 molecular diagnosis: what can NGS do for you when you have a large gene with loss of function mutations? Eur J Hum Genet. 2015;23(5):596–601.
22. Zhang J, Tong H, Fu X, Zhang Y, Liu J, Cheng R, et al. Molecular characterization of *NF1* and neurofibromatosis type 1 genotype-phenotype correlations in a Chinese population. Sci Rep. 2015;5:11291.

23. Calì F, Chiavetta V, Ruggeri G, Piccione M, Selicorni A, Palazzo D, Bonsignore M, Cereda A, et al. Mutation spectrum of *NF1* gene in Italian patients with neurofibromatosis type 1 using Ion Torrent PGM™ platform. Eur J Med Genet. 2017;60(2):93–9.
24. De Raedt T, Maertens O, Serra E. Legius E. In: Kaufmann D, editor. Neurofibromatoses. Monographs in Human Genetics, vol. 16. Basel: Karger; 2008. p. 142–53.
25. Stevenson DA, Zhou H, Ashrafi S, Messiaen LM, Carey JC, D'Astous JL, et al. Double inactivation of *NF1* in tibial pseudarthrosis. Am J Hum Genet. 2006;79(1):143–8.
26. Brekelmans C, Hollants S, De Groote C, Sohier N, Maréchal M, Geris L, Luyten FP, et al. Neurofibromatosis type 1-related pseudarthrosis: beyond the pseudarthrosis site. Hum Mutat. 2019;40(10):1760;[Epub ahead of print].
27. De Schepper S, Maertens O, Callens T, Naeyaert JM, Lambert J, Messiaen L. Somatic mutation analysis in *NF1* café au lait spots reveals two *NF1* hits in the melanocytes. J Invest Dermatol. 2007;128(4):1050–3.
28. Ruggieri M, Huson S. The clinical and diagnostic implications of mosaicism in the neurofibromatoses. Neurology. 2001;56(11):1433–43.
29. Lázaro C, Ravella A, Gaona A, Volpini V, Estivill X. Neurofibromatosis type 1 due to germline mosaicism in a clinically normal father. N Engl J Med. 1994;331(21):1403–7.
30. Bottillo I, Torrente I, Lanari V, Pinna V, Giustini S, Divona L, et al. Germline mosaicism in neurofibromatosis type 1 due to a paternally derived multi-exon deletion. Am J Med Genet A. 2010;152A(6):1467–73.
31. Trevisson E, Forzan M, Salviati L, Clementi M. Neurofibromatosis type 1 in two siblings due to maternal germline mosaicism. Clin Genet. 2014;85(4):386–9.
32. Wernstedt A, Schatz UA, Laccone F, Krogsdam A, TinschertS, Zschocke J, et al. Third case of genetically confirmed paternal *NF1* germ cell mosaicism. Abstractbook 2018 Joint Global Neurofibromatosis Conference Paris, November 2-6, 2018.
33. Callum P, Messiaen LM, Bower PV, Skovby F, Iger J, Timshel S, et al. Gonosomal mosaicism for an *NF1* deletion in a sperm donor: evidence of the need for coordinated, long-term communication of health information among relevant parties. Hum Reprod. 2012;27(4): 1223–6.
34. Tinschert S, Naumann I, Stegmann E, Buske A, Kaufmann D, Thiel G, et al. Segmental neurofibromatosis is caused by somatic mutation of the neurofibromatosis type 1 (*NF1*) gene. Eur J Hum Genet. 2000;8(6):455–9.
35. Maertens O, De Schepper S, Vandesompele J, Brems H, Heyns I, Janssens S, et al. Molecular dissection of isolated disease features in mosaic neurofibromatosis type 1. Am J Hum Genet. 2007;81(2):243–51.
36. Serra E, Rosenbaum T, Winner U, Aledo R, Ars E, Estivill X, et al. Schwann cells harbor the somatic *NF1* mutation in neurofibromas: evidence of two different Schwann cell subpopulations. Hum Mol Genet. 2000;9(20):3055–64.
37. Maertens O, Brems H, Vandesompele J, De Raedt T, Heyns I, Rosenbaum T, et al. Comprehensive *NF1* screening on cultured Schwann cells from neurofibromas. Hum Mutat. 2006;27(10):1030–40.
38. Messiaen LM, Wimmer K. Pitfalls of automated comparative sequence analysis as a single platform for routine clinical testing for *NF1*. J Med Genet. 2005;42(5):e25.
39. Koczkowska M, Chen Y, Callens T, Gomes A, Sharp A, Johnson S, et al. Genotype-phenotype correlation in *NF1*: evidence for a more severe phenotype associated with missense mutations affecting *NF1* codons 844-848. Am J Hum Genet. 2018;102(1):69–87.
40. Richards S, Aziz N, Bale S, Bick D, Das S, Gastier-Foster J, et al. Standards and guidelines for the interpretation of sequence variants: a joint consensus recommendation of the American College of Medical Genetics and Genomics and the Association for Molecular Pathology. Genet Med. 2015;17(5):405–24.
41. Uusitalo E, Leppävirta J, Koffert A, Suominen S, Vahtera J, Vahlberg T, et al. Incidence and mortality of neurofibromatosis: a total population study in Finland. J Investig Dermatol. 2015;135(3):904–6.
42. Neurofibromatosis: conference statement: National Institutes of Health Consensus Development Conference. Arch Neurol. 1988;45(5):575–8.

43. Wimmer K, Rosenbaum T, Messiaen L. Connections between constitutional mismatch repair deficiency syndrome and neurofibromatosis type 1. Clin Genet. 2017;91(4):507–19.. Review
44. Guerrini-Rousseau L, Suerink M, Grill J, Legius E, Wimmer K, Brugières L. Patients with high-grade gliomas and café-au-lait macules: is neurofibromatosis type 1 the only diagnosis? Am J Neuroradiol. 2019;40(6):E30.
45. DeBella K, Szudek J, Friedman JM. Use of the National Institutes of Health criteria for diagnosis of neurofibromatosis 1 in children. Pediatrics. 2000;105(3 Pt 1):608–14.
46. Brems H, Chmara M, Sahbatou M, Denayer E, Taniguchi K, Kato R, et al. Germline loss-of-function mutations in *SPRED1* cause a neurofibromatosis 1-like phenotype. Nat Genet. 2007;39(9):1120–6.
47. Messiaen L, Yao S, Brems H, Callens T, Sathienkijkanchai A, Denayer E, et al. Clinical and mutational spectrum of neurofibromatosis type 1-like syndrome. JAMA. 2009;302(19):2111–8. Erratum in: JAMA. 2010;303(24):2477.
48. Muram-Zborovski TM, Stevenson DA, Viskochil DH, Dries DC, Wilson AR, Mao R. *SPRED1* mutations in a neurofibromatosis clinic. J Child Neurol. 2010;25(10):1203–9.
49. Upadhyaya M, Huson SM, Davies M, Thomas N, Chuzhanova N, Giovannini S, et al. An absence of cutaneous neurofibromas associated with a 3-bp inframe deletion in exon 17 of the *NF1* gene (c.2970-2972 delAAT): evidence of a clinically significant *NF1* genotype–phenotype correlation. Am. J Hum Genet. 2007;80(1):140–51.
50. Koczkowska M, Callens T, Gomes A, Sharp A, Chen Y, Hicks AD, et al. Expanding the clinical phenotype of individuals with a 3-bp in-frame deletion of the *NF1* gene (c.2970_2972del): an update of genotype-phenotype correlation. Genet med. 2019;21(4):867–76. Erratum in: Genet Med 2019;21(3):764–765
51. Pinna V, Lanari V, Daniele P, Consoli F, Agolini E, Margiotti K, et al. p.Arg1809Cys substitution in neurofibromin is associated with a distinctive NF1 phenotype without neurofibromas. Eur J Hum Genet. 2015;23(8):1068–71.
52. Rojnueangnit K, Xie J, Gomes A, Sharp A, Callens T, Chen Y, et al. High incidence of Noonan syndrome features including short stature and pulmonic stenosis in patients carrying *NF1* missense mutations affecting p.Arg1809: genotype-phenotype correlation. Hum Mutat. 2015;36(11):1052–63.
53. Nyström AM, Ekvall S, Allanson J, Edeby C, Elinder M, Holmström G, et al. Noonan syndrome and neurofibromatosis type I in a family with a novel mutation in *NF1*. Clin Genet. 2009;76(6):524–34.
54. Trevisson E, Morbidoni V, Forzan M, Daolio C, Fumini V, Parrozzani R, et al. The Arg1038Gly missense variant in the *NF1* gene causes a mild phenotype without neurofibromas. Mol Genet Genomic Med. 2019;7(5):e616.

Diagnosis in NF1, Old and New

4

Gianluca Tadini

Contents

Neurofibromatosis 1 (NF1) is a "ras-opathy" inherited in a dominant way, caused by mutations of Neurofibromin gene. Since the publication of NIH Consensus Conference results in 1988 [1], the medical knowledge of the disease is dramatically improved, both molecularly and clinically, especially in past few years [2, 3].

Due to the fact that NF1 is one of the more frequent genetic diseases (1/2500–1/3000, see Chap. 1), in the last 20 years dedicated centers for diagnosis and follow-up of these patients have been established allowing clinicians to acquire noteworthy clinical experience [4]. Moreover, diagnostic laboratories are now able to provide molecular analyses with a detection rate that reach 95% of patients affected by NF1 [5].

Thus, there is an increasing need for a critical review of the diagnostic approach to this neurocutaneous genodermatosis leading to a revision of the NIH diagnostic criteria that take into account the new clinical features [6–9] as well as the availability of new generation molecular testing [10, 11].

G. Tadini (✉)
Pediatric Dermatology Unit, Fondazione IRCCS Ca' Granda, Ospedale Maggiore Policlinico, Department of Physiopathology and Transplantation, Milan, Italy

Paediatric Highly Intensive Care Unit, Fondazione IRCCS Ca' Granda Ospedale Maggiore Policlinico, Milan, Italy

Center for Inherited Cutaneous Diseases, University of Milan, Milan, Italy
e-mail: gtadinicmce@unimi.it

G. Tadini et al. (eds.), *Multidisciplinary Approach to Neurofibromatosis Type 1*,
https://doi.org/10.1007/978-3-319-92450-2_4

We try to discuss "old," well-established, diagnostic criteria, and classification of Neurofibromatosis type 1 comparing them to the "new" knowledge.

4.1 Old Diagnostic Criteria

Physicians are suggested to suspect NF1 in patients having the signs reported in Table 4.1 and the diagnosis is confirmed in probands having two or more of the features listed in Table 4.1.

Based to this list, the diagnosis is established within the first year of life in 50% of subjects in sporadic cases and in nearly 100% of patients with positive family history of NF1.

On the contrary, in sporadic cases, the diagnosis will be confirmed only within the eighth year of life for almost all subjects! [12]. These data mean that for a huge number of individuals the correct diagnosis is dramatically delayed.

Friedman in a recent brilliant review [2] argues that the reason for this delayed diagnosis is "…because many features of NF1 increase in frequency with age." Clinical signs of NF1 have a different age of onset, in other words they are age-dependent. These statements express two deeply different concepts and only the second holds true: each clinical sign of NF1 is not increasing in frequency with age but has its own specific age of onset (see Figs. 4.1 and 4.2). We have to remind at this point that clinicians are used to deal with age-dependent symptoms and signs. It is obvious to cite here that clinical signs of Tuberous Sclerosis are in the same way "age-dependent" and this information is worldwide accepted [13, 14]. From the practical point of view, it will be relevant that the "age-dependence" will be well integrated in the knowledge of NF1, avoiding in example to search for Lisch nodules or neurofibromas examining a newborn with café au lait macules.

Table 4.1 NIH 1988 consensus conference – clinical diagnostic criteria for NF1 [1]

Diagnostic criteria of NF1
Two or more of the following:
At least six café-au-lait macules (> 5 mm in greatest diameter in prepuberal individuals and > 15 mm in greatest diameter in postpuberal individuals)
Freckling in the axillary or inguinal region
Optic glioma
Two or more Lisch nodules (iris hamartomas)
Two or more neurofibromas of any type or one plexiform neurofibroma
A distinctive osseous lesion such as sphenoid dysplasia or thinning of long bone cortex with or without pseudarthrosis
A first-degree relative (parent, sibling, or offspring) with NF-1 by the above criteria

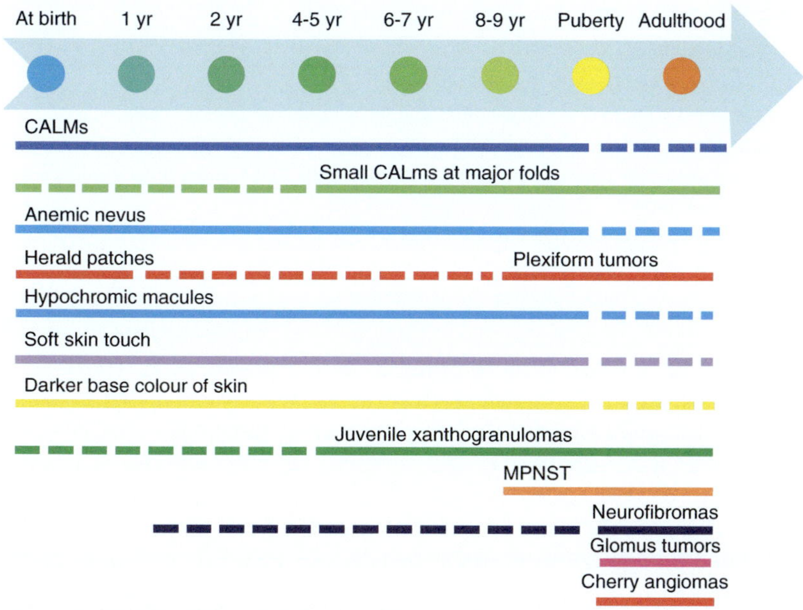

Fig. 4.1 Age-dependency cutaneous signs

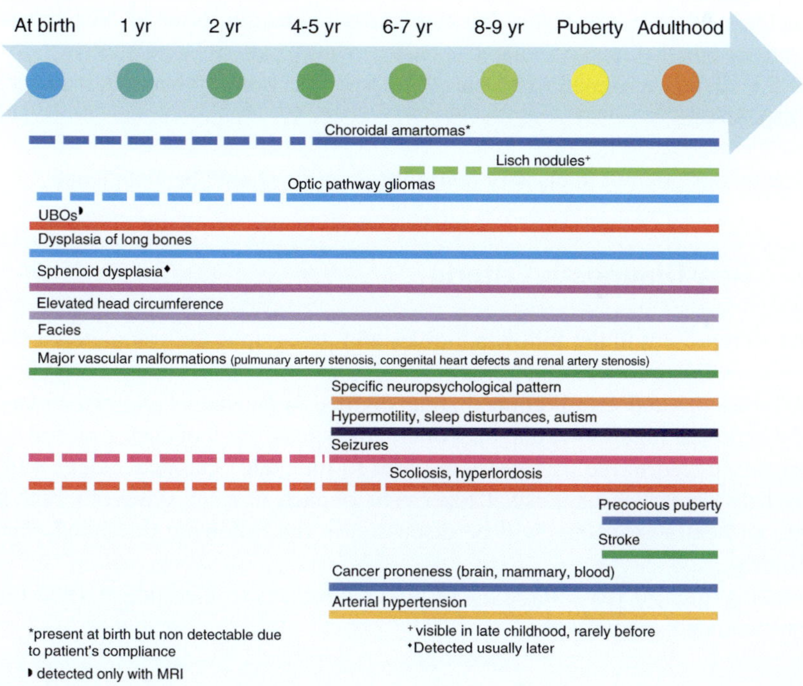

Fig. 4.2 Age-dependency extracutaneous signs

Table 4.2 NF clinical subtypes according to Riccardi [15]

Type	Clinical findings
NF1	Classic type Von Recklinghausen's disease
NF2	Associated with acoustic neurinomas and intracranial tumors (Schwannomas)
NF3	Mixed form between NF1 and NF2 subtypes
NF4	Diffuse neurofibromas and cafè-au-lait pigmentation, but without other clinical features
NF5	Segmental form
NF6	Prominent cafè-au-lait pigmentation only
NF7	Late onset type
NF8	Miscellaneous group, not categorized elsewhere

It seems to be too easy to move criticism to this classification. Thirty-six years ago, clinical and molecular knowledge were so elementary that the effort to classify in any way this complex matter must be only praised Table 4.2.

Nevertheless, it is mandatory to analyze each one of the subtypes in this list:

- NF1 has remained the classical neurofibromatosis type 1 that we are now dealing as well as NF2 that is a well-established disease, clinically and molecularly different from NF1.
- NF3 clearly does not exist anymore as well as NF7 and NF8. These latter, together with NF4 and NF6, reflects only the extreme clinical variability of neurofibromatosis type 1. In particular NF6 may have represented at that time patients with Legius syndrome (see Chap. 16) or olygosymptomatic forms of NF1 or mosaic forms of NF1 having generalized (non-segmental) pattern (see Chap. 15).
- NF5 is clearly assigned to Mosaic NF1 that is a well-known matter today (see Chap. 15).

Finally, this attempt to classify neurofibromatosis should be abandoned.

4.2 New Diagnostic Criteria

We try to represent in the following tables and paragraphs the completely contemporary knowledge concerning NF1.

In Tables 4.3 and 4.4 all clinical signs divided in cutaneous and extracutaneous will be exposed. Figures 4.1 and 4.2 contain the age of onset of each sign and symptom that emerged in the past years in order to integrate "classical" signs with the aim to help for earlier diagnosis. Closer view of each sign and symptom, both skin-related and extracutaneous, will be discussed in the following dedicated chapters (see Index).

Looking after 30 years at the list of NIH Consensus Conference of 1988 further major comments are needed:

1. The only genetic consideration included is: "a first degree relative with NF1 as defined by the above criteria." Just few years after, in 1990 the group of

Table 4.3 Cutaneous signs (see also Chap. 5)

Pigmentary anomalies	Neurofibromas (80% of patients)	Vascular lesions	Other skin anomalies
– Café au Lait macules (CALMs) (almost in 100% of patients) – "smaller" CALMs at major folds (former "freckling") (nearly in 90%) – Darker color of the skin compared with healthy family members or normal population (50%) – Hypopigmented ovalar or roundish spots (10–15%) – Soft skin touch (nearly 50% in pediatric age, less common in adulthood) – "Herald Patch" of plexiform neurofibromas (10–20%) – Some cases (about 5%) with a diffuse small lentiginous-like pattern involving the entire skin intermingled with more classical CALMs	– Sessile – Pedunculated "Button-hole" lesions (20%) – Plexiform Neurofibromas (50%) – MPNST	– Nevus anemicus (20–50%) – Blue-red macules (5%) – Precocious or ectopic cherry angiomas (5%) – Glomus tumors (3%)	– Juvenile xanthogranulomas (10–15%) – Itch (30%) – Disorders of cutaneous adnexa (rare, such hypohidrosis and alopecia) – Mucosal lesions (rare, neurofibromas and plexiform neurofibromas)

Viskochil cloned the NF1 gene on chromosome 17 [13] and nowadays the molecular diagnosis has reached an accuracy of about 95% of patients (see Chaps. 3 and 15), claiming for the introduction of molecular diagnosis as a diagnostic criterion, as occurs for other groups of genodermatoses such as Ichthyoses [16], and Epidermolysis Bullosa [17].

2. We are well aware that availability of molecular diagnosis in different countries may be an obstacle for molecular diagnosis but we cannot deny the relevance of this issue for early diagnosis.
3. There is a different position for "Café au lait macules" and "Freckling." Histological and molecular characterizations of "freckles" revealed that do not differ from café au lait macules [18] and they should therefore not to be considered as different entities and as a separate diagnostic criterion. "Freckles" are "smaller" café au lait macules exceptionally present at birth, usually arising later in childhood (often after the fourth or fifth years of life), located at major folds and possibly with a peculiar clinical presentation (minor dimension) due to their anatomic site. Clinicians are well aware that many skin diseases (e.g., psoriasis) have a different clinical presentation when they are located at major folds.

Table 4.4 Extracutaneous signs

Ocular manifestations	– Lisch Nodules (90% in adulthood but only 50% in late childhood) – Choroidal Hamartomas (>50–70% overall, but visible at 4–5 years of age) – Optic ways gliomas (up to 10%) – Retinal vasoproliferative tumors (hood, Parozzani) (rare) – Neovascular glaucoma (rare) – Scleral CALMs (rare) – Decreased lacrimation (rare)
Neurological manifestations	– Learning disabilities and/or behavioral problems, including social competence (50–80%) (Lehtonen) – Intellectual disability (5–7%) (pride and north) – Autism (up to 30%) – Dyslexia, dyscalculia, other language and memory disorders (20%) – Hypermobility, motor and executive functions, including visual-spatial performances – Sleep disturbances – Polyneuropathy (related to multiple nerve root tumors) and related pain – Risk developing MPNST (5–7%) – Epilepsy (up to 10%) – Headache and migraine (20%) – "Unidentified bright objects" (UBOs) at MRI
Skeletal and structural abnormalities	– Low 25-OH vitamin D levels (up to 40%) – Increased bone resorption – Osteopenia and osteoporosis – Dysplasia of long bones (1–4&) – Sphenoid wing dysplasia (3–7%) – Scoliosis, hyperlordosis (10%) – Elevated head circumference (and related hypertelorism) – Reduced muscle strength
Vascular features	– Arterial hypertension – Malformations, aneurism or stenosis of medium-sized and large arteries (aorta, renal, coronary, cerebral arteries) – Stroke – "Moya-Moya disease"
Cardiologic involvement	– Pulmonary artery stenosis – Other congenital heart defects – Intracardiac neurofibromas (rare)
Cancer-related features	– MPNST (10%) – (Optic pathway gliomas 5–20%) – Brain tumors, benign or malignant – Leukemias, myelodisplasias, lymphomas – Pheochromocytoma – Rhabdomyosarcoma – Cancer proneness (increased risk especially for mammary cancer)
Endocrine pattern	– Precocious puberty (primary or more frequently related to chiasmal tumors) (2–5%) – Vitamin 25-OH deficiency

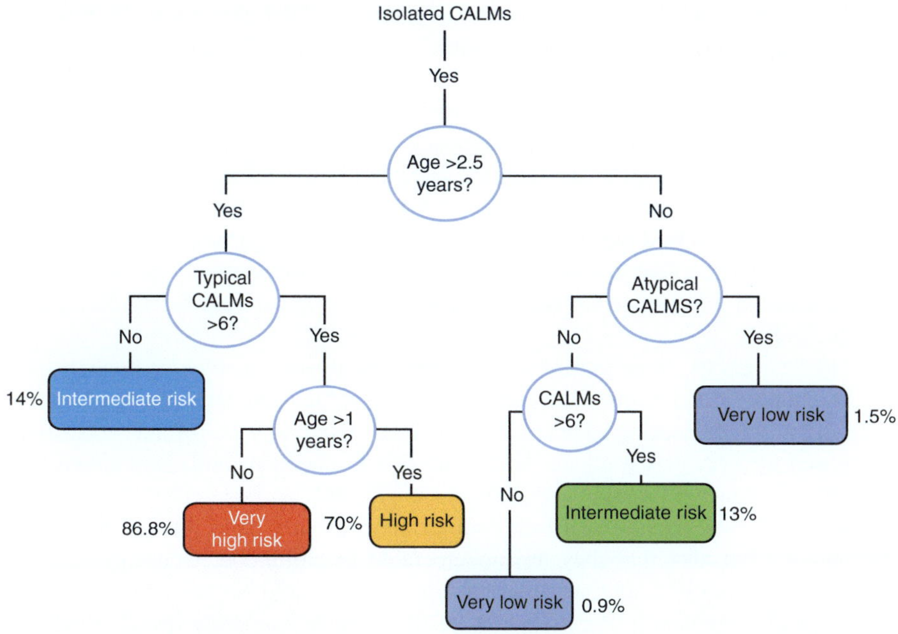

Fig. 4.3 Algorithm predicting NF1

4. Overall, isolated CALMs are visible in about 3% of neonates and about 28% of primary school aged children; they may be multiple in 1% of children and up to 10% of adults. They are not a pathognomonic sign of NF1 but are a hallmark of NF1. It is estimated that at least 5% of individuals with multiple CALMS may not have NF1 (see Table 5.1 in Chap. 5). Furthermore, clinical experience in large cohort of patients shows clearly that the dimensions of cafè au lait macules do not have a high statistical significance as a further specification of a diagnostic criterion. For the same reason, the number of 6 CALMs necessary to be considered as a diagnostic sign may be not so relevant, given the existence of patients with a causal mutation in NF1 gene who do not reach the count of six CALMs, at least for patients under the first 2 years of life [18].
5. In attempt to integrate and improve NIH CC diagnostic criteria, Ben-Schachar et al. in 2017 proposed a simple algorithm (see Fig. 4.3, based on the differences between typical and atypical CALMs) that enables the subdivision of children with isolated CALMs as being at low or high risk to develop constitutional NF1, prior to perform molecular diagnosis [19].
6. The presence of hypochromic macules in 10–15% of NF1 patients adds a further diagnostic sign. They are visible since early childhood intermingled with CALMs in any site of the skin.
7. Recent clinical studies [20–23] have added the Anemic Nevus as a new potential and useful diagnostic criterion for NF1. This sign, often present at birth or visible in early childhood, is a rare occasional finding in healthy controls. In

large cohorts AN is found in 20–40% of patients in NF1 population. Preliminary data have shown that it often correlates with positive NF1 genetic tests.

8. In the same perspective the presence of Juvenile Xanthogranulomas in 10–15% of patients with CALMs in early childhood, compared to 1–2% in normal population, is a new clue for early diagnosis.
9. A tendency to generalized increase in skin pigmentation, probably due to a "one-hit" mutation in melanocytes and a particular soft skin touch complete the new cutaneous findings and may be useful to early diagnosis.
10. Neurofibromas, Lisch nodules, and Optic gliomas are relatively late signs, even specific, of the disease but are rarely found in patients during first childhood [2, 20, 24].
11. On the contrary, bone lesions such as Sphenoid dysplasia and long bone dysplasia, mainly tibial, seem to be pathognomonic of NF1, the latter being present at birth and representing an abnormality of bone itself, and the former rarely diagnosed at birth or within the first years of life and constantly associated to a plexiform neurofibroma and dural ectasia [25, 26].
12. It is well established that Lisch nodules are present in over 90% of NF1 adult patients but also that they are undetectable in childhood. Consequently, the recently described ophthalmological sign of Choroidal Nodules could be diagnostically relevant in the first years of life. One recent study revealed that the prevalence of near-infrared reflectance detected choroidal nodules was 71% in pediatric NF1 group, a much higher figure than 43% prevalence of Lisch nodules in the same group of patients [7, 8].
13. 43 to 93% of NF1 patients show focal areas of high signal intensity (the so-called Unidentified Bright Objects (UBOs) on cerebral magnetic resonance). DeBella proposed this finding in the year 2000 as a new diagnostic sign [27]. (See Chap. 13).
14. Emerging data show a peculiar neuropsychological pattern in children with NF1. Impairment of cognitive and executive functions, attention, emotion, and social competence may be noted in nearly 40% of individuals in pre-scholar and scholar age [28]. (See Chap. 14).
15. Among the structural abnormalities observed in NF1 patients, elevated head circumference and related hypertelorism is frequent and affects about 50% of cases [29–31]. A particular "facies" characterized by upper face predominance and "gross" facial appearance may also be noted in NF1 patients.

Finally, the NIH Consensus Conference Diagnostic Criteria fitted perfectly for at least 20 years, reaching a widespread consensus throughout the world and we are very grateful to Vincent Riccardi and coworkers for this highly qualitative performance. Nevertheless, we believe that, supported by new findings, nowadays we are able to make earlier diagnosis, I mean within the first year of life, which is quite impossible considering only the list of diagnostic criteria established by Riccardi and Colleagues in 1988.

Diagnostic communication to parents of an affected individual in pediatric age is becoming more and more difficult because: (a) the clinical presentation of the disease can vary from exclusively cutaneous involvement to the complete expression of the various signs in different organs, making its course unpredictable and the prognosis uncertain; (b) as it is now an easy access to medical websites that often describe NF1 mainly in its worst presentation, patients and their families understandably become anxious about its prognosis and claim for a prompt diagnosis.

Furthermore, correct communication is only possible if physicians are perfectly aware of the characteristics of the disease, its course and prognosis but, with some exceptions represented by clinicians working in dedicated diagnostic Centers, there seems to be considerable "confusion" about this topic.

Funding Sources None.

Conflict of Interest None declared.

References

1. National Institute of Health Consensus Development Conference Statement. Neurofibromatosis. Arch Neurol (Chic). 1988;45:575–8.
2. Friedman JM. Neurofibromatosis 1. In: Adam MP, Ardinger HH, Pagon RA, Wallace SE, LJH B, Stephens K, Amemiya A, editors. GeneReviews® [Internet]. Seattle: University of Washington; 1998. p. 1993–2020.
3. Sabbagh A, Pasmant E, Imbard A, Luscan A, Soares M, Blanché H, Laureandeau I, Ferkal S, Vidau M, Pinson S, Bellané-Chantelot C, Vidau D, Parfait B, Wolkestein P. NF1 molecular characterization and neurofibromatosis type I genotype-phenotype correlation:the French experience. Hum Mutat. 2013;34:1510–8.
4. Nunley KS, Gao F, Albers AC, Bayliss SJ, Gutmann DH. Predictive value of café au lait macules at initial consultation in the diagnosis of neurofibromatosis type 1. Arch Dermatol. 2009;145:883–7.
5. Curless RG, Siatkowski M, Glaser JS, Shatz NJ. MRI diagnosis of NF-1 in children without café-au-lait skin lesions. Pediatr Neurol. 1998;18:269–71.
6. Tadini G, Milani D, Menni F, Pezzani L, Sabatini C, Esposito S. Is it time to change the neurofibromatosis 1 diagnostic criteria? Eur J Intern Med. 2014;25:506–10.
7. Viola F, Villani E, Natacci F, Selicorni A, Melloni G, Vezzola D, et al. Choroidal abnormalities detected by near-infrared reflectance imaging as a new diagnostic criterion for neurofibromatosis 1. Ophthalmogy. 2012;119:369–75.
8. Parrozzani R, Clementi M, Frizziero L, Miglionico G, Perrini P, Caverzan F, Kotsafti O, Comacchio F, Trevisson E, Convento E, Fusetti S, Midena E. In vivo detection of chroidal abnormalities related to NF1: feasibility and comparison with standard NIH diagnosis criteria in pediatric patients. Invest Ophthalmol Vis Sci. 2015;56:6036–42.
9. Evans DG, Bowers N, Burkitt-Wright E, Miles E, Garg S, Scott-Kitching V, Penman-Splitt M, Dobbie A, Howard E, Ealing J, Vassalo G, Wallace AJ, Newman W, Northen UK, NF1 Research Network, Huson SM. Comprehensive RNA analysis of the NF1 gene in classically affected NF1 affected individuals meeting NIH criteria has high sensitivity and mutation negative testing is reassuring in isolated cases with pigmentary features only. EBioMedicine. 2016;7:212–20.
10. Koczkowska M, Chen Y, Callens T, Gomes A, Sharp A, Johnson S, Hsiao MC, Chen Z, Balasubramanian M, Barnett CP, Becker TA, Ben-Shachar S, Bertola DR, Blakeley JO, Burkitt-Wright EMM, Callaway A, Crenshaw M, Cunha KS, Cunningham M, D'Agostino MD, Dahan K, De Luca A, Destrée A, Dhamija R, Eoli M, Evans DGR, Galvin-Parton P, George-Abraham JK, Gripp KW, Guevara-Campos J, Hanchard NA, Hernández-Chico C, Immken L, Janssens S, Jones KJ, Keena BA, Kochhar A, Liebelt J, Martir-Negron A, Mahoney MJ, Maystadt I, McDougall C, McEntagart M, Mendelsohn N, Miller DT, Mortier G, Morton J, Pappas J, Plotkin SR, Pond D, Rosenbaum K, Rubin K, Russell L, Rutledge LS, Saletti V, Schonberg R, Schreiber A, Seidel M, Siqveland E, Stockton DW, Trevisson E, Ullrich NJ,

Upadhyaya M, van Minkelen R, Verhelst H, Wallace MR, Yap YS, Zackai E, Zonana J, Zurcher V, Claes K, Martin Y, Korf BR, Legius E, Messiaen LM. Genotype-phenotype correlation in NF1: evidence for a more severe phenotype associated with missense mutations affecting NF1 CODONS 844-848. Am J Hum Genet. 2018;102(1):69–87.
11. DeBella K, Szudek J, Friedman JM. Use of the national institutes of health criteria for diagnosis of neurofibromatosis 1 in children. Pediatrics. 2000;105(3 Pt 1):608–14.
12. Tadini G, Brena M, Gelmetti C, Pezzeni L. Atlas of genodermatoses. Second ed. Boca Raton: CRC Press, Taylor & Francis Group; 2015. ISBN 9781466598355.
13. Viskochil D, Buchberg AM, Xu G, Cawthon RM, Stevens J, Wolff RK, Culver M, Carey JC, Copeland NG, Jenkins NA, et al. Deletions and a translocation interrupt a cloned gene at the neurofibromatosis type 1 locus. Cell. 1990;62(1):187–92.
14. Oji V, Tadini G, Akiyama M, et al. Revised nomenclature and classification of inherited ichthyoses: results of the first ichthyoses consensus in Sorèze 2009. J Am Acad Dermatol. 2010;63(4):607–41.
15. Riccardi VM. Neurofibromatosis: clinical heterogeneity. Curr Probl Cancer. 1982;7(2):1–34.
16. Fine JD, Bruckner-Tuderman L, Eady RA, et al. Inherited epidermolysis bullosa: updated recommendations on diagnosis and classification. J Am Acad Dermatol. 2014;70(6):1103–26.
17. Maertens O, De Schepper S, Vandesompele J, Brems H, Heyns I, Janssen S, Speleman F, Legius E, Messiaen L. Molecular dissection of isolated features in mosaic neurofibromatosis type 1. Am J Hum Genet. 2007;81:243–51.
18. Tadini G, Personal observations. Unpublished.
19. Ben-Shachar S, Constantini S, Hallevi H, Sach EK, Upadhyaya M, Evans GD, Huson SM. Increased rate of missense/in-frame mutations in individuals with NF1-related pulmonary stenosis: a novel genotype-phenotype correlation. Eur J Hum Genet. 2013;21:535–9.
20. Tadini G, Brena M, Pezzani L, et al. Nevus anemicus in neurofibromatosis type 1: a potential new diagnostic criterion. J Am Acad Dermatol. 2013;69:768–75.
21. Ferrari F, Masurel A, Olivier-Faivre L, et al. Juvenile xanthogranuloma and nevus anemicus in the diagnosis of neurofibromatosis type 1. JAMA Dermatol. 2014;150:42–6.
22. Hernández-Martín A, García-Martínez FJ, Duat A, López-Martín I, Noguera-Morel L, Torrelo A. Nevus anemicus: a distinctive cutaneous finding in neurofibromatosis type 1. Pediatr Dermatol. 2015;32:342–7.
23. Tadini G, Brena M. Anemic nevus is a new diagnostic criterion for neurofibromatosis type 1. G Ital Dermatol Venereol. 2017;152(5):548–549.
24. Ragge NK, Falk RE, Cohen WE, Murphree AL. Images of Lisch nodules across the spectrum. Eye (Lond). 1993;7:95–101.
25. Arrington DK, Danehy AR, Peleggi A, Proctor MR, Irons MB, Ullrich NJ. Calvarial defects and skeletal dysplasia in patients with neurofibromatosis type 1. J Neurosurg Pediatr. 2013;11:410–6.
26. Hu Z, Liu Z, Qiu Y, Xu L, Yan H, Zhu Z. Morphological differences in the vertebrae of scoliosis secondary to neurofibromatosis type I are caused by mutations in the NF1 gene. Am J Med Genet A. 2006;140:2749–56.
27. DeBella K, Poskitt K, Szudek J, Friedman JM. Use of "unidentified bright objects" on MRI for diagnosis of neurofibromatosis 1 in children. Neurology. 2000;54(8):1646–51.
28. Lehtonen A, Howie E, Trump D, Huson SM. Behaviour in children with neurofibromatosis type 1: cognition, executive function, attention, emotion, and social competence. Dev Med Child Neurol. 2013;55:111–25.
29. Steen RG, Taylor JS, Langston JW, Glass JO, Brewer VR, Reddick WE, Mages R, Pivnick EK. Prospective evaluation of the brain in asymptomatic children with neurofibromatosis type 1: relationship of macrocephaly to T1 relaxation changes and structural brain abnormalities. AJNR Am J Neuroradiol. 2001;22(5):810–7.
30. Margariti PN, Blekas K, Katzioti FG, Zikou AK, Tzoufi M, Argyropoulou MI. Magnetization transfer ratio and volumetric analysis of the brain in macrocephalic patients with neurofibromatosis type 1. Eur Radiol. 2007;17(2):433–8.
31. Gutmann DH, Parada LF, Silva AJ, Ratner N. Neurofibromatosis type 1: modeling CNS dysfunction. J Neurosci. 2012;32(41):14087–93.

Clinical Features of NF1 in the Skin

5

Michela Brena, Francesca Besagni,
Angela Hernandez-Martin, and Gianluca Tadini

Contents

M. Brena (✉) · G. Tadini
Pediatric Dermatology Unit, Fondazione IRCCS Ca' Granda, Ospedale Maggiore Policlinico, Department of Physiopathology and Transplantation, Milan, Italy

Paediatric Highly Intensive Care Unit, Fondazione IRCCS Ca' Granda Ospedale Maggiore Policlinico, Milan, Italy

Center for Inherited Cutaneous Diseases, University of Milan, Milan, Italy
e-mail: michela.brena@policlinico.mi.it

F. Besagni
Independent Contractor, Santa Caterina Health Center, Parma, Italy

A. Hernandez-Martin
Hospital Infantil Universitario Nino Jesus, Madrid, Spain

G. Tadini et al. (eds.), *Multidisciplinary Approach to Neurofibromatosis Type 1*,
https://doi.org/10.1007/978-3-319-92450-2_5

5.1 Café-Au-Lait Macules (CALMs) [1]

CALMs are, probably, the most important clinical sign in children, both because they are present in almost all patients with NF1, and because they are usually the first visible sign of the disease. CALMs are commonly present at birth or they become evident shortly afterwards. Although café-au-lait macules are usually readily diagnosed on examination, they may be overlooked or, in fair-skinned infants, difficult to appreciate on physical examination [2]. The appearance of multiple café-au-lait macules is an early sign of the condition, which often alerts physicians to follow-up and further examine the patient for the possibility of NF1.

Typical CALMs have a variable color, homogenous tone, and a smooth, regular border (Figs. 5.1 and 5.2). They also considerably vary in size, from a few millimeters to several centimeters. Their size increases in proportion with the growth of the child, and they take on a darker tone during childhood, before lightening again during adulthood. Although they can be found anywhere on the body, even if more common on the torso, buttocks, and lower extremities, they do not usually appear on

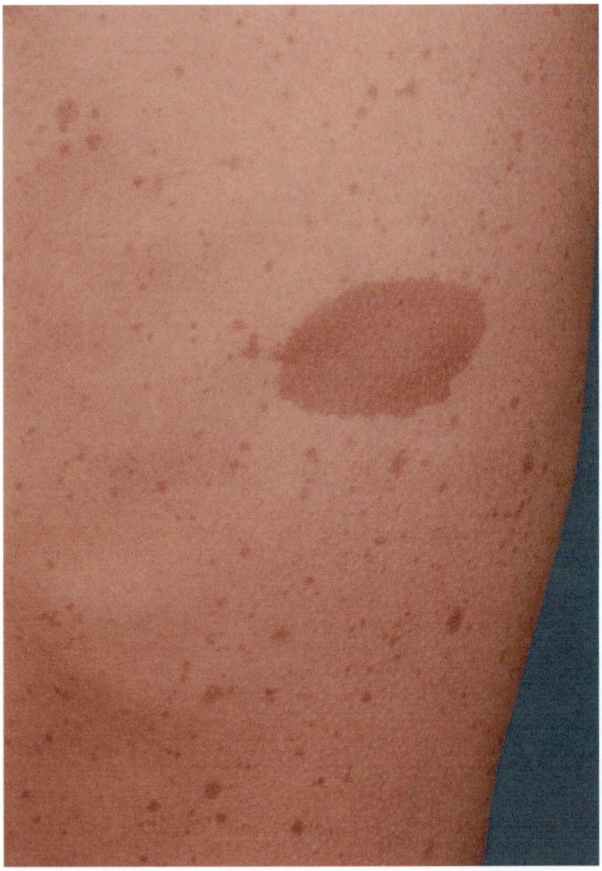

Fig. 5.1 Typical CALMs

Fig. 5.2 Typical CALMs

the face, suggesting that sunlight exposure is not involved in the pathogenesis [3]. Atypical CALMs, indeed, have jagged contours and irregular shape (Figs. 5.3 and 5.4), resembling the "coast of Maine" [2].

Histologically, CALMs show increased melanin in melanocytes and basal keratinocytes, but no melanocyte proliferation. The presence of macromelanosomes has also been observed, along with a greater concentration of melanin in CALMs of patients with NF1 than in NF1-unrelated CALMs. From the molecular point of view, it has been demonstrated that melanocytes of CALMs have a second NF1 mutation in the gene on the other allele [4].

However, although CALMs are very suggestive of NF1, they are not pathognomonic; non-related NF1 CALMs are visible in about 3% of neonates and about 28% of primary school aged children, they may be multiple in 1% of children and up to 10% of adults. On the contrary, in our opinion, these high percentages of patients are due to the scarce diffusion of NF1 molecular detection. The more typical the morphology of CALMs, the greater probability that NF1 is confirmed, whereas there is no association between number of CALMs and severity of NF1 [2, 3].

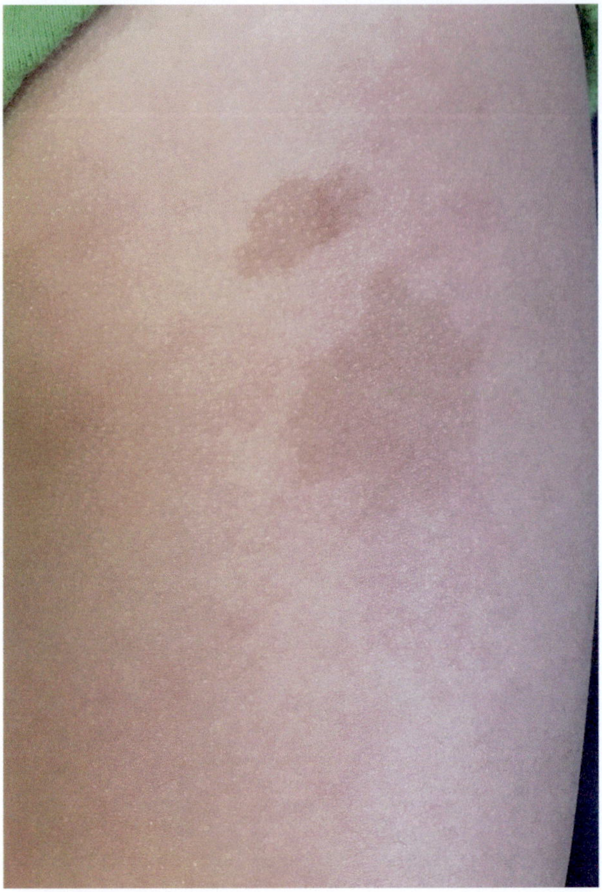

Fig. 5.3 Atypical CALMs

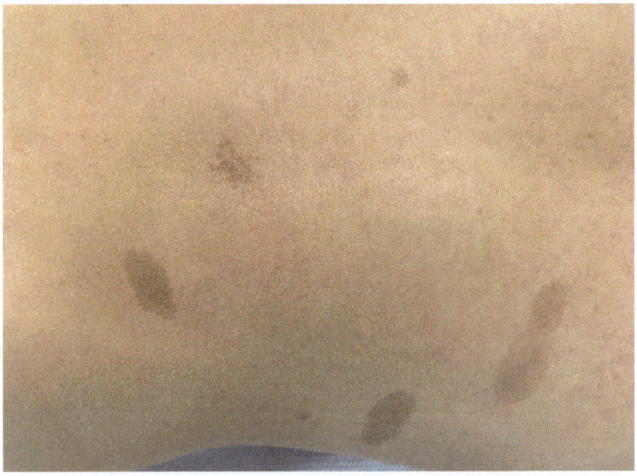

Fig. 5.4 Atypical CALMs

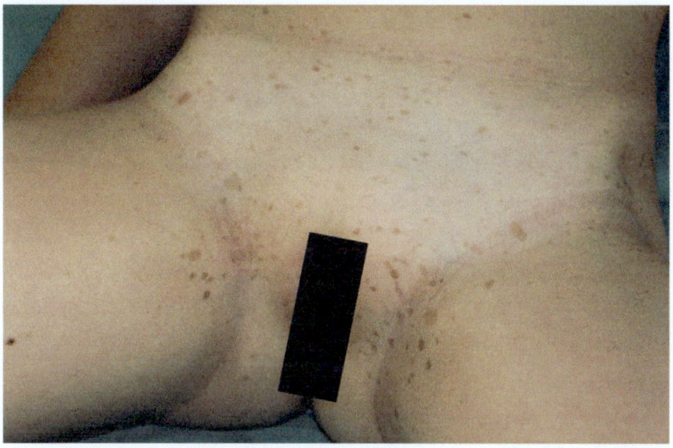

Fig. 5.5 Small CALMs distributed on large folds

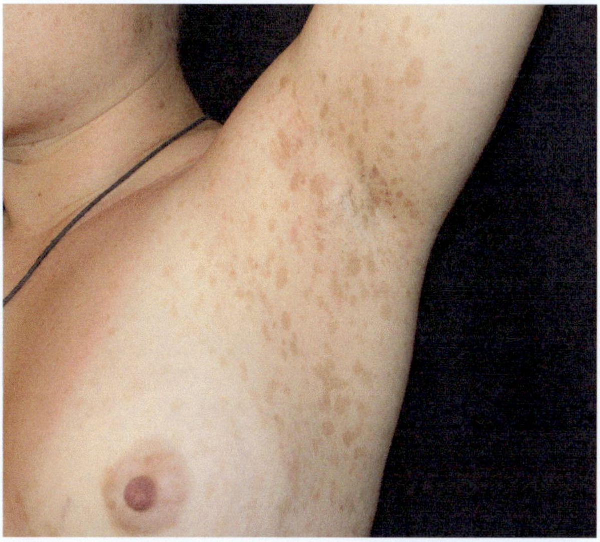

Fig. 5.6 Small CALMs distributed on large folds

CALMs of minor dimensions are visible as small pigmented lesions (1 or 2 mm) of light brown color, preferentially distributed on large folds that are not usually present at birth but rather develop during childhood, usually from the age of 2 years onwards (Figs. 5.5 and 5.6). This sign has been traditionally called “freckling” or “Crowe’s sign,” but the histological and ultrastructural findings are identical to those of CALMs, confirming being the same entity. Because of that, they should, therefore, not be considered as a separate criterion but as “small café-au-lait spots” that appear later in childhood (often after the age of 4–5 years) and have a particular presentation possibly because of their anatomic site [5]. In some cases (about 5% of patients) they have a diffuse small lentiginous-like pattern involving the entire skin, intermingled with more classical CALMs.

Café-au-lait macules are often the only NF1 presentation, which is shown in 99% of NF1 patients at 1 year of age [6].

Segmental lentiginosis is characterized by pinpoint to small pigmented macules in a mosaic pattern (checkerboard), especially located in the upper part of the body with or without intermingled café-au-lait macules; true melanocytic nevi may be scattered in association with segmental lentiginosis (Fig. 5.7), see Chap. 15. The distinction between true lentiginous mosaicism and mosaic forms of neurofibromatosis type 1, however, is still to be explained and elucidated by molecular analysis [7]. It is very important to differentiate these lesions from others such as hyperchromic nevi, pigmentary mosaicisms, congenital melanocytic nevi, nevus spilus, macular urticaria pigmentosa, and post inflammatory hyperpigmentation.

Several diseases may be associated with CALMs, mainly Legius syndrome, an autosomal dominant human disorder caused by mutations in SPRED1 (Sprouty Related, EVH1 domain containing I) gene, characterized by partial clinical overlap with NF1 (Table 5.1) (see Chap. 16).

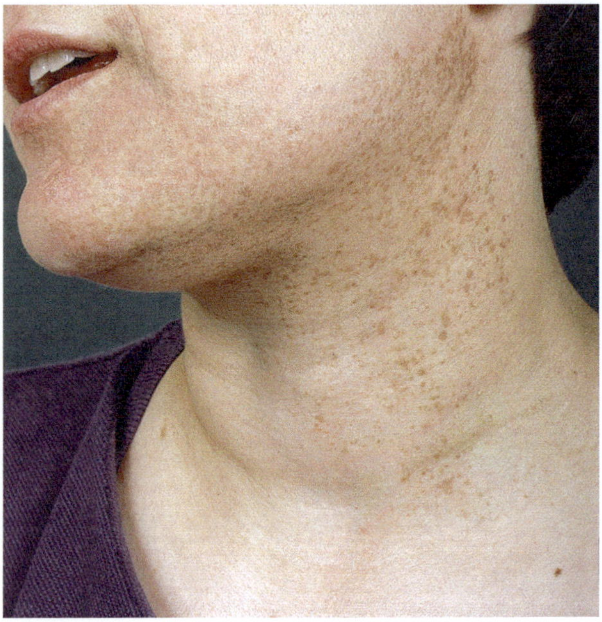

Fig. 5.7 Segmental lentiginosis

Table 5.1 Major other diseases with cafè-au-lait macules

Legius syndrome
McCune-Albright syndrome
Noonan-CFC syndrome
LEOPARD syndrome
Neurofibromatosis type 2
Ataxia–telangiectasia
Ringed chromosome disease
Mismatch-repair syndromes
Tuberous sclerosis
Turner syndrome
Gorlin syndrome
Bloom's syndrome

Segmental NF1 is a variant of NF1 that results from somatic mosaicism arising from postzygotic mutations in the NF1 gene, such that the clinical manifestations of the disease are present only in a localized body segment: due to this reason, it should be called mosaic NF1 (MNF1) (see Chap. 15). The involved area can be one or more segments or even half of the body, in a symmetrical or asymmetrical arrangement, the phenotype depending on the timing and cell lines affected by the mosaic mutation [8, 9] (Figs. 5.8 and 5.9). According to a recent review by Vàzquez-Osorio and colleague, no patient with juvenile xanthogranulomas in MNF1 has been reported, and only one patient with MNF1 and anemic nevus has been published [10]. Individuals with MNF have milder phenotypes and present with fewer clinical manifestations and complications than individuals with complete NF1, which may lead to under recognition [11–13].

The calculated prevalence of MNF1 in the general population is 1 in 36,000–40,000 individuals (0.0006–0.0027%), although it is probably underreported [13]. Individuals with MNF1 are also at risk of gonadal mosaicism and thus having offspring with complete NF1 and its associated complications [12, 13]. There is a risk of malignancy associated with the mutation, and there are

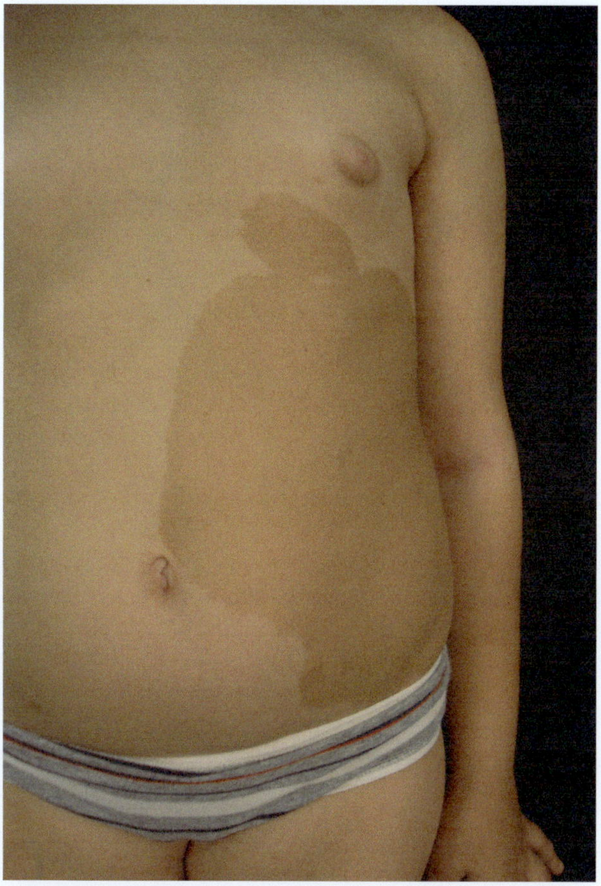

Fig. 5.8 Mosaic NF1

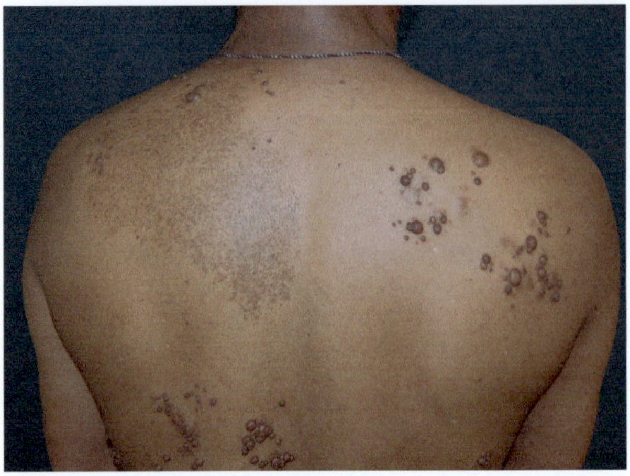

Fig. 5.9 Mosaic NF1

several reports of patients with malignant tumors associated with MNF1 [14, 15], although the risk is lower than in complete NF1. Individuals with MNF1 should receive appropriate genetic counseling because they may have gonadal mosaicism and could have children with complete NF1, even if they have a mild localized phenotype. This might be particularly true for individuals with pigmentary changes only.

Very few patients with MNF1 underwent genetic testing, which is important information to further expand the knowledge of the disease. Genetic testing should be conducted on blood and skin biopsies of lesional and unaffected skin, in order to find the somatic mutation and to improve the yield of the disease [10].

5.2 Diffuse Hyperpigmentation

Patients with NF1 have diffuse generalized hyperpigmentation that becomes evident by comparing the tone of their skin with that of unaffected family members, and this explains the underlying hyperpigmentation often seen in segmental forms of NF1 [5].

It has been shown that melanocytes from some patients with NF1 contain giant pigment granules known as macromelanosomes in both CALMs and non-CALM-derived melanocytes [16]. More recently, it was reported that a loss of neurofibromin expression in human primary cultures of melanocytes derived from healthy patients led to aberrant subcellular localization of melanosomes [17]. Jennifer Allouche et al. highlighted the functional consequences of decreased neurofibromin expression on melanosome maturation. They showed that in melanocytes, decreased expression of neurofibromin on signaling pathways is characterized by an increase in the MEK/MAPK and cAMP-mediated PKA pathways, involved in melanin biosynthesis and pigmentation of melanosomes, leading in overexertion of melanogenic enzymes [18].

5.3 Neurofibromas [1]

Neurofibromas are benign tumors that originate from the neural sheath of the peripheral nerves. They are composed of a heterogeneous mixture of Schwann cells, fibroblasts, perineural cells, mastocytes, axons, endothelial cells and abundant extracellular matrix. It seems that the cells that begin to proliferate are Schwann cells and that these cells harbour mutations of NF1 gene in both alleles [3].

Neurofibromas are further characterized as cutaneous (dermal), subcutaneous, and plexiform.

Cutaneous neurofibromas appear as rubbery, exophytic soft papules and nodules ranging from 2–3 mm to 1–2 cm in dimension, flesh colored, randomly distributed anywhere in the body, focused along the course of peripheral nerves (Fig. 5.10). Less frequently they are soft subcutaneous small masses, slightly protruding with a dome-shaped appearance, easily pressable with palpable borders (buttonholes neurofibromas) (Fig. 5.11). These lesions usually present during adolescence and increase in number during adulthood; they may cause significant disfigurement and pruritus, which is attributed to abundance of mastocytes that infiltrate the lesions [2, 3]. There are two critical periods of development, adolescence and pregnancy, and therefore these lesions are thought to be hormone-dependent and, in fact, it has been shown that they have progesterone receptors [19, 20]. At times, they may need to be surgically removed when they cause esthetic or functional problems due to their number or size, although malignant transformation is very rare. Even with complete surgical resection, however, recurrence is expected in approximately 20% of cases [21]. From the histological point of view, cutaneous neurofibromas are unencapsulated tumors characterized by a mixture of Schwann cells, fibroblasts, mastocytes, and perineural cells nestled in a collagen stroma of variable myxoid component.

Subcutaneous neurofibromas appear as rubbery subcutaneous masses: the diffuse lesions are manifest as subcutaneous masses of greater or lesser extension, with poorly defined borders and elastic consistency. They are often painful, and those that involve the dorsal root ganglia may cause symptoms of spinal cord compression. Subcutaneous neurofibromas can be nodular or diffuse on palpation, whereas

Fig. 5.10 Cutaneous neurofibromas

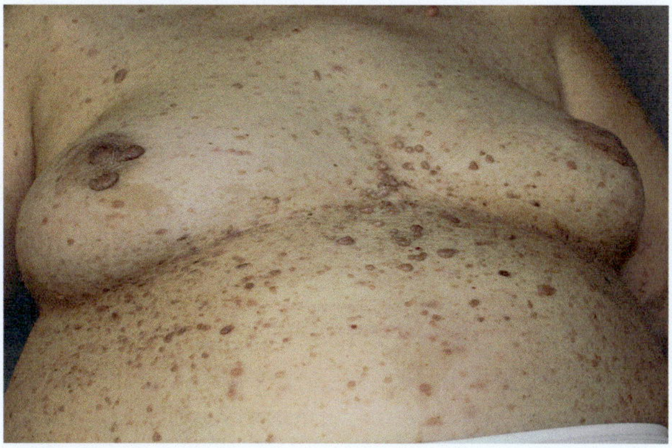

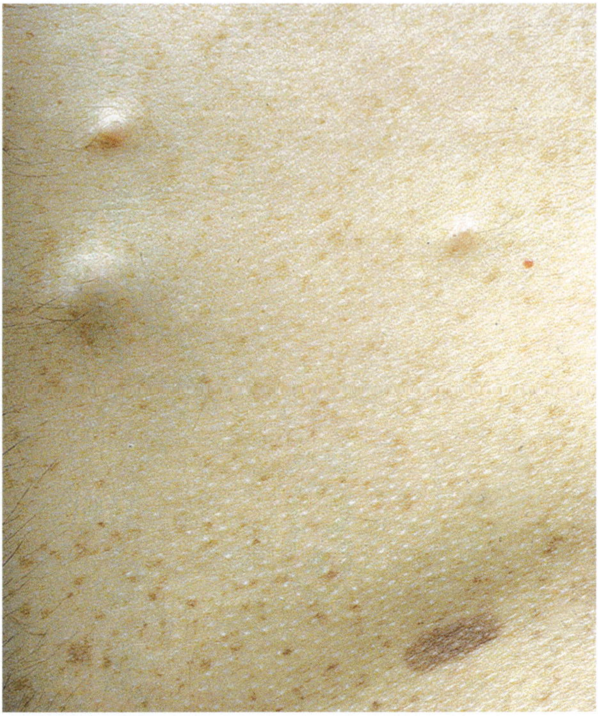

Fig. 5.11 Buttonholes neurofibromas

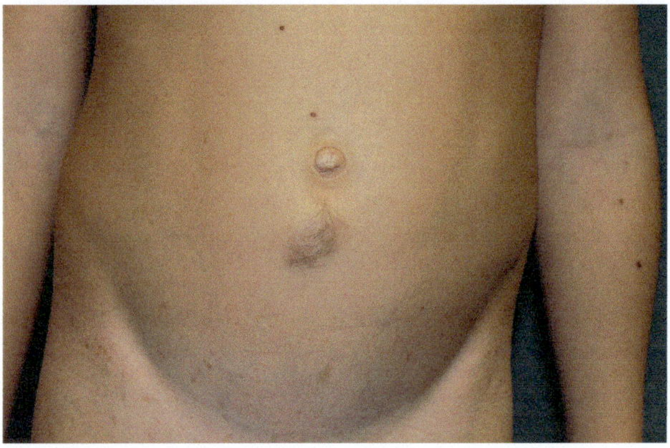

Fig. 5.12 Subcutaneous neurofibromas

the deeper lesions are not usually palpable and require imaging tests to be visualized (Fig. 5.12). A recent research by Riccardi, in which he treated a NF1 patient with oral ketotifen for 30 years since infancy, showed an arrest of the growth of neurofibromas at a very early stage of development: these data suggested a distinctive benefit to treat an NF1 patient with a mast cell degranulation inhibitor before cutaneous neurofibromas are clinically apparent [22]. Further studies and research are, however, still required to confirm this observation.

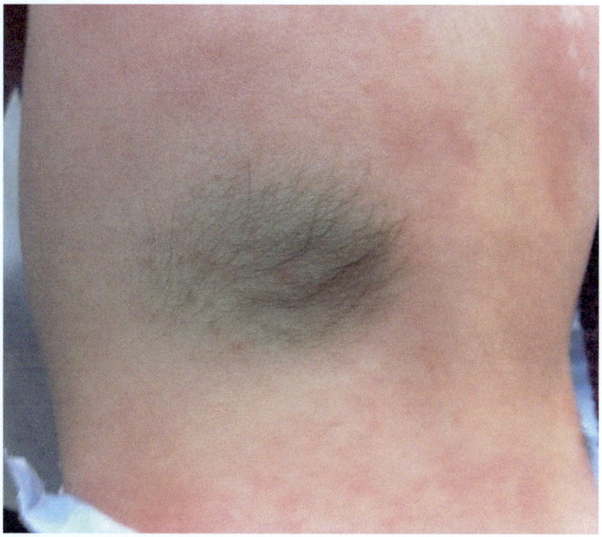

Fig. 5.13 "Herald patch" of plexiform neurofibroma

Plexiforms neurofibromas (PN) are usually present at birth as hyperpigmented and often hairy lesions ("herald patch," Figs. 5.13 and 5.14), although they may not become clinically apparent until later childhood or adulthood, growing progressively as large subcutaneous soft tumors showing mosaic distribution, with a particular full bag texture, located elsewhere on the skin and potentially reaching huge dimensions, becoming the so-called "tumeurs royales" (Figs. 5.15 and 5.16). Plexiform tumors arise from bi-allelic inactivation of NF1 gene (loss of heterozygosity—LOH). Histologically, PN are similar to solitary neurofibromas and are composed of myxoid stroma and a cellular component; in neurofibromas, the Schwann cell is the primary neoplastic cell and is the only cell to harbor a "second hit" in the NF1 gene. It appears that inactivation of NF1 is enough to plexiform neurofibromas initiation, whereas a series of additional mutations is likely required for subsequent malignant transformation [23]. Rarely, plexiform tumors are only part of an overgrowth syndrome involving soft tissues and bones [1, 3]. The size increases from adolescence onwards and, although this change is more marked in females, no hormonal markers have been found to explain the change [19, 24]. Several studies have shown a prevalence of these lesions of approximately 10% in children, which arises to 30–50% in adult patients [25–27].

Large, diffuse plexiform neurofibromas may cause significant pain, disfigurement and compression of the skin, subcutis, and associated viscera. These tumors are associated with the development of malignant peripheral nerve sheath tumors (MPNST), an aggressive soft tissue sarcoma (see Chap. 9), which are relatively resistant to chemo- and radiotherapies and carry a dismal prognosis. Although plexiform neurofibromas are often noted to grow during childhood, the development of sudden, rapid growth, associated pain or neurologic deficit should alert the clinician to the possibility of malignant transformation.

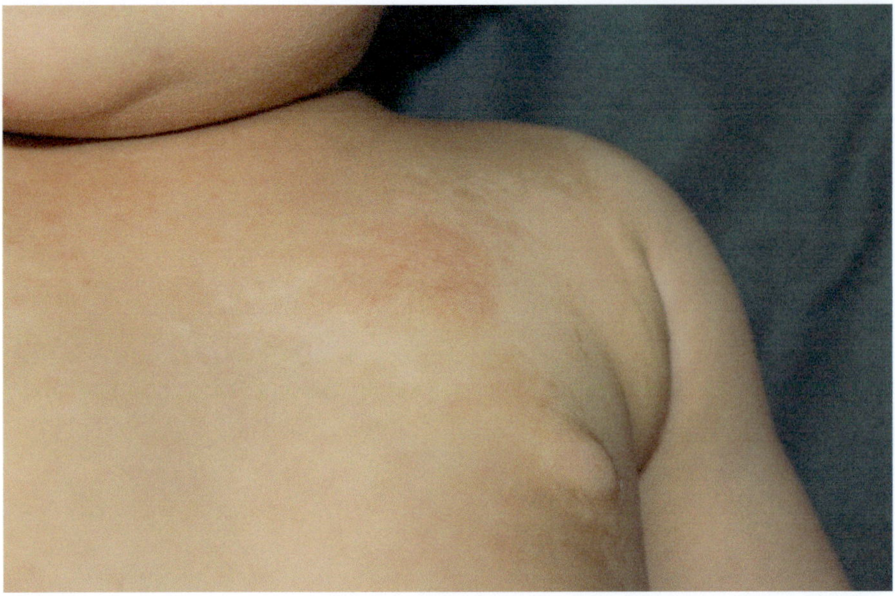

Fig. 5.14 "Herald patch" of plexiform neurofibroma

Fig. 5.15 Plexiform tumor (plexiform neurofibroma)

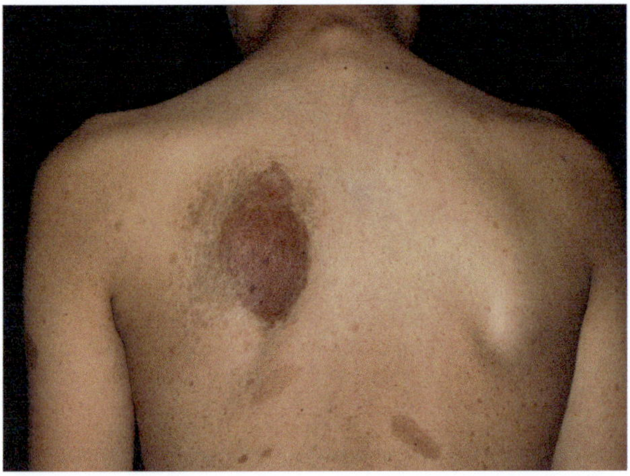

Massive, growing neurofibromas, for which surgery is impractical, are responsible for significant morbidity in patients with NF1. Clinical trials are ongoing, and animal models are under development to assess the efficacy of MEF1/2 inhibitors in these tumors [28].

Blue-red macules are characteristic skin lesions of neurofibromatosis that have been infrequently mentioned and can arise before or during puberty. Initially, the

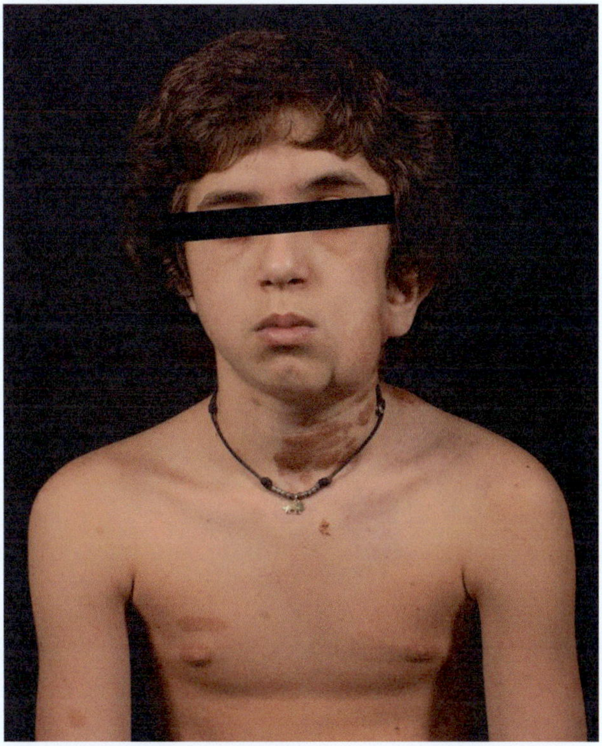

Fig. 5.16 Plexiform tumor (plexiform neurofibroma)

lesions are macular and subsequently may become elevated or dome-shaped while the overlying skin remains blue-red (Figs. 5.17 and 5.18). These lesions are made up of proliferating small blood vessels localized in the upper dermis, which give the skin a red color or a more blue appearance when there is stasis of blood or cold temperature. The histologic characteristics of blue-red macules show thick-walled blood vessels located mainly in the upper dermis and often overlying subcutaneous neurofibromatous tissue.

The pseudoatrophic macules can appear at birth or in early childhood and are slightly depressed, roughly ovalar shaped lesions, ranging from 5 to 10 cm, softer than nearer skin. On palpation, the underlying subcutaneous tissue appears partially absent. The lesions grow harmoniously with the body development and the atrophic aspect may be attributed to a reduction of normal collagen bundles in the reticular dermis caused by the proliferation of neuroid tissue around blood vessels. The histologic characteristics of the pseudoatrophic macules show a collagen reduction in the reticular dermis, with diffuse replacement by neuroid tissue. These clinical signs represent peculiar types of neurofibromas, can be detected early in the course of the disease, and are useful for establish an early diagnosis [29, 30].

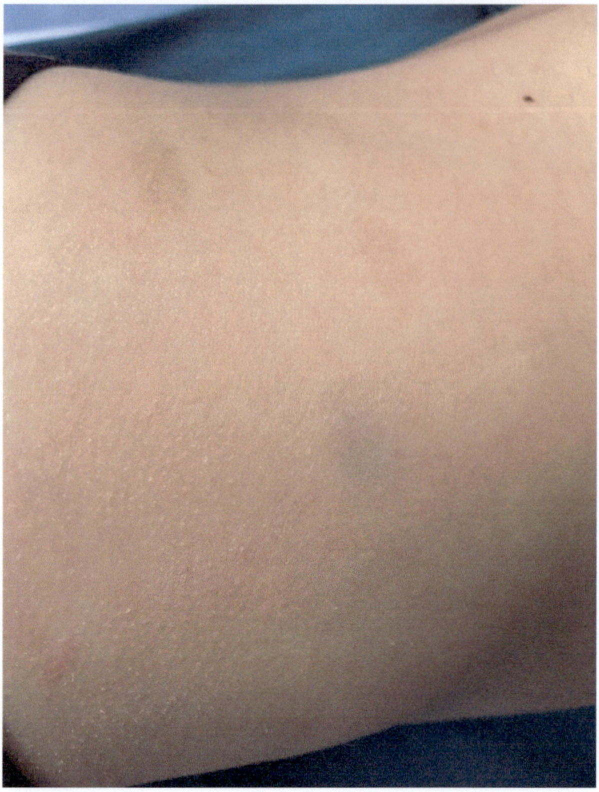

Fig. 5.17 Blue-red macules

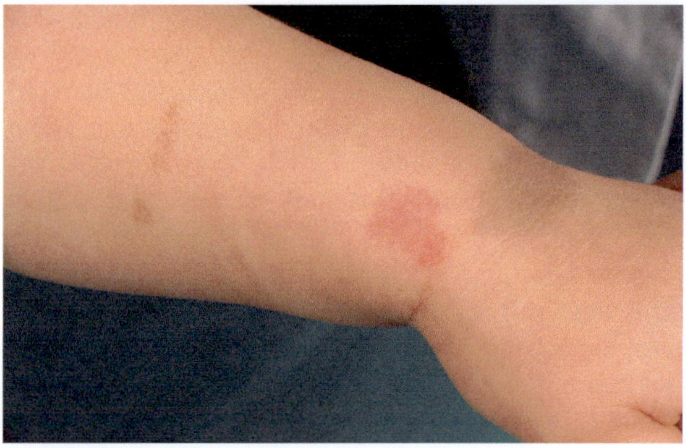

Fig. 5.18 Blue-red macules

5.4 Anemic Nevus (AN)

It is a congenital non-progressive vascular skin anomaly described by Voerner in 1906 [31]. It is characterized by pale, sharply bordered, well-defined macular skin area, often with polycyclic borders, caused by vasoconstriction in the superficial dermis, while surrounding skin become erythematous (Fig. 5.19). AN may be single or multiple and may appear as a confluent lesion and it is spontaneously visible under emotional or temperature stress, or evoked by rubbing the skin (Fig. 5.20). In general, this asymptomatic lesion tends to appear at birth (Fig. 5.21) or early childhood. Histological examination of the affected skin shows a normal epidermis, with no abnormality in either the size or structure of dermal blood vessels.

An association between NF1 and AN was first suggested in 1915 [32] and was later confirmed [33, 34]. According to these older references, AN can appear in up to 15% of individuals with NF1. AN did not receive further attention in the literature until 2013, when four group of experts assessed large series of individuals with NF1 and associated AN [35–39]. Retrospective studies provided much lower estimates than prospective assessments, 8.85% against 51%, respectively, probably because AN is clinically subtle and may be easily overlooked unless purposely searched for. Furthermore, the first study investigated that AN was most frequently localized on

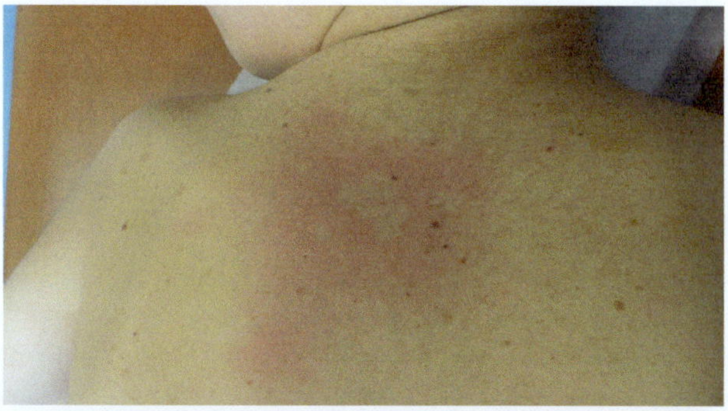

Fig. 5.19 Anemic nevus

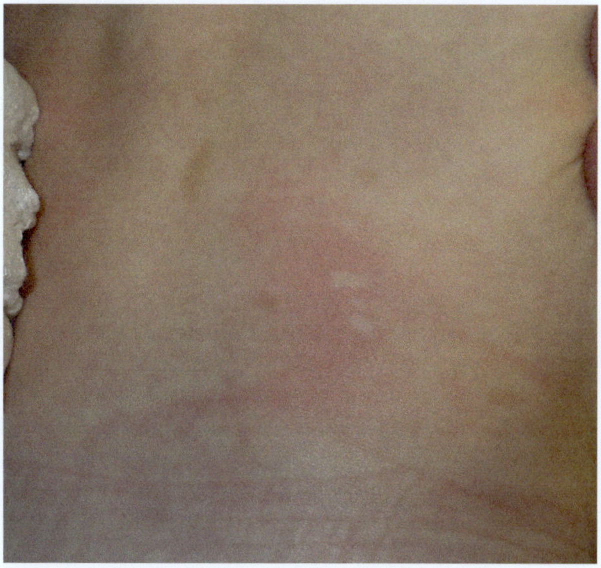

Fig. 5.20 Multiple anemic nevi

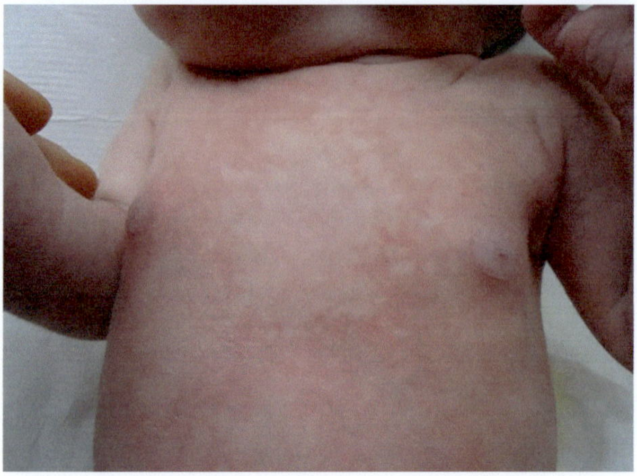

Fig. 5.21 Anemic nevus at birth

the upper half on the back and the neck, compared to the second, in which the most common location was the anterior chest wall, particularly the sternal or parasternal area, and more rarely on the face or other districts. AN equally appears in both sexes and is more prevalent in patients with NF1 under the age of 18 than in adults, respectively, 59% and 36% [36] and more and more in younger ages with average of 7–10 years. The possibility of a spontaneous regression of AN with age cannot be excluded [37].

Pathogenesis of AN is found in a local hypersensitivity to the action of catecholamines on the alpha1-adrenergic receptor sites of papillary dermal blood vessels by sustained vasoconstriction [40, 41]. A further confirmation of this last hypothesis comes from histological, pharmacological, and exchange transplant studies on a patient with AN. The AN plug that had been transplanted into normal skin retained its pale appearance, whereas the graft of normal skin transferred into the nevus remained pink and easily identifiable against the pale background, showing donor dominance of all exchange grafts [42].

Alpha-1-adrenergic receptors belong to the 7-transmembrane-domain receptor superfamily of G protein-coupled receptors, predominantly linked to the Gq/11 family [43]. Targeted studies focus on additional function of neurofibromin, the protein encoded by NF1, about the ability to regulate the G protein-stimulated adenylyl cyclase/cyclic adenosine monophosphate pathway, either directly by the guanosine triphosphatase activating protein-related domain or indirectly through other signal mediators in mammals and flies [44]. AN may result from defective neurofibromin-induced regulation of adenylyl cyclase and/or cyclic adenosine monophosphate activity associated with G protein-coupled receptors- alpha1-, leading to a permanent activation of alpha- adrenergic signaling and enhanced vasoconstriction of skin vessels. The localized and multifocal cutaneous distribution of AN could be explained by a somatic or second-hit mutation, similarly to what is observed with CALMs, glomus tumors, or neurofibromas [45].

5.5 Juvenile Xanthogranuloma

Juvenile xanthogranuloma (JXG) is the most common non-Langerhans cell histiocytosis and begin as an asymptomatic, red-brown, rubbery papule that rapidly becomes a yellow-orange papule or nodule, usually solitary, preferentially located on the head and neck (Fig. 5.22). It appears in early childhood, in 45–70% of cases in the first year of life, and up to 35% of patients at birth [46]. The lesions heal spontaneously, some with atrophic scars. JXGs occur in approximately 5–10% of patients with neurofibromatosis type 1 (NF1) and are common in children with NF1 under 2 years of age [47]. Its association with NF1 was first reported in 1937 by Lamb and Lain [48]; since then, multiple additional cases have been reported [49–56]. Male predominance was found (sex ratio: 2.5) and patients with NF1 had multiple lesions, often found in genital areas, whereas JXG lesions are usually solitary papules or nodules in patients without NF1.

Relationship between JXG and NF1 is unclear but the presence of a defect in the Ras pathway in JXG has not been investigated, although a study found recurrent Ras mutations in Erdheim–Chester disease, which is also a non-Langerhans cell histiocytosis [57]. It might be that JXGs are associated with NF1 because of a loss of heterozygosity of the NF1 gene, as in the case of other skin manifestations of NF1 [58].

The presence of JXG in patients with NF1 is considered a warning sign for juvenile chronic myelomonocytic leukemia (JCMML) [59–65].

Fig. 5.22 Juvenile xanthogranuloma (JXG)

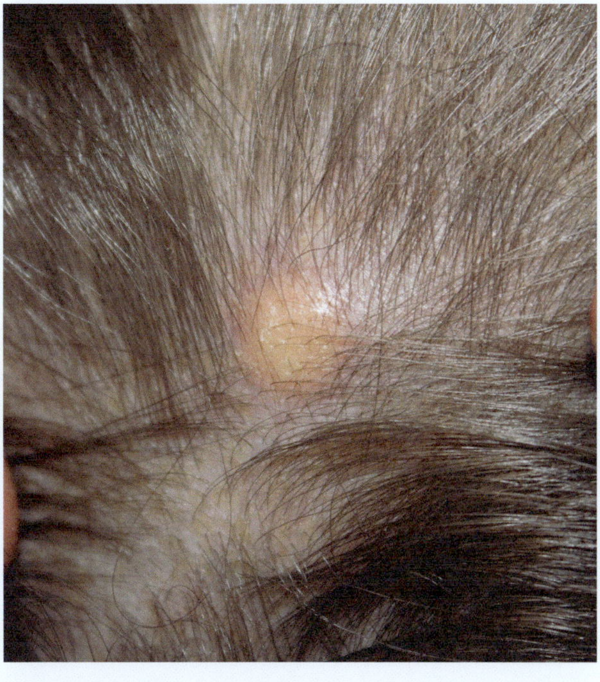

The coincidence of NF1, JXG, and JCMML is relatively rare, with approximately 20 reports in the literature and the first case was reported in 1958 [66]. In 1995, Zvulunov et al. concluded that this triple association is 30–40 times more common than expected by chance and estimated a 20–32 times higher risk of developing JCMML in children with NF-1 and JXG than in those with NF-1 alone [67]. Methodological and statistical limitations, however, might have resulted in overestimation of the association [63]. No increased incidence of JMML was found in at least two other retrospective case series on JXG in patients with NF-1. JXG was found in 30% of 20 children under 2 years with NF-1, but no patient with NF-1 and JXG had JCMML at the time of diagnosis or during follow-up [37, 47]. These authors assume that previous articles about JXG associated with JCMML may have included patients with NF1 features who actually may have had a cancer prone syndrome associated with a deficiency of mismatch-repair genes, such as MSH6 [58]. Recently, another retrospective case-control study compared children with NF-1 and malignancy with sex- and age-matched children with NF-1 without malignancy: this study did not find an increased risk for malignancy associated with JXG in children with neurofibromatosis type 1. Because both JXG and malignancy are associated with NF-1, their coexistence in the same patient might be coincidental. Patients with NF-1 should be monitored for malignancy regardless of the presence or absence of JXG [68].

5.6 Glomus Tumors

Glomus tumors are benign neoplasms that arise from the glomus body, a specialized thermoregulatory shunt concentrated in the fingers and toes (Fig. 5.23) [69]. The lesions are usually located in acral regions, particularly below the nails, and they are characterized by paroxysmal pain on applying pressure or temperature changes. The glomus body is a highly innervated structure containing an afferent arteriole, an anastomotic Suquet-Hoyer canal and an efferent venule. The canal is surrounded by concentric layers of contractile alpha smooth muscle actin (αSMA)-positive glomus cells. Heat-induced contraction of the glomus body causes closure of the

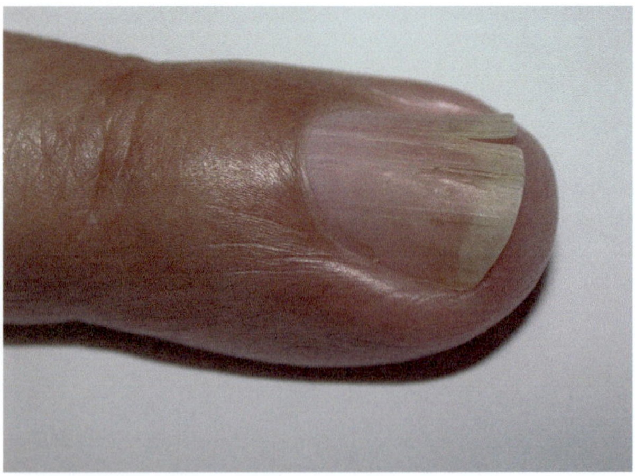

Fig. 5.23 Glomus tumor

arteriovenous anastomosis and forces blood flow through the capillary network of the distal phalanx, causing heat loss [70]. Cold temperatures cause prompt relaxation of the glomus body, opening the anastomosis and conserving body heat.

The first association of NF1 and glomus tumors was published in 1938 by Klaber R. et al. [71] and thanks to Brems H. et al. the first genetic and molecular proof of an association of glomus tumors of the fingers and toes with NF1 was definitively confirmed [72].

Bi-allelic inactivation of NF1 is a common pathogenic mechanism of NF1-associated tumors; these mechanisms lead to an increased activation of the MAPK pathway as observed in other tumor cells with bi-allelic inactivation of NF1 [73, 74]. In patients with NF1, these lesions are usually multiple and recurring but rare in children, with an estimated prevalence of 5% in adult patients with NF1 [75].

5.7 Other Skin Findings

Pruritus affects 20% of patients with NF1 and considerably influences their quality of life. Itching has been attributed to increased mastocytes in the skin, but there doesn't seem to be any differences in plasma levels of histamine in patients with itch compared to the general population. Many patients, however, have pruritus localized in the neurofibromas, where elevated mastocytes have been detected; administration of ketotifen can suppress itching [76].

Hypopigmented ovalar spots similar to those occurring in tuberous sclerosis can be noticed in 10% of patients, but to date there are no studies that have characterized their prevalence, number, and morphology (Fig. 5.24) [77].

Skin softness in patients with NF1 is a subjective perception that is detectable in over 40% of patients [5].

Gingival enlargement refers to the overgrowth of the attached gingiva due to an increase in the number of cells and is a common manifestation in patients, particularly children, with NF-1. The patient usually presents with non-tender unilateral swelling of the gums without signs of inflammation. The patients may present with absent, impacted, and/or malpositioned teeth. In rare cases, patients with NF-1 may present with melanin pigmentation of the gingivae. The pigmentation is symmetric and persistent and can occur at any age in all races, without association between age, race, and gender [78].

Neurofibromas of oral and perioral soft tissues with subsequent periodontitis, impacted and supernumerary teeth, enlarged alveolar process with dental spacing, morphological changes in teeth, and class III molar relationship have been reported in NF-1 patients (Fig. 5.25). Plexiform neurofibromas were reported in oral soft tissue, maxilla, and mandible with evidence of malignant transformation in 8–13% of cases [79]. In addition to the presence of neurofibromas within the tongue musculature, macroglossia due to plexiform neurofibromas and enlargement of fungiform papillae have also been reported [80, 81]. Facial skeletal abnormalities, including enlargement of mandibular foramen, increased dimensions of the coronoid and sigmoid notches and indentation of the posterior border of the mandible have also been reported. Association between dental caries and NF-1 remains unclear, but it is surely related to poor oral hygiene due to dental abnormalities in these patients [78].

Fig. 5.24 Hypopigmented spots

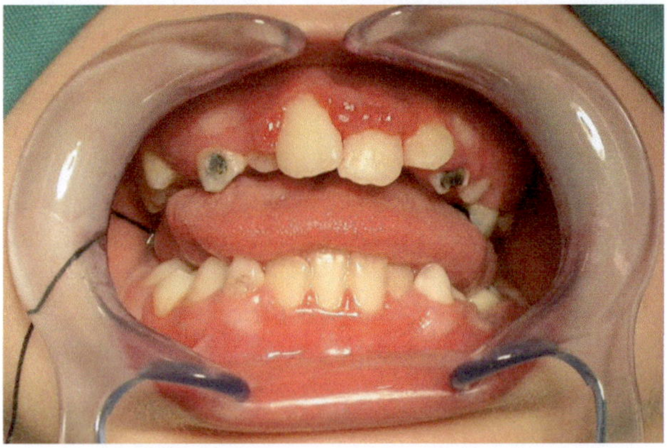

Fig. 5.25 Neurofibromas of oral soft tissues

The association of poliosis with solitary neurofibromas has been reported in three patients by Koplon BS et al., Kwon IH et al., and Sandoval-Tress C [82–84], showing histological changes consisting of a neurofibroma with a marked reduction of the melanocyte number and melanin pigment in the hair follicles. It has been proposed that hair depigmentation in patients with a scalp neurofibroma is the consequence of an autoimmune mechanism in which cytotoxic T-cells for neurofibroma could crossreact with the melanocytes of the hair bulbs overlying the neurofibroma and thus result in the destruction of the latters [83]. Neri et al. recently reported a familial case with two brothers affected by NF1 and poliosis overlying plexiform neurofibromas on the scalp: the peculiarity of these cases was the familiarity and the same location of the poliosis [85].

A study by Madeira LG et al. identified markedly reduced thermoregulatory capacity in NF1 patients, which could contribute to their reduced aerobic capacity and daily physical activities as well as increasing their risk of heat injury and illnesses. The results suggested an autonomic neuropathy as the main mechanism for reduced heat and exercise tolerance in NF1 patients [86].

Cherry angiomas, with precocious appearance and often ectopic distribution on arms and legs (Fig. 5.26), are significantly more common in NF1 patients rather than

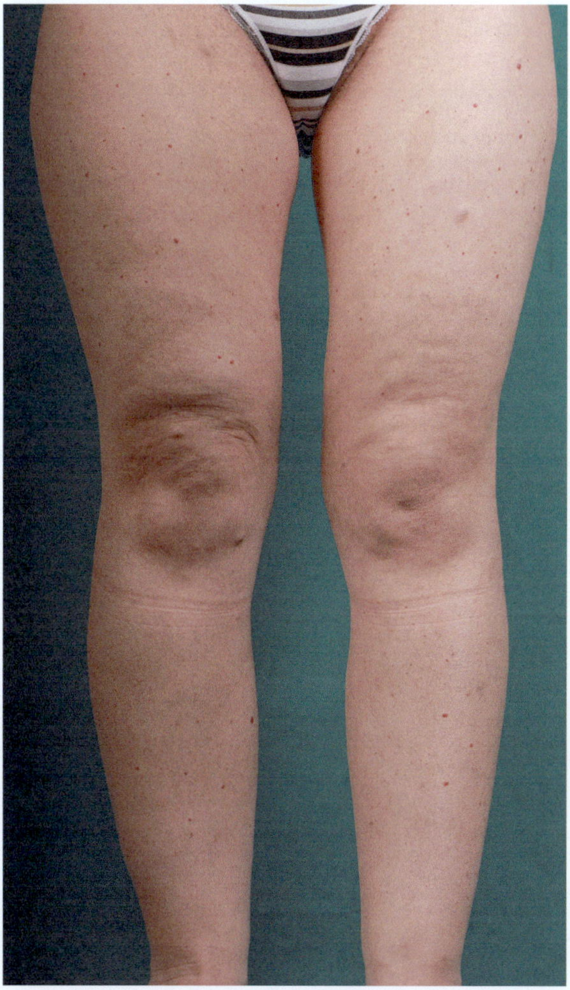

Fig. 5.26 Cherry angiomas

in unaffected relatives or general population: this personal observation has not been published yet [1].

Funding Sources None.

Conflict of Interest None declared.

References

1. Tadini G, Brena M, Gelmetti C, Pezzani L. Chapter 11: Neurocutaneous syndromes. In: Atlas of genodermatoses. 2nd ed. Boca Raton: CRC Press/Taylor & Francis Group; 2015. ISBN 9781466598355.
2. Shah KN. The diagnostic and clinical significance of café-au-lait macules. Pediatr Clin N Am. 2010;57(5):1131–53.
3. Hernández-Martín A, Duat-Rodríguez A. An update on neurofibromatosis type 1: not just Café-au-Lait spots, freckling, and neurofibromas. An update. Part I. dermatological clinical criteria diagnostic of the disease. Actas Dermosifiliogr. 2016;107(6):454–64.
4. Maertens O, de Schepper S, Vandesompele J, Brems H, Heyns I, Janssens S, et al. Molecular dissection of isolated disease features in mosaic neurofibromatosis type 1. Am J Hum Genet. 2007;81:243–51.
5. Tadini G, Milani D, Menni F, Pezzani L, Sabatini C, Esposito S. Is it time to change the neurofibromatosis 1 diagnostic criteria? Eur J Intern Med. 2014;25(6):506–10.
6. Yao R, Wang L, Yu Y, Wang J, Shen Y. Diagnostic value of multiple café-au-lait macules for neurofibromatosis 1 in Chinese children. J Dermatol. 2016;43(5):537–42.
7. Tadini G, Brena M, Gelmetti C, Pezzani L. Chapter 17 disorders of pigmentation. In: Atlas of genodermatoses. 2nd ed. Boca Raton: CRC Press/Taylor & Francis Group; 2015. ISBN 9781466598355.
8. Ruggieri M, Huson SM. The clinical and diagnostic implications of mosaicism in the neurofibromatoses. Neurology. 2001;56:1433–43.
9. Ruggieri M, Pavone P, Polizzi A, et al. Ophthalmological manifestations in segmental neurofibromatosis type 1. Br J Ophthalmol. 2004;88:1429–33.
10. Vázquez-Osorio I, Duat-Rodríguez A, García-Martínez FJ, Torrelo A, Noguera-Morel L, Hernández-Martín A. Cutaneous and systemic findings in mosaic neurofibromatosis type 1. Pediatr Dermatol. 2017;34(3):271–6.
11. Adigun CG, Stein J. Segmental neurofibromatosis. Dermatol Online J. 2011;17:25. 14.
12. Moss C, Green SH. What is segmental neurofibromatosis? Br J Dermatol. 1994;130:106–10.
13. García-Romero MT, Parkin P, Lara-Corrales I. Mosaic neurofibromatosis type 1: a systematic review. Pediatr Dermatol. 2016;33(1):9–17.
14. Dang JD, Cohen PR. Segmental neurofibromatosis of the distal arm in a man who developed Hodgkin lymphoma. Int J Dermatol. 2009;48:1105–9.
15. Kajimoto A, Oiso N, Fukai K, et al. Bilateral segmental neurofibromatosis with gastric carcinoma. Clin Exp Dermatol. 2007;32:43–4.
16. Martuza RL, Philippe I, Fitzpatrick TB, Zwaan J, Seki Y, Lederman J. Melanin macroglobules as a cellular marker of neurofibromatosis: a quantitative study. J Invest Dermatol. 1985;85(4):347–50.
17. De Schepper S, Boucneau JM, Westbroek W, Mommaas M, Onderwater J, Messiaen L, Naeyaert JM, Lambert JL. Neurofibromatosis type 1 protein and amyloid precursor protein interact in normal human melanocytes and colocalize with melanosomes. J Invest Dermatol. 2006;126(3):653–9.
18. Allouche J, Bellon N, Saidani M, Stanchina-Chatrousse L, Masson Y, Patwardhan A, et al. In vitro modeling of hyperpigmentation associated to neurofibromatosis type 1 using melano-

cytes derived from human embryonic stem cells. Proc Natl Acad Sci U S A. 2015;112(29): 9034–9.
19. Tucker T, Friedman JM, Friedrich RE, Wenzel R, Funsterer C, Mautner VF. Longitudinal study of neurofibromatosis 1 associated plexiform neurofibromas. J Med Genet. 2009;46:81–5.
20. McLaughlin ME, Jacks T. Neurofibromatosis type 1. Methods Mol Biol. 2003;222:223–37.
21. Haworth KB, Arnold MA, Pierson CR, Choi K, Yeager ND, Ratner N, Roberts RD, Finlay JL, Cripe TP. Immune profiling of NF1-associated tumors reveals histologic subtype distinctions and heterogeneity: implications for immunotherapy. Oncotarget. 2017;8(47):82037–48.
22. Riccardi VM. Ketotifen suppression of NF1 neurofibroma growth over 30 years. Am J Med Genet A. 2015;167(7):1570–7.
23. Pemov A, Li H, Patidar R, Hansen NF, Sindiri S, Hartley SW, Wei JS, Elkahloun A, Chandrasekharappa SC, Boland JF, Bass S, Mullikin JC, Khan J, Widemann BC, Wallace MR, Stewart DR, NISC Comparative Sequencing Program, CI DCEG Cancer Genomics Research Laboratory. The primacy of NF1 loss as the driver of tumorigenesis in neurofibromatosis type 1-associated plexiform neurofibromas. Oncogene. 2017;36(22):3168–77.
24. Dagalakis U, Lodish M, Dombi E, Sinaii N, Sabo J, Baldwin A, et al. Puberty and plexiform neurofibroma tumor growth in patients with neurofibromatosis type I. J Pediatr. 2014;164:620–4.
25. Duat Rodriguez A, Martos Moreno GA, Martin Santo-Domingo Y, Hernandez Martin A, Espejo-Saavedra Roca JM, Ruiz-Falco Rojas ML, et al. Phenotypic and genetic features in neurofibromatosis type 1 in children. An Pediatr (Barc). 2015;83:173–82.
26. Duong TA, Bastuji-Garin S, Valeyrie-Allanore L, Sbidian E, Ferkal S, Wolkenstein P. Evolving pattern with age of cutaneous signs in neurofibromatosis type 1: a cross-sectional study of 728 patients. Dermatology. 2011;222:269–73.
27. Hirbe AC, Gutmann DH. Neurofibromatosis type 1: a multidisciplinary approach to care. Lancet Neurol. 2014 Aug;13(8):834–43.
28. Rauen KA, Huson SM, Burkitt-Wright E, Evans DG, Farschtschi S, Ferner RE, et al. Recent developments in neurofibromatoses and RASopathies: management, diagnosis and current and future therapeutic avenues. Am J Med Genet A. 2015;167A:1–10.
29. Westerhof W, Konrad K. Blue-red macules and pseudoatrophic macules: additional cutaneous signs in neurofibromatosis. Arch Dermatol. 1982;118:577–81.
30. Zeller J, Wechsler J, Revuz J, Wolkenstein P. Blue-red macules and pseudoatrophic macules in neurofibromatosis 1. Ann Dermatol Venereol. 2002;129(2):180–1.
31. Voerner H. Über Naevus anaemicus. Arch Dermatol Syph. 1906;82:391–8.
32. Naegeli O. Naevi anaemici und Reckinghausensche Krankheit. Arch Dermatol Syph. 1915;121:742–5.
33. Fleisher TL, Zeligman I. Nevus anemicus. Arch Dermatol. 1969;100:750–5.
34. Degos R, Schnitzler L, Barrau-Fusade C. Anemic nevus and Recklinghausen's neurofibromatosis. Apropos of a case. Bull Soc Fr Dermatol Syphiligr. 1970;77:800–2.
35. Tadini G, Brena M, Pezzani L, et al. Anemic nevus in neurofibromatosis type 1. Dermatology. 2013;226:115–8.
36. Marque M, Roubertie A, Jaussent A, et al. Nevus anemicus in neurofibromatosis type 1: a potential new diagnostic criterion. J Am Acad Dermatol. 2013;69:768–75.
37. Ferrari F, Masurel A, Olivier-Faivre L, et al. Juvenile xanthogranuloma and nevus anemicus in the diagnosis of neurofibromatosis type 1. JAMA Dermatol. 2014;150:42–6.
38. Hernández-Martín A, García-Martínez FJ, Duat A, López-Martín I, Noguera-Morel L, Torrelo A. Nevus anemicus: a distinctive cutaneous finding in neurofibromatosis type 1. Pediatr Dermatol. 2015;32(3):342–7.
39. Tadini G, Brena M. Anemic nevus is a new diagnostic criterion for neurofibromatosis type 1. G Ital Dermatol Venereol. 2017;152(5):548–549.
40. Greaves MW, Birkett D, Johnson C. Nevus anemicus: a unique catecholamine-dependent nevus. Arch Dermatol. 1970;102:172–6.
41. Mountcastle EA, Diestelmeier MR, Lupton GP. Nevus anemicus. J Am Acad Dermatol. 1986;14:628–32.

42. Daniel RH, Hubler WR Jr, Wolf JE Jr, Holer WR. Nevus anemicus: donor-dominant defect. Arch Dermatol. 1977;113:53–6.
43. Graham RM, Perez DM, Hwa J, Piascik MT. Alpha 1-adrenergic receptor subtypes: molecular structure, function and signaling. Cir Res. 1996;78:737–49.
44. Tong J, Hannan F, Zhu Y, Bernards A, Zhong Y. Neurofibromin regulates G protein-stimulated adenylyl cyclase activity. Nat Neurosci. 2002;5:95–6.
45. Jouhilahti EM, Peltonen S, Heape AM, Peltonen J. The pathoetiology of neurofibromatosis 1. Am J Pathol. 2011;178:1932–9.
46. Jansen D. Juvenile xanthogranuloma in childhood and adolescence: a clinicopathologic study of 129 patients from the Kiel pediatric tumor registry. Am J Surg Pathol. 2005;29(8):1118.
47. Cambiaghi S, Restano L, Caputo R. Juvenile xanthogranuloma associated with neurofibromatosis 1:14 patients without evidence of hematologic malignancies. Pediatr Dermatol. 2004;21(2):97–101.
48. Lamb JH, Lain ES. Nevo xanthoendothelioma: its relationship to juvenile xanthoma. South Med J. 1937;30:585–94.
49. Nomland R. Nevo xanthro-endothelioma; a benign xanthromatous disease of infants and children. J Invest Dermatol. 1954;22(3):207–15.
50. Marten R. Naevo xanthoendothelioma with pigmentary abnormalities. Br J Dermatol. 1960;72:308.
51. Jensen NE, Sabharwal S, Walker AE. Naevoxanthoendothelioma and neurofibromatosis. Br J Dermatol. 1971;85(4):326–30.
52. Sourreil P, Beylot C, Bioulac P. Xanthogranulome juvénile associé à la maladie de Recklinhausen: a propos de 3 cas. J Med Lyon. 1972;53(232):1165–71.
53. Newell GB, Stone OJ, Mullins JF. Juvenile xanthogranuloma and neurofibromatosis. Arch Dermatol. 1973;107(2):262.
54. Smitt JH. Juvenile xanthogranuloma in neurofibromatosis type I. Br J Dermatol. 1991;125(4):390.
55. Ackerman CD, Cohen BA. Juvenile xanthogranuloma and neurofibromatosis. Pediatr Dermatol. 1991;8(4):339–40.
56. Tan HH, Tay YK. Juvenile xanthogranuloma and neurofibromatosis 1. Dermatology. 1998;197(1):43–4.
57. Emile JF, Diamond EL, Helias-Rodzewicz Z, et al. Recurrent RAS and PIK3CA mutations in Erdheim–Chester disease. Blood. 2014;124:3016–9.
58. Paulus S, Koronowska S, Folster-Holst R. Association between juvenile myelomonocytic leukemia, juvenile xanthogranulomas and neurofibromatosis type 1: case report and review of the literature. Pediatr Dermatol. 2017;34(2):114–8.
59. Dehen L, Zeller J, Cosnes A, Bernaudin F, Roujeau JC, Revuz J. Xanthogranulomes, neurofibromatose de type 1 et leucémie myélomonocytaire spontanément résolutive. Ann Dermatol Venereol. 1990;117(11):812–4.
60. Morier P, Mérot Y, Paccaud D, Beck D, Frenk E. Juvenile chronic granulocytic leukemia, juvenile xanthogranulomas, and neurofibromatosis: case report and review of the literature. J Am Acad Dermatol. 1990;22(5, pt 2):962–5.
61. Song M, Gheeraert P, Jonckheer T, Otten J, Achten G. Xanthomes, neurofibromatose et leucémie chez l'enfant. Dermatologica. 1984;168(3):138–40.
62. Raygada M, Arthur DC, Wayne AS, Rennert OM, Toretsky JA, Stratakis CA. Juvenile xanthogranuloma in a child with previously unsuspected neurofibromatosis type 1 and juvenile myelomonocytic leukemia. Pediatr Blood Cancer. 2010;54(1):173–5.
63. Gutmann DH, Gurney JG, Shannon KM. Juvenile xanthogranuloma, neurofibromatosis 1 and juvenile chronic myeloid leukemia. Arch Dermatol. 1996;132(11):1390–1.
64. Benessahraoui M, Aubin F, Paratte F, Plouvier E, Humbert P. Leucémie myélomonocytaire ju-vénile, xanthomes et neurofibromatose de type 1. Arch Pediatr. 2003;10(10):891–4.
65. Shin HT, Harris MB, Orlow SJ. Juvenile myelomonocytic leukemia presenting with features of hemophagocytic lymphohistiocytosis in association with neurofibromatosis and juvenile xanthogranulomas. J Pediatr Hematol Oncol. 2004;26(9):591–5.

66. Royer P, Blondet C, Guihard J. Xantho-leukemia in infants & Recklinghausen's neurofibromatosis. Sem Hop. 1958;34:1504–13.
67. Zvulunov A, Barak Y, Metzker A. Juvenile xanthogranuloma, neurofibromatosis, and juvenile chronic myelogenous leukemia. World statistical analysis. Arch Dermatol. 1995;131(8):904–8.
68. Liy-Wong C, Mohammed J, Carleton A, Pope E, Parkin P, Lara-Corrales I. The relationship between neurofibromatosis type 1, juvenile xanthogranuloma, and malignancy: a retrospective case-control study. J Am Acad Dermatol. 2017;76(6):1084–7.
69. Rettig AC, Strickland JW. Glomus tumor of the digits. J Hand Surg [Am]. 1977;2:261–5.
70. McDermott EM, Weiss AP. Glomus tumors. J Hand Surg [Am]. 2006;31:1397–400.
71. Klaber R. Morbus Recklinghausen with glomoid tumors. Proc Roy Soc Med. 1938;31:347.
72. Brems H, Park C, Maertens O, Pemov A, Messiaen L, Upadhyaya M, et al. Glomus tumors in neurofibromatosis type 1: genetic, functional, and clinical evidence of a novel association. Cancer Res. 2009;69:7393–401.
73. Maertens O, Prenen H, Debiec-Rychter M, et al. Molecular pathogenesis of multiple gastrointestinal stromal tumors in NF1 patients. Hum Mol Genet. 2006;15:1015–23.
74. Cichowski K, Santiago S, Jardim M, Johnson BW, Jacks T. Dynamic regulation of the Ras pathway via proteolysis of the NF1 tumor suppressor. Genes Dev. 2003;17:449–54.
75. Kumar MG, Emnett RJ, Bayliss SJ, Gutmann DH. Glomus tumors in individuals with neurofibromatosis type 1. J Am Acad Dermatol. 2014;71:44–8.
76. Yoshida Y, Adachi K, Yamamoto O. Local mast cell histamine and plasma histamine levels in neurofibromatosis type 1. Acta Derm Venereol. 2010;90(6):637–9.
77. Hernández-Martín A, Duat-Rodríguez A. An update on neurofibromatosis type 1: not just Café-au-Lait spots and freckling. part II. Other skin manifestations characteristic of NF1. NF1 and Cancer. Actas Dermosifiliogr. 2016;107(6):465–73.
78. Javed F, Ramalingam S, Ahmed HB, Gupta B, Sundar C, Qadri T, Al-Hezaimi K, Romanos GE. Oral manifestations in patients with neurofibromatosis type-1: a comprehensive literature review. Crit Rev Oncol Hematol. 2014;91(2):123–9.
79. Evans DG, Baser ME, McGaughran J, Sharif S, Howard E, Moran A. Malignant peripheral nerve sheath tumours in neurofibromatosis 1. JMed Genet. 2002;39:311–4.
80. Neville BW, Damm DD, Allen CM, Bouquot JE. Oral and maxillofacialpathology. 2nd ed. Philadelphia: Elsevier; 2002. p. 457–61.
81. Kumar CA, Jagat Reddy RC, Gupta S, Laller S. Oral hamartomas with von Recklinghausen disease. Ann Saudi Med. 2011;31:428–30.
82. Koplon BS, Shapiro L. Poliosis overlying a neurofibroma. Arch Dermatol. 1968;98:631–3.
83. Kwon IH, Cho YJ, Lee SH, Lee JH, Cho KH, Kim JA, Moon SE. Poliosis circumscripta associated with neurofibroma. J. Dermatol. 2005;32:446–9. 14.
84. Sandoval-Tress C, Nava-Jiménez G. Poliosis circumscripta associated with neurofibromatosis 1. Australas J Dermatol. 2008;49(3):167–8.
85. Neri I, Liberati G, Piraccini BM, Patrizi A. Poliosis and neurofibromatosis type 1: two familiar cases and review of the literature. Skin Appendage Disord. 2017;3(4):219–21.
86. Madeira LG, Passos RL, Souza JF, Rezende NA, Rodrigues LO. Autonomic thermoregulatory dysfunction in neurofibromatosis type 1. Arq Neuropsiquiatr. 2016;74(10):796–802.

Ocular Manifestations in Neurofibromatosis Type 1

6

Maura Di Nicola and Francesco Viola

Contents

6.1 Introduction

Neurofibromatosis type 1 (NF1), also known as von Recklinghausen disease, is a genetic disease caused by a defect in a single gene encoding for neurofibromin, a cytoplasmic protein involved in control of the cell cycle [1–3]. More specifically, neurofibromin acts as a negative regulator of the *Ras* protoncogene, which represents a key molecule in cell growth [4, 5].

NF1 has a classic Mendelian inheritance pattern, autosomal dominant with complete penetrance but variable expression [2]. It affects 1:2500–3500 people throughout the world, with no gender or ethnicity predilection [1–3]. Around 50% of cases are caused by sporadic mutations, given the high rate of spontaneous mutation of the NF1 gene (about 1:10,000) [1]. Less frequently, somatic mosaicism may also occur leading to segmental NF1 in which characteristic features of the disease are displayed only in certain body segments, including the eye [6]. Genetic testing is

M. Di Nicola · F. Viola (✉)
Università degli Studi di Milano, UO Oculistica, Fondazione IRCCS Cà Granda Ospedale Maggiore Policlinico, Milan, Italy
e-mail: francesco.viola@unimi.it

G. Tadini et al. (eds.), *Multidisciplinary Approach to Neurofibromatosis Type 1*,
https://doi.org/10.1007/978-3-319-92450-2_6

currently available to identify specific mutations in the NF1 gene and confirm the diagnosis. However, diagnosis remains a clinical decision due to the complexity of genetic testing considering the large size of the gene, the variety and lack of clustering of possible defects and the existence of pseudogenes [1].

In order to guide clinicians in the recognition of the disease, in 1998 the National Institutes of Health (NIH) established the following clinical criteria for diagnosis of this disorder [7]:

1. Six or more café-au-lait macules >5 mm in greatest diameter in children and >15 mm in greatest diameter in adults
2. Two or more neurofibromas or one plexiform neurofibroma
3. Axillary or inguinal freckling
4. Optic pathway glioma
5. Two or more Lisch nodules
6. Characteristic skeletal dysplasia (sphenoid wing, long bones)
7. First-degree relative with NF1 diagnosed by the above criteria

The presence of at least 2 of the above-mentioned criteria is sufficient for the diagnosis. Most of these clinical features are age dependent, so the vast majority of patients (around 95%) meet diagnostic criteria by age 8 and virtually all of them do so by their 20s [8]. The most common ocular manifestations are Lisch nodules (50–90% of patients), [9] followed by optic pathway gliomas (around 15% of patients) [10] and plexiform neurofibromas (less than 10% of patients) [11]. These entities represent hallmark lesions of NF1, indicating the pivotal role ophthalmologists may have in the diagnosis of this disorder.

6.2 Ocular Adnexa

The most common ocular adnexal finding in NF1 is plexiform neurofibromas (PNs), even though their overall incidence is fairly low as previously mentioned (less than 10% of children affected by NF1) [11]. PNs are complex nerve sheath tumors that follow multiple nerve branches and are at risk for malignant transformation. In contrast, discrete neurofibromas (dermal or subcutaneous) arise from small nerves or nerve endings, appear later in life and have no risk for malignant transformation [11].

Most PNs are identified in early childhood (usually before age 5 years) and may grow rapidly during this period, as well as during puberty and pregnancy. Clinically they commonly present with ptosis (“S-shaped ptosis” in cases of predominantly lateral infiltration of upper eyelid), proptosis, eyelid swelling, orbital dystopia, and strabismus [1, 11, 12]. PNs can involve the upper eyelid, brow, orbit, and temple and may grow to the point that they become disfiguring for patients [1, 11]. In addition to affecting children’s aesthetic appearance, decreased visual acuity and deprivational, refractive or strabismic (less frequently) amblyopia may occur in up to 50% of cases [13].

One of the rare secondary complications of PNs is sphenoid wing dysplasia, defined as absence or marked thinning of the sphenoid bone that comprises the posterolateral wall of the orbit. It has been found in 1–6% of children with NF1 and is usually found ipsilateral to the plexiform neurofibroma [14]. This dysplasia allows protrusion of the anterior temporal lobe into the orbit, causing proptosis, pulsatile exophthalmos, strabismus, and optic nerve compression [11].

Biopsy for tissue diagnosis is usually unnecessary in patients with NF1. However, all children with newly diagnosed PNs should undergo magnetic resonance imaging (MRI) of the brain and orbits regardless of whether a diagnosis of NF1 has been confirmed [11].

Surgery is the mainstay of treatment for PNs, but a detailed discussion of surgical techniques is beyond the scope of this chapter. However, it is important to highlight that the non-encapsulated and highly vascular tumor has an infiltrative nature, which increases the potential for recurrence and complications such as bleeding, in response to surgical intervention [1, 15]. Some authors suggest that conservative management via close observation with serial MRIs might be an acceptable alternative in selected cases [11]. The main indications for surgery include clinical progression causing anatomical and functional damage (amblyopia, optic neuropathy, corneal exposure) or facial disfigurement [15].

Given the variety of opinions on timing and selection of treatment, a multidisciplinary task force of experts from tertiary care centers proposed a consensus statement for ophthalmic monitoring and management of PNs as outlined below [11]:

1. Adoption of the uniform terminology "Orbital-Periorbital Plexiform Neurofibroma" or OPPN for plexiform neurofibromas involving the eyelid, orbit, periorbital, and facial structures.
2. Children with OPPN are at highest risk for rapid growth of OPPN before the age of 8. Comprehensive ophthalmic evaluation is recommended every 6 months until visual maturity. After that, frequency of examination should be guided by the clinical course.
3. Patients with OPPN confined to the upper eyelid may not need to undergo neuroimaging. For patients with orbital, periorbital, or facial involvement, high resolution MRI scanning with and without contrast of the orbit, face, and cavernous sinus should be performed.
4. Treatment for related ophthalmic issues, such as ptosis, lacrimal involvement, or amblyopia is supportive. Early intervention is recommended with the exception of strabismus surgery. Strabismus caused by orbital or periorbital tumor involvement while the tumor is in its rapid growth phase carries a high risk for recurrence after strabismus surgery. Associated problems such as amblyopia and refractive error should be managed aggressively and surgery deferred until the tumor growth has stabilized, if clinically appropriate to do so.
5. Debulking surgery may be indicated for the following:
   (a). Visual decline.
   (b). Progressive tumor growth involving a vital structure.
   (c). Progressive disfigurement or functional decline.

Debulking is more successful in older patients and adults. Younger patients have a high risk of recurrent progression and need for more surgery.

6. Clinical trials using biologic agents (i.e., MEK inhibitors) are underway but no definitive recommendations can be made at this time.

6.3 Anterior Segment

Lisch nodules (Fig. 6.1) represent the most common finding of NF1 in the anterior segment and they are specific to the disease, thus qualifying as one of its hallmark manifestations [1]. These lesions are melanocytic hamartomas of the iris, consisting of a condensation of spindle cells on the anterior surface of the iris [16]. They may be visualized without the aid of a microscope occasionally, but slit-lamp examination is frequently required to assess the exact number and location of the nodules. In adults, Lisch nodules lack intrinsic vasculature and present as multiple, bilateral elevated nodules located in the inferior half of the iris, ranging from white to yellow or brown in color [8, 9, 17].

Lisch nodules might not be evident in early years, but they become apparent later in life, as their prevalence is known to correlate with age, but not with the severity of the disease or the number of café-au-lait macules or neurofibromas [1, 17]. Several studies have investigated the prevalence of Lisch nodules by age groups.

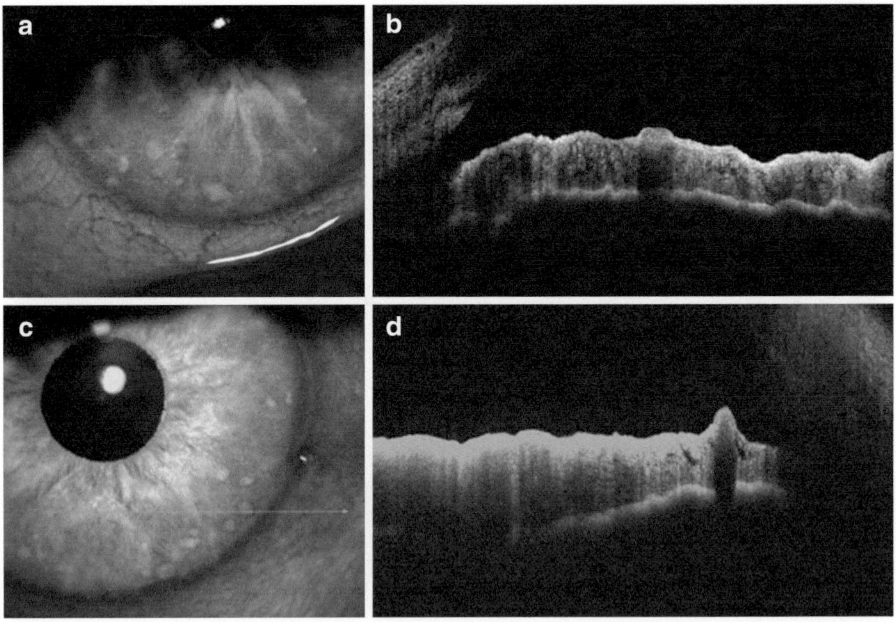

Fig. 6.1 NIR (near infrared) anterior segment picture of a 53-year-old man (**a**) and a 64-year-old woman (**c**) affected by NF1 showing multiple Lisch nodules. AS-OCT (anterior segment optical coherence tomography) scans demonstrate the iris lesions casting a shadow posteriorly (**b**, **d**)

According to Beauchamp, they are found in virtually all adults with a confirmed diagnosis of NF1, while their prevalence in children is lower (around 53% in patients under the age of 10 years) [9]. In another work by Lubs and colleagues, the prevalence of Lisch nodules was studied by age group and was found to be only 5% in children under 3 years of age, 42% in children between 3 and 4 years of age (the largest incremental increase among age subdivisions), 55% in children between 5 and 6 years of age, and 100% among adults over 21 years of age [17]. Furthermore, the prevalence of Lisch nodules was greater than that of neurofibromas in all but the youngest age group (under 3 years of age) [17]. These findings indicate that the lack of these nodules in young children does not rule out NF1, as they may present at a later age.

In terms of management, Lisch nodules are not correlated with ocular complications, visual impairment or ocular morbidity of any sort; therefore, they do not require any treatment [1, 17]. However, careful clinical examination is essential to differentiate these lesions from other conditions with similar presentations, such as iris nevi, which usually appear as flat or variably elevated darkly pigmented lesions with ill-defined margins and iris mammillations, a condition associated with ocular melanocytosis that presents as uniformly distributed nipple-like protuberances in the anterior part of a deeply pigmented iris [1, 17].

Juvenile xanthogranuloma (JXG) is a benign histiocytic proliferation that occurs in young children most frequently in the skin but can manifest in the eye also. Ocular involvement typically occurs with adnexal involvement, as a circumscribed iris nodule that can occasionally lead to hyphema and elevated intraocular pressure and rarely as a diffuse iris infiltration [18]. Several reports have suggested an association between NF1 and JXG, with the latter manifesting as the initial presenting feature of NF1. In a series of 288 patients, 17 of 77 patients under 3 years of age with NF1 had JXG [19]. Furthermore, an association between JXG with NF1 and a particular kind of leukemia called juvenile myelomonocytic leukemia (JMML) has been described. More specifically, the presence of both NF1 and JXG seems to create a 20–30 times higher risk for developing JMML compared to NF1 alone [20]. However, the existence of this relationship has been disputed in a recent study [21]. Therefore, it is questionable whether or not children diagnosed with NF1 and clinical evidence of JXG benefit from a hematological evaluation to rule out JMML.

Other very rare anterior segment findings reported in the literature include conjunctival neurofibromas and diffuse hypertrophy of corneal stromal nerves ("lignes grise") [1, 8].

6.4 Retina

Retinal abnormalities associated with NF1 are not very common and range from retinal vascular abnormalities (RVAs) to several benign retinal tumors.

RVAs were first described in 2002 in a cohort of 12 patients out of 32 subjects affected by NF1 (37.5%) [22]. The anomalies described in this paper ranged from a single affected vessel ("forme fruste") to the full-blown manifestation ("complete form"). The most common finding consisted of minuscule second or third order tortuous venules called "corkscrew vessels," usually one to two disc diameters in dimensions, isolated and most often located temporally. Fluorescein angiography (FA) better characterized these lesions but showed no leakage. Less common vascular abnormalities included a venous-venous anastomosis that was found in the nasal retina in one patient and an extensive arteriovenous malformation associated with an epiretinal membrane that was detected in another patient [22].

More recently, a series of 17 NF1 patients was reported in which 6 patients (35%) presented with distinctive microvascular abnormalities, consisting of small tortuous "spiral" or "corkscrew" vessels, often located overlying choroidal alterations that were visible with near infrared reflectance (NIR) [23].

Interestingly, in a much bigger series of 294 patients affected by NF1 only 18 patients (6.1%) presented with RVAs, defined as small, tortuous retinal vessels with a "spiral/corkscrew" appearance originating from small tributaries of retinal veins [24]. RVAs were mostly unilateral (94%) and single (83%), located along the temporal vascular arcades in two third of cases and at the posterior pole in the remaining one thirds of cases. On FA, RVAs were first visible during the arteriovenous phase and did not develop late leakage. On optical coherence tomography angiography (OCTA), RVAs were located in the superficial vascular plexus in all cases, with associated localized abnormal congested capillary networks in the deep vascular plexus [24]. Also of interest, the presence of RVAs did not correlate with the presence of other specific ocular or systemic NF1 features [24].

In terms of benign neoplastic lesions associated with NF1, several entities have been described [25]. Astrocytic hamartomas in neurofibromatosis present as small whitish to yellowish masses with a "mulberry-like" appearance usually involving the optic nerve, similar to lesions most commonly seen in tuberous sclerosis. Combined hamartomas of the retina and retinal pigment epithelium and retinal capillary hemangiomas have also been associated with NF1. Occasionally, these lesions might cause vision-threatening complications such as massive exudation, retinal detachment, neovascular glaucoma, and vitreous hemorrhage [25]. Finally, in a more recent series of 275 patients with retinal vasoproliferative tumors, 6 (2.2%) were found to have NF1 [26]. The tumors were located between the equator and the ora serrata in all cases and were variably associated with subretinal fluid and exudation, epiretinal membrane, retinal and vitreous hemorrhage, retinal neovascularization, and cystoid macular edema [26].

6.5 Choroid

Choroidal neurofibromatosis was once considered a rare variant of NF1, but is now known to be a common feature of the disease. Improved imaging modalities such as indocyanine-green fundus angiography and confocal microscopy using infrared light can penetrate the retinal pigment epithelium (RPE), which allows imaging of the choroid [1, 27, 28]. Histopathologic examination of enucleated eyes with choroidal neurofibromatosis revealed choroidal thickening with ovoid bodies and proliferation of connective tissue with pigment-containing cells and ganglion-like cells, features consistent with choroidal ganglioneuroma [29].

In 1998, Rescaldani and colleagues were the first to use indocyanine-green angiography (ICGA) to investigate the choroidal features of 2 cases of NF1 [30]. In both cases, early phases of the examination showed multiple extensive areas of hypofluorescence, that became smaller in the late phases. The authors speculated that the early hypofluorescence could be due to slow choroidal filling caused by alterations to the walls of the choroidal arterioles induced by the disease. Late hypofluorescent areas were presumed to be either persistent nonperfused lobules of choriocapillaris or choroidal nodules [30].

Later, Yasunari and colleagues investigated the use of infrared monochromatic light examination by confocal scanning laser ophthalmoscope (cSLO) in 33 eyes of 17 patients with NF1 [27]. They detected multiple bright patchy regions at and around the posterior pole of all 33 eyes examined, which corresponded to the hypofluorescent areas on ICGA. No abnormalities were noted at corresponding areas under conventional ophthalmoscopic examination or FA [27]. The authors pointed out that bright patchy regions under infrared light may indicate the presence of refractile tissue or material in the choroid, corresponding to choroidal neurofibromas, which are thought to be refractile in nature [27].

Another study from 2012 used cSLO to examine 95 consecutive adult and pediatric patients (190 eyes) [28]. Bright patchy choroidal nodules (Fig. 6.2) were detected by NIR in 79 (82%) patients, including 15 children (71%), while conventional fundus ophthalmoscopy, fundus autofluorescence, and red-free imaging did not disclose any abnormalities in the corresponding areas. Lesions were more frequently located in the posterior pole, but occurred diffusely throughout the fundus. Optical coherence tomography (OCT) showed irregular hyperreflective foci located under the RPE, corresponding to the alterations detected by NIR imaging [28]. Interestingly, the authors found no significant correlation between Lisch nodules and choroidal nodules, but a correlation was found between increased patient age

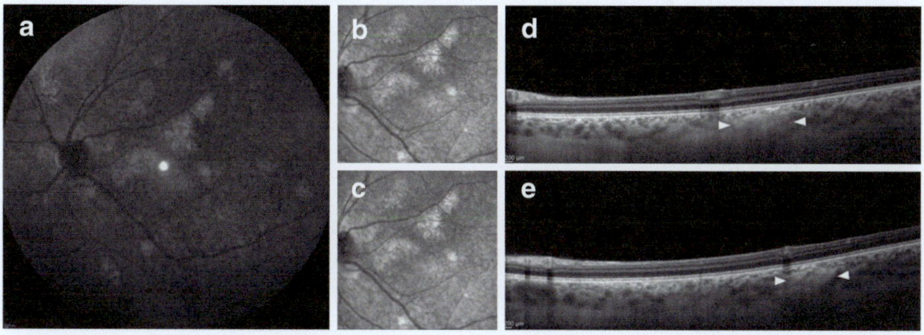

Fig. 6.2 NIR (near infrared) fundus picture of the left eye (OS) of a 16-year-old boy with NF1 discloses multiple bright patches at the posterior pole and along the arcades (**a**). OCT (optical coherence tomography) scans through 2 of these lesions show that the bright areas correspond to choroidal nodules (**b–e**, arrowheads)

and more diffused involvement of the fundus [28]. The prevalence of choroidal nodules detected by NIR in the overall NF1 population (82%) was similar to the average prevalence of the 4 most common NIH diagnostic criteria (cafè-au-lait, freckling, Lisch nodules, and neurofibromas). In the pediatric population, choroidal nodules were present in a much higher frequency (71%) than that of the NIH diagnostic criteria of for iris Lisch nodules (43%) [28]. Therefore, the authors suggested the presence of choroidal abnormalities detected by NIR imaging should be used as an additional diagnostic criterion for NF1.

Following this observation, Parrozzani and colleagues evaluated the diagnostic performance of NF1-related choroidal abnormalities detected by NIR as a diagnostic criterion in the pediatric population [31]. They evaluated 140 consecutive pediatric patients aged 0–16 years old and found choroidal abnormalities in 72 affected (61%) and 1 suspected (2%) children. Compared with standard NIH criteria, the presence of choroidal abnormalities detected by NIR was the third parameter for positive predictive value and the fourth for sensitivity, specificity, and negative predictive value. Compared with Lisch nodules, this criterion had higher specificity and positive predictive value [31].

A similar study by Vagge and colleagues investigated the presence of choroidal abnormalities detected by NIR in pediatric patients with NF1 and documented similar findings [32]. Choroidal abnormalities were found in 54 patients (69%), were most frequently located at the posterior pole and the number of involved areas correlated with patient age [32].

Finally, NIR and OCT imaging modalities have been useful in detecting other interesting choroidal findings. In a series of 34 eyes of 17 patients with NF1 and typical choroidal nodules, bilateral anomalous choroidal vessels were observed with NIR in 4 patients. Enhanced depth imaging (EDI)-OCT revealed unusually dilated choroidal vessels and an absence of the choriocapillaris or Sattler's layer above the dilated vessels [33]. In another study EDI-OCT was able to identify 2 distinctive morphologies of choroidal nodules detected by NIR imaging, "dome-shaped" or "placoid" [34]. In the same study, authors reported a reduction in the mean choroidal thickness in patients with NF1, as well as in the neuroepithelium, photoreceptor-retinal pigment epithelium, and outer nuclear layer thickness [34].

6.6 Optic Nerve

Optic pathway gliomas (OPGs) occur in 15–20% of patients, and they represent the most common orbital and intracranial manifestation of NF1, as well as the most common central nervous system tumor in children with NF1 [35]. They can affect any part of the visual pathway from the pre-chiasmatic tracts of the optic nerves to the chiasmatic-hypothalamic region to the posterior optic pathway (Fig. 6.3) [1, 36]. Rarely, gliomas in the brainstem may also occur in children with NF1 [1]. Histologically, they are classified as grade I astrocytomas or juvenile pilocytic astrocytomas according to the World Health Organization [37].

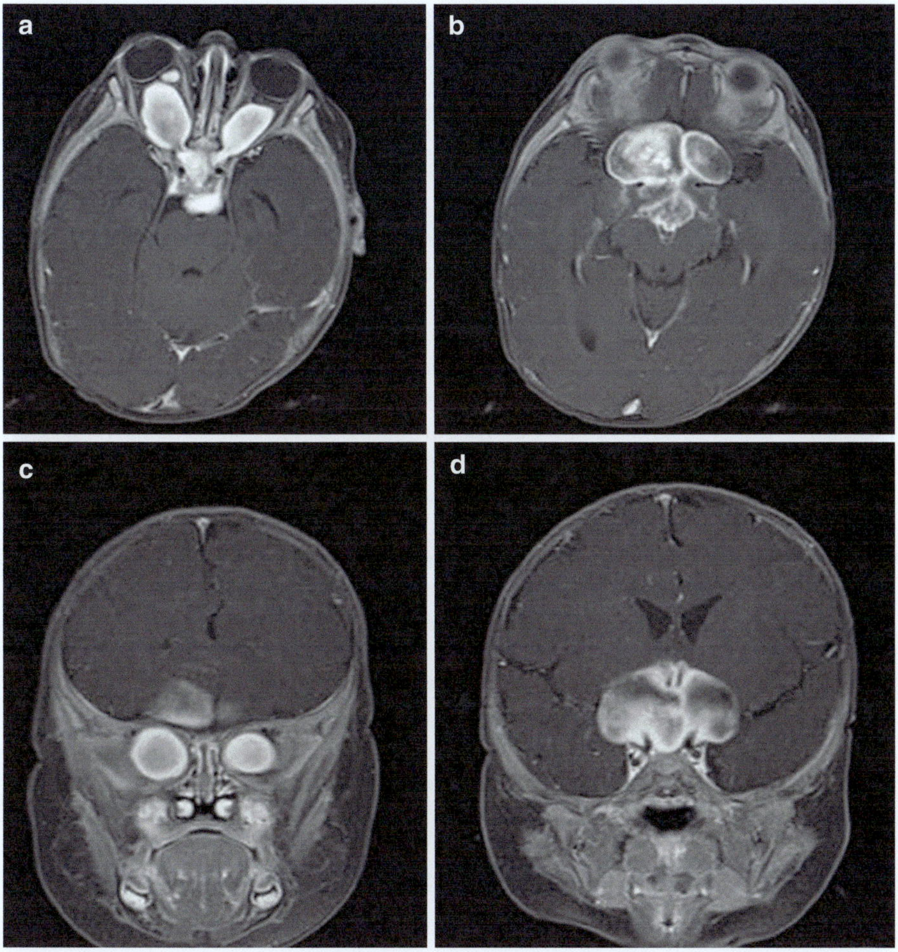

Fig. 6.3 Axial scans (**a**, **b**) and coronal scans (**c**, **d**) of MRI of the brain and orbits disclose large bilateral fusiform optic nerve masses with extension into the suprasellar region and extending posteriorly to involve the chiasm and hypothalamus. The lesions are compatible with optic pathway gliomas found in NF1

OPGs usually develop during the first decade of life (with children aged 6 years or younger at greatest risk), even though later onset has been described in the literature [35]. They are usually unilateral, but bilateral presentation has been described in about one third of cases [10]. Clinical symptoms at time of diagnosis have been reported in about 60% of cases, with clinical presentation varying according to tumor location [38]. Clinical behavior of OPGs is highly variable [35]. For tumors located in the optic nerve, typical presentation is with gradual onset of painless unilateral loss of vision, with visual acuity ranging from 20/20 to no light perception. Clinical examination may disclose a combination of dyschromatopsia, centrocecal scotoma on visual field (VF) testing, and/or a relative afferent pupillary defect.

The optic nerve may appear normal, swollen or atrophic. Proptosis, nystagmus or strabismus can also occur. Other rare findings include headaches and papilledema secondary to high intracranial pressure in larger chiasmal-hypothalamic gliomas that are more likely to occur in sporadic cases [1, 2, 39–41]. If the location of the tumor is in the chiasm, bilateral visual loss, bilateral swelling or atrophy of the optic nerves, and bitemporal hemianopsia on VF might occur [42]. Finally, if the hypothalamus is invaded, precocious puberty can be seen in up to 40% of patients older than 6 years of age. This finding can represent the presenting symptom or the first sign of progression of the disease [35].

In terms of natural history, OPGs are usually benign and show a more indolent course compared to sporadic cases. However, hazardous evolution with significant morbidity, vision loss, and endocrine abnormalities has been reported in one third of cases [36, 38, 43]. In a recent study on 414 consecutive patients with NF1 referred before age 6, 52 (13%) developed OPGs during follow-up, with females more commonly affected [36]. OPGs were more frequently detected in patients with suggestive symptoms compared to patients who underwent an MRI for screening purposes. Clinical management was conservative in most patients, with only 8 (2%) requiring therapy due to visual deterioration [36]. This study confirmed findings from previous studies, in which the presence of symptoms at the time of diagnosis was shown to be the best predictor of the need for treatment, with asymptomatic children rarely requiring treatment [2, 38].

The preferred screening protocol for asymptomatic children affected by NF1 is controversial. Some centers prefer performing more frequent examinations in the first year of life and then gradually increasing the intervals between visits [35, 40, 41]. However, the recommendations from the American Academy of Pediatrics (AAP) indicate annual ophthalmic examinations from ages 1 to 7 years and then every 2 years from ages 8 to 18 years [44]. Several papers indicate that visual deterioration is considered the best indicator of presence or progression of OPGs, therefore visual acuity should be quantitatively assessed at every visit [35, 39]. When visual deterioration (defined as a 2 line decrease in visual acuity) not attributable to other causes is detected, prompt MRI of the brain and orbits should be performed [35].

The role of systematic MRI screening for OPGs in children with NF1 has been widely discussed in the literature. In 1997, the OPG Task Force determined that there was no conclusive evidence that early detection of asymptomatic gliomas led to reduced vision loss [40]. These findings, combined with the potential neurotoxic effects of repeated sedation in children, led the AAP not to recommend routine MRI screening for asymptomatic NF1 patients. However, in a more recent study on 826 individuals with NF1, Prada and colleagues found that chiasmatic and postchiasmatic OPGs carried the highest risk for progression and vision loss and that early identification with MRI screening in asymptomatic cases may lead to improved visual outcomes [45]. Nevertheless, current indications identify MRI of the brain and orbits as the preferred imaging modality to confirm the diagnosis of OPG once an abnormal ophthalmological evaluation has been documented [35]. Neuroradiological appearance is fairly typical: OPGs appear as fusiform masses in the optic nerve and chiasm region, hypointense or isointense on T1 images, and hyperintense in T2 images [46].

Other screening modalities for OPGs in older and more cooperative children include VF testing and OCT. Kinetic (Goldmann) VF testing can be easier for younger children, however, VF testing can be difficult to perform in a repeatable and reliable way [35]. It has been found that subjects with NF1 and OPGs have a thinner retinal nerve fiber layer (RNFL) on OCT [47]. Interestingly, Parrozzani and colleagues found that RNFL assessment using spectral domain OCT can be superior to visual function assessment and optic nerve evaluation as a screening tool for OPGs [48].

As previously mentioned, the clinical course of OPGs can be varied and unpredictable, making the management quite challenging. In a large study from 2003, no single specific epidemiological factor that could serve as a predictor of the need for future treatment was identified [41]. Also, there is still debate about the optimal choice and timing of treatment. Generally speaking, most authors agree that documented clinical decline and/or radiographic progression represent the main indications for treatment [35, 38, 40, 42]. Clinical progression includes decreased visual acuity or color vision, VF defect progression, progressive proptosis or endocrine, and neurological dysfunctions [38, 42]. Radiographic progression is defined as tumor enlargement, change in enhancement or progressive involvement of the posterior visual pathway [35]. It is important to keep in mind that initial management often involves careful observation, as about one half of OPGs do not cause clinical symptoms.

A detailed discussion about different treatment protocols for OPGs in NF1 patients is beyond the scope of this chapter. However, it is important to mention that chemotherapy currently represents the first-line treatment for all age groups [35, 42]. Standard combination includes vincristine and carboplatin. This regimen is overall well tolerated, does not carry significant long-term toxicity and is effective in the control of both newly diagnosed and recurrent OPGs [49]. However, there is a risk of acute toxicity (myelosuppression). Radiotherapy was once considered the first-line treatment in children older than 6 years of age, but a risk for secondary tumors and unacceptable complications have been identified [35, 42]. This is particularly dangerous in patients with NF1, that are already predisposed to both benign and malignant lesions. Finally, surgery has very limited role in OPGs from NF1. It is reserved for biopsies in atypical cases or when the mass effect causes painful and disfiguring proptosis associated with corneal exposure of a blind eye [35, 39, 42].

6.7 Glaucoma

Glaucoma rarely occurs in patients with NF1 (about 1–2%), but these patients are at increased risk of developing elevated intraocular pressure for multiple reasons [1].

Patients with NF1 and orbitofacial involvement (mainly plexiform neurofibroma of the upper lid) have a higher incidence of glaucoma, found in up to 23% of these patients [50]. In this subset of NF1 patients, glaucoma seems to be associated with poor visual outcomes and surgical intervention is often required [50]. More specifically, unilateral glaucoma associated with buphthalmos can be found in patients with NF1 and ipsilateral plexiform neurofibroma of the upper eyelid [51]. The association of unilateral buphthalmos, ipsilateral plexiform neurofibroma, and ipsilateral facial hemihypertrophy is referred to as François syndrome [1].

Potential mechanisms of increased intraocular pressure include angle abnormalities such as abundant iris processes, anteriorization of angle insertion, pigmentary disturbances, secondary angle closure from synechiae formation, and angle infiltration by Lisch nodules or neurofibromas [52].

Assessment for glaucoma, including gonioscopy, intraocular pressure evaluation, visual field testing, and optic nerve assessment is, therefore, advised in patients with NF1 [8].

References

1. Kinori M, Hodgson N, Zeid JL. Ophthalmic manifestations in neurofibromatosis type 1. Surv Ophthalmol. 2018;63:518.
2. Savar A, Cestari DM. Neurofibromatosis type I: genetics and clinical manifestations. Semin Ophthalmol. 2008;23(1):45–51.
3. Friedman JM. Neurofibromatosis : phenotype, natural history, and pathogenesis. Baltimore: Johns Hopkins University Press; 1999.
4. DeClue JE, Cohen BD, Lowy DR. Identification and characterization of the neurofibromatosis type 1 protein product. Proc Natl Acad Sci U S A. 1991;88(22):9914–8.
5. Gutmann DH, Collins FS. The neurofibromatosis type 1 gene and its protein product, neurofibromin. Neuron. 1993;10(3):335–43.
6. Tinschert S, Naumann I, Stegmann E, Buske A, Kaufmann D, Thiel G, et al. Segmental neurofibromatosis is caused by somatic mutation of the neurofibromatosis type 1 (NF1) gene. Eur J Hum Genet. 2000;8(6):455–9.
7. National Institutes of Health Consensus Development Conference Statement: neurofibromatosis. Bethesda, Md., USA, July 13–15, 1987. Neurofibromatosis. 1988;1(3):172–8.
8. Abdolrahimzadeh B, Piraino DC, Albanese G, Cruciani F, Rahimi S. Neurofibromatosis: an update of ophthalmic characteristics and applications of optical coherence tomography. Clin Ophthalmol. 2016;10:851–60.
9. Beauchamp GR. Neurofibromatosis type 1 in children. Trans Am Ophthalmol Soc. 1995;93:445–72.
10. Listernick R, Charrow J, Greenwald MJ, Esterly NB. Optic gliomas in children with neurofibromatosis type 1. J Pediatr. 1989;114(5):788–92.
11. Avery RA, Katowitz JA, Fisher MJ, Heidary G, Dombi E, Packer RJ, et al. Orbital/periorbital plexiform neurofibromas in children with neurofibromatosis type 1: multidisciplinary recommendations for care. Ophthalmology. 2017;124(1):123–32.
12. Chaudhry IA, Morales J, Shamsi FA, Al-Rashed W, Elzaridi E, Arat YO, et al. Orbitofacial neurofibromatosis: clinical characteristics and treatment outcome. Eye. 2012;26(4):583–92.
13. Oystreck DT, Morales J, Chaudhry I, Alorainy IA, Elkhamary SM, Pasha TM, et al. Visual loss in orbitofacial neurofibromatosis type 1. Ophthalmology. 2012;119(10):2168–73.
14. Hirbe AC, Gutmann DH. Neurofibromatosis type 1: a multidisciplinary approach to care. Lancet Neurol. 2014;13(8):834–43.
15. Keren S, Dotan G, Ben-Cnaan R, Leibovitch L, Leibovitch I. A combined one-stage surgical approach of orbital tumor debulking, lid reconstruction, and ptosis repair in children with orbitotemporal neurofibromatosis. J Plast Reconstr Aesthet Surg. 2017;70(3):336–40.

16. Williamson TH, Garner A, Moore AT. Structure of Lisch nodules in neurofibromatosis type 1. Ophthalmic Paediatr Genet. 1991;12(1):11–7.
17. Lubs ML, Bauer MS, Formas ME, Djokic B. Lisch nodules in neurofibromatosis type 1. N Engl J Med. 1991;324(18):1264–6.
18. Sanders TE. Intraocular juvenile xanthogranuloma (nevoxanthogranuloma): a survey of 20 cases. Trans Am Ophthalmol Soc. 1960;58:59–74.
19. Cambiaghi S, Restano L, Caputo R. Juvenile xanthogranuloma associated with neurofibromatosis 1: 14 patients without evidence of hematologic malignancies. Pediatr Dermatol. 2004;21(2):97–101.
20. Zvulunov A, Barak Y, Metzker A. Juvenile xanthogranuloma, neurofibromatosis, and juvenile chronic myelogenous leukemia. World statistical analysis. Arch Dermatol. 1995;131(8):904–8.
21. Liy-Wong C, Mohammed J, Carleton A, Pope E, Parkin P, Lara-Corrales I. The relationship between neurofibromatosis type 1, juvenile xanthogranuloma, and malignancy: a retrospective case-control study. J Am Acad Dermatol. 2017;76(6):1084–7.
22. Muci-Mendoza R, Ramella M, Fuenmayor-Rivera D. Corkscrew retinal vessels in neurofibromatosis type 1: report of 12 cases. Br J Ophthalmol. 2002;86(3):282–4.
23. Abdolrahimzadeh S, Felli L, Piraino DC, Mollo R, Calvieri S, Recupero SM. Retinal microvascular abnormalities overlying choroidal nodules in neurofibromatosis type 1. BMC Ophthalmol. 2014;14:146.
24. Parrozzani R, Pilotto E, Clementi M, Frizziero L, Leonardi F, Convento E, et al. Retinal vascular abnormalities in a large cohort of patients affected by neurofibromatosis type 1: a study using optical coherence tomography angiography. Retina. 2018;38(3):585.
25. Destro M, D'Amico DJ, Gragoudas ES, Brockhurst RJ, Pinnolis MK, Albert DM, et al. Retinal manifestations of neurofibromatosis. Diagnosis and management. Arch Ophthalmol. 1991;109(5):662–6.
26. Shields JA, Pellegrini M, Kaliki S, Mashayekhi A, Shields CL. Retinal vasoproliferative tumors in 6 patients with neurofibromatosis type 1. JAMA Ophthalmol. 2014;132(2):190–6.
27. Yasunari T, Shiraki K, Hattori H, Miki T. Frequency of choroidal abnormalities in neurofibromatosis type 1. Lancet. 2000;356(9234):988–92.
28. Viola F, Villani E, Natacci F, Selicorni A, Melloni G, Vezzola D, et al. Choroidal abnormalities detected by near-infrared reflectance imaging as a new diagnostic criterion for neurofibromatosis 1. Ophthalmology. 2012;119(2):369–75.
29. Woog JJ, Albert DM, Craft J, Silberman N, Horns D. Choroidal ganglioneuroma in neurofibromatosis. Graefes Arch Clin Exp Ophthalmol. 1983;220(1):25–31.
30. Rescaldani C, Nicolini P, Fatigati G, Bottoni FG. Clinical application of digital indocyanine green angiography in choroidal neurofibromatosis. Ophthalmologica. 1998;212(2):99–104.
31. Parrozzani R, Clementi M, Frizziero L, Miglionico G, Perrini P, Cavarzeran F, et al. In vivo detection of choroidal abnormalities related to NF1: feasibility and comparison with standard NIH diagnostic criteria in pediatric patients. Invest Ophthalmol Vis Sci. 2015;56(10):6036–42.
32. Vagge A, Camicione P, Capris C, Sburlati C, Panarello S, Calevo MG, et al. Choroidal abnormalities in neurofibromatosis type 1 detected by near-infrared reflectance imaging in paediatric population. Acta Ophthalmol. 2015;93(8):e667–71.
33. Abdolrahimzadeh S, Parisi F, Abdolrahimzadeh B, Cruciani F. Unusual choroidal vessels in neurofibromatosis type 1 observed with near-infrared reflectance and spectral domain optical coherence tomography. Acta Ophthalmol. 2016;94(8):e815–e6.
34. Abdolrahimzadeh S, Felli L, Plateroti R, Plateroti AM, Giustini S, Calvieri S, et al. Morphologic and vasculature features of the choroid and associated choroid-retinal thickness alterations in neurofibromatosis type 1. Br J Ophthalmol. 2015;99(6):789–93.
35. Listernick R, Ferner RE, Liu GT, Gutmann DH. Optic pathway gliomas in neurofibromatosis-1: controversies and recommendations. Ann Neurol. 2007;61(3):189–98.
36. Trevisson E, Cassina M, Opocher E, Vicenzi V, Lucchetta M, Parrozzani R, et al. Natural history of optic pathway gliomas in a cohort of unselected patients affected by Neurofibromatosis 1. J Neuro-Oncol. 2017;134(2):279–87.

37. Kleihues P, Louis DN, Scheithauer BW, Rorke LB, Reifenberger G, Burger PC, et al. The WHO classification of tumors of the nervous system. J Neuropathol Exp Neurol. 2002;61(3):215–25; discussion 26-9.
38. Thiagalingam S, Flaherty M, Billson F, North K. Neurofibromatosis type 1 and optic pathway gliomas: follow-up of 54 patients. Ophthalmology. 2004;111(3):568–77.
39. Avery RA, Fisher MJ, Liu GT. Optic pathway gliomas. J Neuroophthalmol. 2011;31(3):269–78.
40. Listernick R, Louis DN, Packer RJ, Gutmann DH. Optic pathway gliomas in children with neurofibromatosis 1: consensus statement from the NF1 Optic Pathway Glioma Task Force. Ann Neurol. 1997;41(2):143–9.
41. King A, Listernick R, Charrow J, Piersall L, Gutmann DH. Optic pathway gliomas in neurofibromatosis type 1: the effect of presenting symptoms on outcome. Am J Med Genet A. 2003;122A(2):95–9.
42. Liu GT. Optic gliomas of the anterior visual pathway. Curr Opin Ophthalmol. 2006;17(5):427–31.
43. Listernick R, Darling C, Greenwald M, Strauss L, Charrow J. Optic pathway tumors in children: the effect of neurofibromatosis type 1 on clinical manifestations and natural history. J Pediatr. 1995;127(5):718–22.
44. Hersh JH. Health supervision for children with neurofibromatosis. Pediatrics. 2008;121(3):633–42.
45. Prada CE, Hufnagel RB, Hummel TR, Lovell AM, Hopkin RJ, Saal HM, et al. The use of magnetic resonance imaging screening for optic pathway gliomas in children with neurofibromatosis type 1. J Pediatr. 2015;167(4):851–6.e1.
46. Mentzel HJ, Seidel J, Fitzek C, Eichhorn A, Vogt S, Reichenbach JR, et al. Pediatric brain MRI in neurofibromatosis type I. Eur Radiol. 2005;15(4):814–22.
47. Chang L, El-Dairi MA, Frempong TA, Burner EL, Bhatti MT, Young TL, et al. Optical coherence tomography in the evaluation of neurofibromatosis type-1 subjects with optic pathway gliomas. J AAPOS. 2010;14(6):511–7.
48. Parrozzani R, Clementi M, Kotsafti O, Miglionico G, Trevisson E, Orlando G, et al. Optical coherence tomography in the diagnosis of optic pathway gliomas. Invest Ophthalmol Vis Sci. 2013;54(13):8112–8.
49. Packer RJ, Lange B, Ater J, Nicholson HS, Allen J, Walker R, et al. Carboplatin and vincristine for recurrent and newly diagnosed low-grade gliomas of childhood. J Clin Oncol. 1993;11(5):850–6.
50. Morales J, Chaudhry IA, Bosley TM. Glaucoma and globe enlargement associated with neurofibromatosis type 1. Ophthalmology. 2009;116(9):1725–30.
51. Greenwald MJ, Paller AS. Ocular and dermatologic manifestation of neurocutaneous syndromes. Dermatol Clin. 1992;10(3):623–39.
52. Grant WM, Walton DS. Distinctive gonioscopic findings in glaucoma due to neurofibromatosis. Arch Ophthalmol. 1968;79(2):127–34.

Skeletal Manifestations in NF1

7

David H. Viskochil and David A. Stevenson

Contents

7.1 Introduction

Skeletal abnormalities have long been recognized as part of the phenotype associated with neurofibromatosis type 1 (NF1) [1–5], and an osseous manifestation has been projected to occur in up to half of the affected individuals. A comprehensive evaluation of 950 individuals with NF1 seen through Dr. Vincent Riccardi's NF Institute Clinical Research Program through 1991 provides an excellent estimate of the incidence of various skeletal manifestations [6]; subsets were definitively scored

D. H. Viskochil (✉)
Department of Pediatrics, Division of Medical Genetics, Stanford University, Stanford, CA, USA
e-mail: Dave.Viskochil@hsc.utah.edu

D. A. Stevenson
The University of Utah, Division of Medical Genetics, Salt Lake City, UT, USA
e-mail: dasteven@stanford.edu

G. Tadini et al. (eds.), *Multidisciplinary Approach to Neurofibromatosis Type 1*,
https://doi.org/10.1007/978-3-319-92450-2_7

for each feature as either having the manifestation or not having the manifestation as follows: short stature (716 patients)-12%; macrocephaly (726 patients)-29%; craniofacial dysplasia (470 patients)-12%; vertebral dysplasia (370 patients)-11%; scoliosis (752 patients)-25%; lumbar scalloping (404 patients)-10%; pseudarthrosis/tibial (909 patients)-3%; pectus excavatum (675 patients)-31%. Thus, when the initial clinical diagnostic criteria were developed in 1988 through an NIH consensus conference, a "distinctive osseous lesion" was listed as one of the seven diagnostic criteria [1]. The presence of these lesions would lead experienced radiologists and orthopedists to search for other signs of NF1. The most distinctive and specific skeletal manifestations of NF1 are tibial pseudarthrosis and sphenoid wing dysplasia, in which the presence of either alone raises the concern for NF1.

Historically, NF1-related research focused on the non-skeletal abnormalities resulting in a relative lack of understanding about the role of neurofibromin in bone development and a dearth of treatment options [7]. However, it is now known that the *NF1* gene product, neurofibromin, acting through the Ras/MAPK signal transduction pathway plays a significant role in bone homeostasis and bone development. This is supported by the observation that other genetic conditions due to mutations in genes whose encoded peptides interact in this pathway also have some overlapping musculoskeletal phenotype [8]. The absence of tumor tissue adjacent to many skeletal manifestations in NF1 supports the contention initially posited by James Hunt in his thesis of 1961 entitled "Skeletal Lesions in Neurofibromatosis" [5] that mesodermal dysplasia is key to the pathogenesis of many of the NF1-related bone abnormalities. The lack of cell material to assess the status of the *NF1* gene and/or signaling through the Ras/MAPK pathway precludes most human studies assessing this potential role in the bone dysplasias of NF1. However, numerous conditional knockout animal models provide evidence that neurofibromin is critical in bone homeostasis and development [9–23]. Animal models have provided insight to the pathophysiology of skeletal abnormalities; however, treatment options are still relatively limited to surgical management. To date, medical therapies targeted to the Ras/MAPK pathway have focused on tumor responses rather than bone. In this chapter, we will provide an overview of the skeletal manifestations of NF1.

7.2 Cranial Bone Abnormalities

Cranial bone dysplasias in NF1 include calvarial defects and dysplasias. Cranial bones are derived from the neural crest; therefore, it should not be surprising that *NF1*-related dysregulation of Ras/MAPK signal transduction in the cranial neural crest has implications for bone development of the head. Calvarial defects involving the lambdoid suture have long been recognized as an association with NF1 [24]. Palpation of the skull can easily detect depressions of the bone that are generally asymptomatic and do not require intervention. Size of the bone deficiency is a concern for meningeal herniation, but this is rare. The most common cranial bone deficiency in NF1 is sphenoid wing dysplasia, seen in up to ~10% of individuals with NF1 [25]. The sphenoid bones coalesce to form the orbits, and deficiency of any of

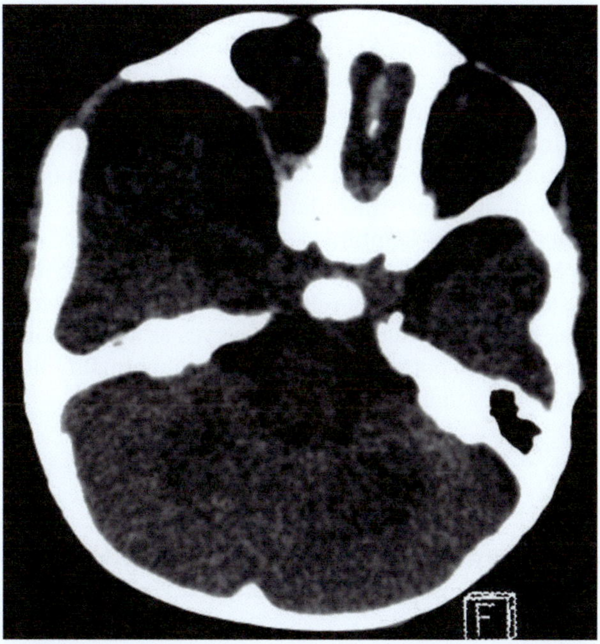

Fig. 7.1 Head CT scan showing deficiency of the sphenoid bone on the right

the bones leads to an asymmetric orbit (see Fig. 7.1). The most common is deficiency of the greater sphenoid wing that is almost invariably unilateral; therefore, visual inspection of the face leads to detection of asymmetry without the need for radiologic assessment. The ipsilateral association of plexiform neurofibroma (>50% of cases) makes it imperative for health care providers to seek soft tissue tumors when sphenoid wing dysplasia is suspected. Soft tissue asymmetry can be subtle and involve the eyelids, forehead, temples, and internal bone structures of the face. Palpation of the zygomatic and temporal regions can potentially detect a fullness and subcutaneous nodularity if neurofibromas are present and strong consideration should be given for MRI assessment of the face and head in those with facial bone asymmetry of the orbits. Deficiency of the sphenoid bone(s) sometimes results in propagation of the brain vascular pulsations to be transmitted to the eye globe.

The pathophysiology of the association of facial neurofibromas with bone defects is controversial. Some speculate that cases where cranial bone dysplasia occurs without adjacent neurofibroma tissue demonstrate that calvarial dysplasia is a primary phenomenon [5], whereas others point out the rarity of sphenoid dysplasia in the absence of adjacent tumor implies that bone dysplasia is a secondary phenomenon [26, 27]. In the cases of large congenital facial plexiform neurofibromas of the cranium, progression of bone loss suggests that the tumors disrupt normal bone remodeling, either through vascular steal phenomenon or possibly paracrine secretion of factors that interfere with normal intramembranous bone homeostasis. In addition to the cranial bone loss associated with plexiform neurofibromas, the mandible can also undergo osteolysis [28] leading to potential problems in mastication.

Surgical correction of calvarial defects and sphenoid wing dysplasia are fraught with complications [27, 29]. In those cases where an adjacent plexiform neurofibroma is implicit in bone erosion, full surgical resection is indicated, but rarely achieved. The advent of MEK inhibitor therapy to decrease the progression and decrease volume of some plexiform neurofibromas [30] may alleviate the bone erosion in some cases. In cases where there is no tumor involvement, a combination of surgical techniques including closure of bone defects in adults with non-biologic material may be helpful.

Macrocephaly is common in NF1 with about 25% having an OFC of greater than the 98th centile [6] and relative macrocephaly much more common. Macrocephaly does not require intervention. It serves as a potential clue to the diagnosis of NF1, but it neither portends an underlying abnormality nor provides insight for altered anticipatory guidance.

7.3 Long Bone Dysplasia

Historically, tibial pseudarthrosis is the term that most physicians associate with the "distinctive" osseous findings of NF1. However, tibial pseudarthrosis is a specific finding that technically means non-union of the tibia. Not all individuals with NF1 who have anterolateral bowing of the tibia progress to fracture and non-union. In addition, multiple long bones have been reported to be dysplastic and lead to pseudarthrosis. Therefore, long bone dysplasia is perhaps a more accurate term to encompass this specific phenotype seen in NF1, and management is different based on whether or not the tibia has sustained a fracture without union versus a dysplastic bowed tibia that has not yet fractured.

For unknown reasons, the tibia is the most common long bone affected in NF1 (≈3–4%) [25]. The clinical presentation is typically an anterolateral bowing of the lower leg with radiographic features showing a thickened cortex with narrowing of the medullary canal in the region of the apex of the bowing occurring around the distal third of the tibia [31] (see Fig. 7.2). In infancy, physiologic bowing can be confused with pathologic bowing associated with NF1, although physiologic bowing is typically a lateral bowing that lacks the anterior bowing. The dysplastic tibia frequently will sustain a fracture, which in many cases leads to non-union (i.e., pseudarthrosis). In one study the average age of fracture was 4.6 years with >50% fracturing prior to 2 years of age, and in >50% the abnormality was identified in infancy [32]. Once there is a fracture with non-union, the tibial segments tend to develop what has been described as a "sucked candy" appearance with narrowing of the fragment ends suggestive of a disordered remodeling process. Surgical samples have shown that the tissue that develops at the fracture site between the fractured bone segments consists of a highly cellular fibrocartilage tissue that lacks markers of a neurofibroma [33–35] and Heerva et al. [36] documented a number of multinuclear osteoclasts embedded within this pseudarthrosis tissue.

The long bone dysplasia is typically unilateral and localized, suggesting stochastic events. Several studies have documented somatic "second hits" in the *NF1* gene

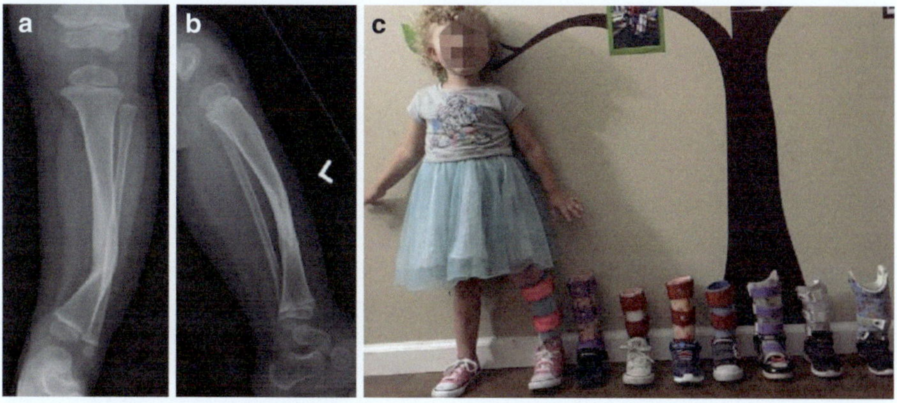

Fig. 7.2 Radiographs of tibial dysplasia showing anterolateral bowing with thickened cortex and narrowing of the medullary canal at the apex of the curve (**a**, **b**). Bracing of lower leg is used in an attempt to protect the dysplastic bone from fracture and progression to pseudarthrosis (**c**)

from tissue extracted from the surgical site of the pseudarthrosis [34, 37]. This, in addition to the congenital onset, suggests that a contributing etiology of long bone dysplasia in NF1 is an early somatic event in the *NF1* gene in osteoprogenitor cells.

The radiographic findings can vary between individuals although they likely can evolve over time, even within the same individual. Multiple radiographic classification systems have been proposed for tibial pseudarthrosis (e.g., Crawford, Boyd, and Anderson systems), but the Crawford classification system, which includes four types [38], has historically been the most widely adopted by the orthopedic community [39]. Tudisco et al. [40] suggested that the Crawford classification may be useful in predicting eventual outcomes in patients with tibial dysplasia, but there is only limited evidence that these radiographic classifications are useful in clinical management decisions.

Treatment of the pseudarthrosis is difficult, generally requiring multiple surgical procedures, and, in some cases, amputation. Stevenson et al. [32] reported an average of 3 surgical procedures in a cohort of individuals with NF1 and tibial pseudarthrosis, with one receiving 13 surgical procedures. Even if union is obtained, function can be limited. Optimal treatment protocols when pseudarthrosis occurs are limited and require careful discussion with an orthopedist as there have been a multitude of surgical approaches reported in the medical literature [41–43] and reports of adjunctive pharmacologic therapies (e.g., BMP) [44]. An NF1 Bone Abnormalities Consortium in 2013 proposed a set of concepts to consider when treating tibial pseudarthrosis that included the following: bone fixation appropriate to achieve rigid stability; debridement of the fibrous pseudarthrosis tissue; creation of a healthy vascular bed for bone repair; promotion of osteogenesis; control of overactive bone resorption; prevention of recurrence of the fibrous pseudarthrosis tissue; and achievement of long-term bone health to prevent recurrence [45].

The tibia is not the only long bone to be affected in NF1. In particular, the fibula can be dysplastic and there is often co-occurrence of both the tibia and fibula [32].

Interestingly it is the distal long bones (tibia, fibula, radius, and ulna) that are most commonly affected bones with only rare reports of the proximal long bones.

7.4 Scoliosis

Although scoliosis may not be considered a "distinctive" osseous finding specific to NF1, it is one of the more common of the skeletal abnormalities observed in NF1 with a wide range of incidences reported in the literature. Scoliosis in NF1 has been typically classified into "dystrophic" and "non-dystrophic," although there are no diagnostic criteria for what constitutes these specific classifications. Durrani et al. [46] provided a description of specific radiographic features that represented a "dystrophic" finding and these included rib penciling, vertebral rotation of Grade 3+, vertebral wedging, spindling of the transverse process, widened interpedicular distance, enlarged intervertebral foramina, and posterior, lateral, or anterior vertebral scalloping (see Fig. 7.3). However, Durrani et al. [46] documented that scoliosis could evolve from a curvature with no "dystrophic" features to the development "dystrophic" features, which was termed modulation.

It is likely that the vertebrae in individuals with NF1 who have scoliosis are intrinsically compromised. One study investigated vertebral samples of individuals with NF1 and showed severe reduction in mineral content [47]. However, paraspinal neurofibromas have been shown to be associated with scoliosis [48, 49] and this non-osseous manifestation likely contributes to progression of scoliosis whether through mass effect, paracrine actions, or other factors. The relationship of scoliosis with paraspinal tumors is still not well understood, but it is clear that the presence of a paraspinal neurofibroma is not required as there are many cases of dystrophic scoliosis in NF1 without an accompanying neurofibroma. It is our experience that individuals with a short segment scoliosis with "dystrophic" radiographic findings typically present early in childhood. This suggests that dystrophic scoliosis likely represents a

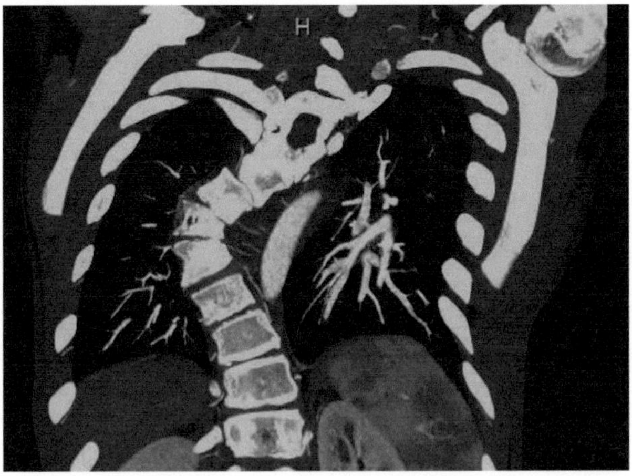

Fig. 7.3 Spine CT demonstrating NF1-related dystrophic scoliosis

congenital osteopathy with a more rapid progression. The "non-dystrophic" scoliosis generally follows a course seen in the general population with a later onset.

The relatively high prevalence of both dystrophic and non-dystrophic forms of scoliosis in the NF1 population requires frequent clinical monitoring for evidence of scoliosis, even early in life. One should be aware that scoliosis can develop over time; one study showed that 18% of young adults in one cohort had developed a scoliosis in adulthood that was not present earlier [50]. Hence, scoliosis needs to continue to be monitored even as an adult, and the American College of Medical Genetics (ACMG) guidelines for adults with NF1 recommend annual clinical evaluation of the back with Adam's forward bend test to screen for scoliosis [51]. Pediatric guidelines are currently in development (in press) [52]. Management by an orthopedist experienced in NF1 is critical given the complexities and co-morbidities (e.g., intraspinal neurofibromas, dural ectasias, dysplastic vertebrae, vertebral pseudarthrosis).

7.5 Vertebral Defects

As observed in NF1-related dystrophic kyphoscoliosis, vertebral bodies and ribs can be dysplastic without adjacent tumor effects. Vertebral scalloping, hypoplasia of transverse processes and pedicles, and proximal rib anomalies are the most common dysplasias [5, 53]. Like other bone abnormalities in NF1, these are likely intrinsic bone anomalies and are associated with the dystrophic form of NF1-related scoliosis. Vertebral scalloping is associated with dural ectasia and meningoceles [49, 54]. Dural ectasia refers to widening of the dural sac (see Fig. 7.4), whereas meningocele refers to a localized protrusion of the spinal meninges through intervertebral

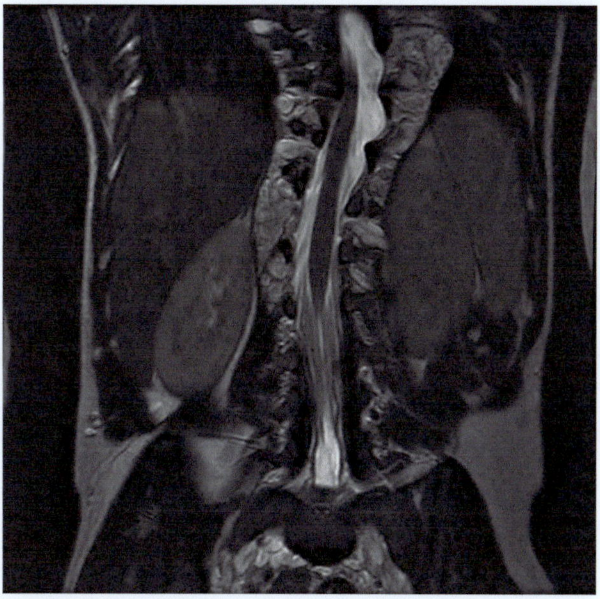

Fig. 7.4 Spine MRI demonstrating paraspinal neurofibromas and dural ectasia

foramena or, in the event of severe dysplasia, through the vertebral body. Typically seen in other connective tissue disorders such as Marfan syndrome, the etiology of dural ectasia is not well understood, and it is not clear if the pathophysiology of dural ectasia is similar between these 2 conditions. Rather than increased CSF pressure eroding bone, an alternate explanation is that as dysplasia of vertebral bodies progresses with scalloping, the dura conforms to the vacated space and CSF follows. Regardless of how dural ectasias and meningoceles form, treatment is difficult and can result in more harm than conservative management.

7.6 Short Stature

About a third of individuals with NF1 are shorter than family background, and NF1-specific growth charts are available as a reference to help determine when intervention is warranted for unexpected growth delay [55–57]. Like other Rasopathies, endocrine assessment is warranted when growth velocity falls off the typical curve and includes thyroid and growth hormone studies. Hormonal replacement guidelines and management is similar to the general population. The implementation of growth hormone replacement therapy requires discussion with families about potential long-term risks for neurofibromas because IGF (insulin growth factor) receptors are present on Schwann cells. Observations of individuals with NF1 and plexiform neurofibromas who have been treated with growth hormone did not show increased tumor progression over a couple of years of observation [58], but there are no long-term studies. Overgrowth in NF1 is typically secondary to hypothalamic gliomas, and if increased growth velocity is noted, with or without precocious puberty, brain MRI is indicated. Usually, the increased growth is secondary to transient elevation of growth hormone secretion that does not require treatment with luteinizing hormone releasing hormone analogue.

7.7 Pectus Anomalies

Chest wall abnormalities are seen in NF1 and can include asymmetry, pectus excavatum, and pectus carinatum. Pectus excavatum and carinatum are seen in other disorders of the Ras/MAPK pathway such as Noonan syndrome and hence suggest that this pathway is involved in their development. The presence of pectus excavatum in particular should raise the question of a Rasopathy such as NF1 and can be helpful in considering NF1 as a diagnosis. Rarely does pectus excavatum or carinatum require surgical intervention in NF1 and it is generally considered a cosmetic manifestation.

7.8 Osteopenia/Osteoporosis

Multiple studies have documented in different NF1 cohorts that there is decreased bone mineral density (BMD) in NF1, in both the adult and pediatric populations [59–68]. The clinical consequences of these decreases in BMD are not well elucidated.

Heerva et al. [69] showed fracture rates to be increased both in the pediatric and older adult population in the Finnish population. Tucker et al. [66] also showed an increased number of fractures in a cohort of adults from Germany. However, George-Abraham et al. [70] did not identify a significant difference in fracture rates in a pediatric cohort of individuals with NF1 in two clinics from the USA.

The etiology of the decreased BMD is subject of debate. In vitro assays from cultured osteoclasts and markers of bone resorption have provided some evidence that osteoclast function is increased in NF1 [21, 36, 68, 71], suggesting a potential intrinsic propensity for decreased BMD. Vitamin D insufficiency, decreased physical activity, and poor motor proficiency have also been proposed as potential contributing factors [61, 66, 70, 72].

7.9 Non-Ossifying Fibromas

Multiple non-ossifying fibromas (NOFs; aka fibrous cortical defects, FSDs) of the distal femur and proximal tibia are often seen in individuals with NF1 [73, 74] and generally do not require intervention (see Fig. 7.5). However, some individuals

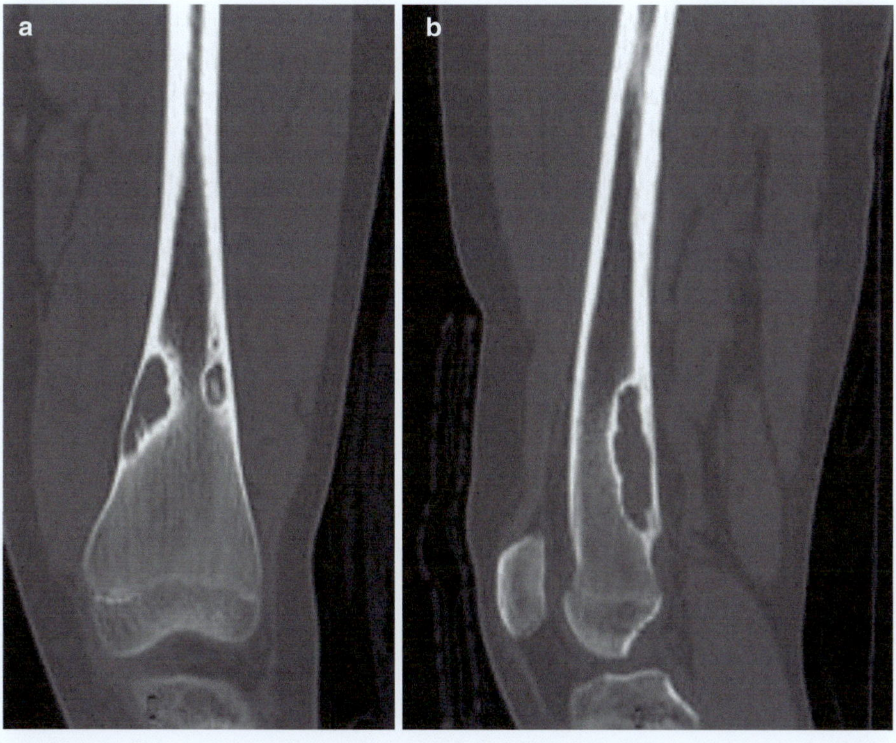

Fig. 7.5 CT scan of distal femur demonstrating cortical bone defects associated with non-ossifying neurofibromas; coronal view (**a**) and sagittal view (**b**)

experience significant knee pain with or without fracture, especially adolescent females with NF1 who benefit from surgical resection. Histologically, non-ossifying fibromas are comprised of hypercellular spindle cells with irregularly distributed multinucleated giant cells and focal hemosiderin deposition [75]. The pathogenesis of NOFs has yet to be elucidated, although a key hypothesis is the "tug" of tendons at insertion sites of the distal femur and proximal tibia [76]. The findings of chromosome changes in NOFs [77], and, in a separate study, *KRAS*, *FGFR1*, and *NF1* mutations in about 80% of NOFs suggest that similar to neurofibromas, activated MAP-kinase signaling plays a significant role in these benign tumors [78]. Regardless of etiology, orthopedic management guidelines have not been established for the NF1 population, and it is not clear that pathogenic fractures are more likely in NF1-NOFs versus NOFs in the non-NF1 population. There is no evidence to suggest NF1-related NOFs should be managed differently than in those without NF1. Individuals with multiple café au lait spots and non-ossifying fibromas (NOFs) have been diagnosed with a condition known as Jaffe–Campanacci syndrome; however, NOFs are now recognized as an associated manifestation of NF1 [79], even though its prevalence has not been formally ascertained.

7.10 Summary

The recognition of potential skeletal manifestations in NF1, beyond those mentioned in the diagnostic criteria (tibial dysplasia and sphenoid wing dysplasia), is key to optimal care for affected individuals. Given the significant skeletal complications that can occur in NF1, close monitoring is important. Referral to orthopedic surgeons with experience with individuals with NF1 is appropriate, although treatment options are not well studied. The pathophysiology of skeletal abnormalities is being explored through animal models and assessment of bone tissue in humans. Similar to random, somatic inactivation of the normal *NF1* allele in melanocytes of café au lait spots and in Schwann cells of neurofibromas, as with double inactivation of *NF1* in tibial psuedarthrosis, the complete loss of neurofibromin in a subset of mesodermal cells could lead to focal skeletal manifestations. However, the association with adjacent tumors in many cases implicates paracrine factors as influential if not causative of the focal bone dysplasias of NF1-related skeletal manifestations. Along these lines, it is important to keep in mind that even though computerized tomography is superior to MRI in bone imaging, the presence of adjacent tumors in the radiation field could increase the risk of inducing additional somatic mutations. Therefore, judicious use of bone imaging for surgical planning is needed lest transformation from plexiform neurofibroma to malignant peripheral nerve sheath tumor ensue.

References

1. Stumpf DA, Alksne JF, Annegers JF, Brown SS, Conneally PM, Housman D, Leppert MF, Miller JP, Moss ML, Pileggi AJ, Rapin I, Strohman RC, Swanson LW, Zimmerman A. Neurofibromatosis conference statement. NIH consensus development conference. Arch Neurol. 1988;45:575–8.

2. Gutmann DH, Aylsworth A, Carey JC, Korf B, Marks J, Pyeritz RE, Rubenstein A, Viskochil D. The diagnostic evaluation and multidisciplinary management of neurofibromatosis 1 and neurofibromatosis 2. JAMA. 1997;278:51–7.
3. Brooks B, Lehman EP. The bone changes in Recklinghausen's neurofibromatosis. Surg Gynec Obstet. 1924;38:587–95.
4. Holt JF, Wright EM. The radiologic features of neurofibromatosis. Radiology. 1948;51:647–64.
5. Hunt JC, Pugh DG. Skeletal lesions in neurofibromatosis. Radiology. 1961;76:1–20.
6. Riccardi VM. Neurofibromatosis. In: Phenotype, natural history, and pathogenesis. 2nd ed. Baltimore: The Johns Hopkins University Press; 1992.
7. Elefteriou F, Kolanczyk M, Schindeler A, Viskochil DH, Hock JM, Schorry EK, Crawford AH, Friedman JM, Little D, Peltonen J, Carey JC, Feldman D, Xijie Y, Armstrong L, Birch P, Kendler DL, Mundlos S, Yang FC, Agiostratidou G, Hunter-Schaedle K, Stevenson DA. Skeletal abnormalities in neurofibromatosis type 1: approaches to therapeutic options. Am J Med Genet A. 2009;149A:2327–38.
8. Stevenson DA, Yang FC. The musculoskeletal phenotype of the RASopathies. Am J Med Genet C. 2011;157:90–103.
9. Elefteriou F, Benson MD, Sowa H, Starbuck M, Liu X, Ron D, Parada LF, Karsenty G. ATF4 mediation of NF1 functions in osteoblast reveals a nutritional basis for congenital skeletal dysplasiae. Cell Metab. 2006;4:441–51.
10. El-Hoss J, Sullivan K, Cheng T, Yu NY, Bobyn JD, Peacock L, Mikulec K, Baldock P, Alexander IE, Schindeler A, Little DG. A murine model of neurofibromatosis type 1 tibial pseudarthrosis featuring proliferative fibrous tissue and osteoclast-like cells. J Bone Miner Res. 2011;27(1):68. [Epub ahead of print].
11. Kolanczyk M, Kossler N, Kühnisch J, Lavitas L, Stricker S, Wilkening U, Manjubala I, Fratzl P, Spörle R, Herrmann BG, Parada LF, Kornak U, Mundlos S. Multiple roles for neurofibromin in skeletal development and growth. Hum Mol Genet. 2007;16:874–86.
12. Kuorilehto T, Nissinen M, Koivunen J, Benson MD, Peltonen J. NF1 tumor suppressor protein and mRNA in skeletal tissues of developing and adult normal mouse and NF1-deficient embryos. J Bone Miner Res. 2004;19:983–9.
13. Schindeler A, Birke O, Yu NY, Morse A, Ruys A, Baldock PA, Little DG. Distal tibial fracture repair in a neurofibromatosis type 1-deficient mouse treated with recombinant bone morphogenetic protein and a bisphosphonate. J Bone Joint Surg Br. 2011;93:1134–9.
14. Schindeler A, Ramachandran M, Godfrey C, Morse A, McDonald M, Mikulec K, Little DG. Modeling bone morphogenetic protein and bisphosphonate combination therapy in wild-type and Nf1 haploinsufficient mice. J Orthop Res. 2008;26:65–74.
15. Schindeler A, Morse A, Harry L, Godfrey C, Mikulec K, McDonald M, Gasser J, Little D. Models of tibial fracture healing in normal and Nf1-deficient mice. J Orthop Res. 2008;26:1053–60.
16. Wang W, Nyman JS, Moss HE, Gutierrez G, Mundy GR, Yang X, Elefteriou F. Local low-dose lovastatin delivery improves the bone-healing defect caused by Nf1 loss of function in osteoblasts. J Bone Miner Res. 2010;25:1658–67.
17. Wang W, Nyman JS, Stevenson DA, Moss H, Yang X, Elefteriou F. Mice lacking Nf1 in osteochondroprogenitor cells display skeletal dysplasia similar to patients with neurofibromatosis type 1. Hum Mol Genet. 2011;20(20):3910. [Epub ahead of print].
18. Wu X, Estwick SA, Chen S, Yu M, Ming W, Nebesio TD, Li Y, Yuan J, Kapur R, Ingram D, Yoder MC, Yang FC. Neurofibromin plays a critical role in modulating osteoblast differentiation of mesenchymal stem/progenitor cells. Hum Mol Genet. 2006;15:2837–45.
19. Wu X, Chen S, He Y, Rhodes SD, Mohammad KS, Li X, Yang X, Jiang L, Nalepa G, Snider P, Robing AG, Clapp DW, Conway SJ, Guise TA, Yang FC. The haploinsufficient hematopoietic microenvironment is critical to the pathological fracture repair in murine models of neurofibromatosis type 1. PLoS One. 2011;6:e24917.
20. Yan J, Chen S, Zhang Y, Li X, Li Y, Wu X, Yuan J, Robling AG, Kapur R, Chan RJ, Yang FC. Rac1 mediates the osteoclast gains-in-function induced by haploinsufficiency of Nf1. Hum Mol Genet. 2008;17:936–48.

21. Yang FC, Chen S, Robling AG, Yu X, Nebesio TD, Yan J, Morgan T, Li X, Yuan J, Hock J, Ingram DA, Clapp DW. Hyperactivation of p21ras and PI3K cooperate to alter murine and human neurofibromatosis type 1 – haploinsufficient osteoclast functions. J Clin Invest. 2006;116:2880–91.
22. Yu X, Chen S, Potter OL, Murthy SM, Li J, Pulcini JM, Ohashi N, Winata T, Everett ET, Ingram D, Clapp WD, Hock JM. Neurofibromin and its inactivation of Ras are prerequisites for osteoblast functioning. Bone. 2005;36:793–802.
23. Zhang W, Rhodes SD, Zhao L, He Y, Zhang Y, Shen Y, Yang D, Wu X, Li X, Yang X, Park SJ, Chen S, Turner C, Yang FC. Primary osteopathy of vertebrae in a neurofibromatosis type 1 murine model. Bone. 2011;48:1378–87.
24. Holt JH. Neurofibromatosis in children. Am J Roentgenol. 1978;130:615–39.
25. Friedman JM, Birch PH. Type 1 Neurofibromatosis: a descriptive analysis of the disorder in 1728 patients. Am J Med Genet. 1997;70:138–43.
26. Jacquemin C, Bosley TM, Liu D, Svedberg H, Buhaliqa A. Reassessment of sphenoid dysplasia associated with neurofibromatosis type 1. Am J Neuroradiol. 2002;23:644–8.
27. Arrington DK, Danehy AR, Peleggi A, Proctor MR, Irons MB, Ullrich NJ. Calvarial defects and skeletal dysplasia in patients with neurofibromatosis type 1. J Neurosurg Pediatr. 2013;11:410–6.
28. Friedrich RE, Scheuer HA. Unilateral creeping destruction of deformed mandibular ramus and angel associated with extensive facial plexiform neurofibroma in neurofibromatosis type 1: a case report with analysis of the literature for diagnosis osteolytic events of the mandible in tumor-suppressor gene syndrome. Anticancer Res. 2018;38:4083–91.
29. Pessis R, Lantieri L, Britto JA, Leguerinel C, Wolkenstein P, Hivelin M. Surgical care burden in orbito-temporal neurofibromatosis: multiple procedures and surgical care duration analysis in 47 consecutive adult patients. J Craniomaxillaofac Surg. 2015;43:1684–93.
30. Dombi E, Baldwin A, Marcus L, Fisher M, Weiss B, Kim A, Whitcomb P, Martin S, Aschbacher-Smith L, Rizvi T, Wu J, Ershler R, Wolters P, Therrien J, Glod J, Belasco J, Schorry E, Brofferio A, Starosta A, Gillespie A, Doyle A, Ratner N, Widemann B. Activity of selumetinib in neurofibromatosis type 1-related plexiform neurofibromas. N Engl J Med. 2016;375:2550–60.
31. Stevenson DA, Viskochil DH, Schorry EK, Crawford AH, D'Astous J, Murray KA, Friedman JM, Armstrong L, Carey JC. The use of anterolateral bowing of the lower leg in the diagnostic criteria for neurofibromatosis type 1. Genet Med. 2007;9:409–12.
32. Stevenson DA, Birch PH, Friedman JM, Viskochil DH, Balestrazzi P, Boni S, Buske A, Korf BR, Niimura M, Pivnick EK, Schorry EK, Short MP, Tenconi R, Tonsgard JH, Carey JC. Descriptive analysis of tibial pseudarthrosis in patients with neurofibromatosis 1. Am J Med Genet. 1999;84:413–9.
33. Cho TJ, Seo JB, Lee HR, Yoo WJ, Chung CY, Choi IH. Biologic characteristics of fibrous hamartoma from congenital pseudarthrosis of the tibia associated with neurofibromatosis type 1. J Bone Joint Surg Am. 2008;90:2735–44.
34. Stevenson DA, Zhou H, Ashrafi S, Messiaen LM, Carey JC, D'Astous JL, Santora SD, Viskochil DH. Double inactivation of NF1 in tibial pseudarthrosis. Am J Hum Genet. 2006;79:143–8.
35. Sakamoto A, Yoshida T, Yamamoto H, Oda Y, Tsuneyoshi M, Iwamoto Y. Congenital pseudarthrosis of the tibia: analysis of the histology and the NF1 gene. J Orthop Sci. 2007;12:361–5.
36. Heervä E, Alanne MH, Peltonen S, Kuorilehto T, Hentunen T, Väänänen K, Peltonen J. Osteoclasts in neurofibromatosis type 1 display enhanced resorption capacity, aberrant morphology, and resistance to serum deprivation. Bone. 2010;47:583–90.
37. Sant DW, Margraf RL, Stevenson DA, Grossmann AH, Viskochil DH, Hanson H, Everitt MD, Rios JJ, Elefteriou F, Hennessey T, Mao R. Evaluation of somatic mutations in tibial pseudarthrosis samples in neurofibromatosis type 1. J Med Genet. 2015;52:256–61.
38. Crawford AH, Schorry EK. Neurofibromatosis in children; the role of the orthopaedist. J Am Acad Orthop Surg. 1999;7:217–30.

39. Hefti F, Bollini G, Dungl P, Fixsen J, Grill F, Ippolito E, Romanus B, Tudisco C, Wientroub S. Congenital pseudarthrosis of the tibia: history, etiology, classification, and epidemiologic data. J Pediatr Orthop. 2000;9:11–5.
40. Tudisco C, Bollini G, Dungl P, Fixen J, Grill F, Hefti F, Romanus B, Wientroub S. Functional results at the end of skeletal growth in 30 patients affected by congenital pseudoarthrosis of the tibia. J Pediatr Orthop. 2000;9:94–102.
41. Weintroub S, Grill F. Editorial. Congenital pseudarthrosis of the tibia: part 1. J Pediatr Orthop. 2000;9:1–2.
42. Grill F, Bollini G, Dungl P, Fixsen J, Hefti F, Ippolito E, Romanus B, Tudisco C, Wientroub S. Treatment approaches for congenital pseudarthrosis of tibia: results of the EPOS multicenter study. J Pediatr Orthop B. 2000;9:75–89.
43. Coleman SS, Coleman DA, Biddulph G. Congenital pseudarthrosis of the tibia: current concepts of treatment. Adv Oper Orthop. 1995;3:121–45.
44. Richards BS, Anderson TD. rhBMP-2 and intramedullary fixation in congenital pseudarthrosis of the tibia. J Pediatr Orthop. 2018;38:230–8.
45. Stevenson DA, Little D, Armstrong L, Crawford AH, Eastwood D, Friedman JM, Greggi T, Gutierrez G, Hunter-Schaedle K, Kendler DL, Kolanczyk M, Monsell F, Oetgen M, Richards BS, Schindeler A, Schorry EK, Wilkes D, Viskochil DH, Yang FC, Elefteriou F. Approaches to treating NF1 tibial pseudarthrosis – consensus from the Children's Tumor Foundation NF1 Bone Abnormalities Consortium. J Pediatr Orthop. 2013;33:269–75.
46. Durrani AA, Crawford AH, Chouhdry SN, Saifuddin A, Morley TR. Modulation of spinal deformities in patients with neurofibromatosis type 1. Spine. 2000;25:69–75.
47. Brunetti-Pierri N, Doty SB, Hicks J, Phan K, Mendoza-Londono R, Blazo M, Tran A, Carter S, Lewis RA, Plon SE, Phillips WA, O'Brian Smith E, Ellis KJ, Lee B. Generalized metabolic bone disease in neurofibromatosis type 1. Mol Genet Metab. 2008;94:105–11.
48. Khong PL, Goh W, Wong VC, Fung CW, Ooi GC. MR imaging of spinal tumors in children with neurofibromatosis 1. AJR Am J Roentgenol. 2003;180:413–7.
49. Tsirikos AI, Ramachandran M, Lee J, Saifuddin A. Assessment of vertebral scalloping in neurofibromatosis type 1 with plain radiography and MRI. Clin Radiol. 2004;59:1009–17.
50. Oates EC, Payne JM, Foster SL, Clarke NF, North KN. Young Australian adults with NF1 have poor access to health care, high complication rates, and limited disease knowledge. Am J Med Genet A. 2013;161A:659–66.
51. Stewart DR, Korf BR, Nathanson KL, Stevenson DA, Yohay K. Care of adults with neurofibromatosis type 1: a clinical practice resource of the American College of Medical Genetics and Genomics (ACMG). Genet Med. 2018;20:671–82.
52. Miller DT, Freedenberg D, Schorry E, Ulrich N, Viskochil D, Korf B. Health supervision for children with neurofibromatosis type 1. Pediatrics. 2019;143:e20190660.
53. Leeds NE, Jacobson HG. Spinal neurofibromatosis. Radiology. 1973;126:617–23.
54. Salerno NR, Edeiken J. Vertebral scalloping in neurofibromatosis. Radiology. 1970;97:509–10.
55. Szudek J, Birch P, Friedman J. Growth in North American white children with neurofibromatosis 1 (NF1). J Med Genet. 2000;37:933–8.
56. Clementi M, Milani S, Mammi I, Boni S, Monciotti C, Tenconi R. Neurofibromatosis type 1 growth charts. Am J Med Genet. 1999;87:317–23.
57. Rafia S, Garcia-Pena J, Lopez-Pison J, Aguirre-Rodriguez J, Ramos-Lizana J, Garcia-Perez A, Martinez-Granero M, Sans A, Campistol J, Pena-Sequra J, Espino-Hernandez. Growth charts for the Spanish population with neurofibromatosis type 1. Rev Neurol. 2004;38:1009–12.
58. Howell SJ, Wilton P, Lindberg A, Shalet SM. Growth hormone replacement and the risk of malignancy in children with neurofibromatosis. J Pediatr. 1998;133:201–5.
59. Illes T, Halmai V, de Jonge T, Dubousset. Decreased bone mineral density in neurofibromatosis-1 patients with spinal deformities. Osteoporos Int. 2001;12:823–7.
60. Kuorilehto T, Pöyhönen M, Bloigu R, Heikkinen J, Väänänen K, Peltonen J. Decreased bone mineral density and content in neurofibromatosis type 1: lowest local values are located in the load-carrying parts of the body. Osteoporos Int. 2005;16:928–396.

61. Lammert M, Kappler M, Mautner VF, Lammert K, Störkel S, Friedman JM, Atkins D. Decreased bone mineral density in patients with neurofibromatosis 1. Osteoporos Int. 2005;16:1161–6.
62. Stevenson DA, Moyer-Mileur LJ, Carey JC, Quick JL, Hoff CJ, Viskochil DH. Case-control study of the muscular compartments and osseous strength in neurofibromatosis type 1 using peripheral quantitative computed tomography. J Musculoskelet Neuronal Interact. 2005;5:145–9.
63. Dulai S, Briody J, Schindeler A, North KN, Cowell CT, Little DG. Decreased bone mineral density in neurofibromatosis type 1: results from a pediatric cohort. J Pediatr Orthop. 2007;27:472–5.
64. Stevenson DA, Moyer-Mileur LJ, Murray M, Slater H, Sheng X, Carey JC, Dube B, Viskochil DH. Bone mineral density in children and adolescents with neurofibromatosis type 1. J Pediatr. 2007;150:83–8.
65. Yilmaz K, Ozmen M, Bora Goksan S, Eskiyurt N. Bone mineral density in children with neurofibromatosis 1. Acta Paediatr. 2007;96:1220–2.
66. Tucker T, Schnabel C, Hartmann M, Friedrich RE, Frieling I, Kruse HP, Mautner VF, Friedman JM. Bone health and fracture rate in individuals with neurofibromatosis 1 (NF1). J Med Genet. 2009;46:259–65.
67. Caffarelli C, Gonnelli S, Tanzilli L, Vivarelli R, Tamburello S, Balestri P, Nuti R. Quantitative ultrasound and dual energy x-ray absorptiometry in children and adolescents with neurofibromatosis of type 1. J Clin Densitom. 2010;13:77–83.
68. Seitz S, Schnabel C, Busse B, Schmidt HU, Beil FT, Friedrich RE, Schinke T, Mautner VF, Amling M. High bone turnover and accumulation of osteoid in patients with neurofibromatosis 1. Osteoporos Int. 2010;21:119–27.
69. Heervä E, Koffert A, Jokinen E, Kuorilehto T, Peltonen S, Aro HT, Peltonen J. A controlled register-based study of 460 neurofibromatosis 1 patients: increased fracture risk in children and adults over 41 years of age. J Bone Miner Res. 2012;27:2333–7.
70. George-Abraham JK, Martin LJ, Kalkwarf HJ, Rieley MB, Stevenson DA, Viskochil DH, Hopkin RJ, Stevens AM, Hanson H, Schorry EK. Fractures in children with neurofibromatosis type 1 from two NF clinics. Am J Med Genet A. 2013;161A:921–6.
71. Stevenson DA, Yan J, He Y, Li H, Liu Y, Jing Y, Guo Z, Zhang Q, Zhang W, Yang D, Wu X, Hanson H, Li X, Staser K, Viskochil DH, Carey JC, Chen S, Miller L, Roberson K, Moyer-Mileur L, Yang FC. Increased multiple osteoclast functions in individuals with neurofibromatosis type 1. Am J Med Genet A. 2011;155:1050–9.
72. Johnson B, MacWilliams B, Carey JC, Viskochil DH, D'Astous JL, Stevenson DA. Examination of motor proficiency in children with neurofibromatosis type 1. Pediatr Phys Ther. 2010;22:344–8.
73. Faure C, Laurent JM, Schmit P, Sirinelli D. Multiple and large non-ossifying fibromas in children with neurofibromatosis. Ann Radiol. 1986;29:369–73.
74. Colby RS, Saul RA. Is Jaffe-Campanacci syndrome just a manifestation of neurofibromatosis type 1? Am J Med Genet A. 2003;123A:60–3.
75. Nielsen GP, Kyriakos M. Non-ossifying fibroma/benign fibrous histiocytoma of bone. In: Fletcher CDM, Bridge JA, Hogendoorn PCW, Mertens F, editors. WHO classification of tumours of soft tissue and bone. 4th ed. Lyon: International Agency for Research on Cancer; 2013.
76. Goldin A, Muzykewicz D, Dwek J, Mubarak S. The aetiology of the non-ossifying fibroma of the distal femur and its relationship to the surrounding soft tissues. J Child Orthop. 2017;11:373–9.
77. Brasseco MS, Valera ET, Engel EE, Nogueira-Barbosa MH, Becker AP, Scrideli CA, Tone LG. Clonal complex chromosome aberration in non-ossifying fibroma. Pediatr Blood Cancer. 2010;54:764–7.
78. Baumhoer D, Kovac M, Sperveslage J, Ameline B, Strobl AC, Krause A, Trautmann M, Wardelmann E, Nathrath M, Holler S, Hardes J, Gosheger G, Krieg AH, Vieth V, Tirabosco

R, Amary F, Flanagan AM, Hartmann W. Activating mutations in the MAP-kinase pathway define non-ossifying fibroma of bone. J Pathol. 2018;248(1):116. [Epub ahead of print].
79. Stewart DR, Brems H, Gomes AG, Ruppert SL, Callens T, Williams J, Claes K, Bober MB, Hachen R, Kaban LB, Li H, Lin A, McDonald M, Melancon S, Ortenbert J, Radtke H, Samson I, Saul RA, Shen J, Siqveland E, Toler TL, van Maarle M, Wallace M, Williams M, Legius E, MessiaenL. Jaffe-Campanacci syndrome, revisited: detailed clinical and molecular analyses determine whether patients have neurofibromatosis type 1, coincidental manifestations, or a distinct disorder. Genet Med. 2014;16:448–59.

NF1 in Other Organs

8

Emma Burkitt Wright, Michael Burkitt, and Hilde Brems

Contents

E. Burkitt Wright (✉)
NHSE Highly Specialised Service for Complex NF1, Manchester Centre for Genomic Medicine, Manchester University NHS Foundation Trust, Manchester Academic Health Sciences Centre, Manchester, UK

Division of Evolution and Genomic Sciences, University of Manchester, Manchester Academic Health Sciences Centre, Manchester, UK
e-mail: emma.burkitt-wright@mft.nhs.uk

M. Burkitt
Gastrointestinal Medicine and Surgery, Manchester University NHS Foundation Trust, Manchester Academic Health Sciences Centre, Manchester, UK

Division of Diabetes, Endocrinology and Gastroenterology, University of Manchester, Manchester Academic Health Sciences Centre, Manchester, UK
e-mail: mike.burkitt@mft.nhs.uk

H. Brems
Clinical Department of Human Genetics, KU Leuven-University of Leuven, University Hospitals Leuven, Leuven, Belgium

Department of Human Genetics, KU Leuven-University of Leuven, Leuven, Belgium
e-mail: hilde.brems@kuleuven.be

G. Tadini et al. (eds.), *Multidisciplinary Approach to Neurofibromatosis Type 1*,
https://doi.org/10.1007/978-3-319-92450-2_8

8.1 Cardiovascular Complications of NF1

Cardiovascular disease is a common cause of mortality in NF1. Cerebrovascular disease can occur at any age, and the risk of childhood stroke, particularly haemorrhagic stroke, is significantly elevated [2]. Hypertension appears a strong risk factor for paediatric stroke in NF1, but less so for adult stroke. Abnormal arterial anatomy with ectatic or stenotic vessels and intracranial aneurysms is frequently seen. The internal carotid, middle cerebral or anterior cerebral arteries are most likely to be involved [3], with the appearance of moya moya a frequent consequence. This may be amenable to treatment by pial synangiosis, with a resultant improvement in outcome [3].

8.1.1 Hypertension

The incidence of hypertension in NF1 is higher than in age-matched general populations. This increase is especially notable in childhood, warranting lifelong 6–12 monthly surveillance from as early as is practicable. Dubov et al. [4] noted blood pressure recordings above the 95th centile for age in 20% of measurements made in a paediatric NF1 cohort, with 6% of patients having persistent hypertension. No association with obesity was identified. Renal artery stenosis and phaeochromocytoma are the most characteristic specific causes of hypertension to occur in association with NF1, but essential hypertension is common, accounting for over 50% of high blood pressure in this patient group. No difference in the management of essential hypertension is recognised between people with or without NF1, once underlying causes have been excluded.

8.1.1.1 Renal Artery Stenosis and Mid-Aortic Syndrome

Renal artery stenosis has been estimated to affect 2% of patients with NF1, and classically presents in childhood. It may be unilateral or bilateral. Renal revascularisation may be effective in managing this condition, which may be due to localised fibromuscular dysplasia as in sporadic cases, or represent a manifestation of a more generalised NF1-associated vasculopathy. Compression of vessels by neurofibroma or diffuse neurofibromatous tissue has also been postulated as a mechanism for renal hypertension. Further manifestations of vasculopathy include aneurysms (in up to 30% of patients [5], with spontaneous rupture of accessory renal artery aneurysm reported [6], for example). Venous aneurysms may also occur [7].

NF1 is the commonest identified genetic cause of mid-aortic syndrome [8], a rare presentation which results from severe narrowing of the abdominal aorta and associated arteries, often associated with extensive vasculopathy elsewhere. Whilst a rare manifestation of NF1, it may be very difficult to treat if multiple vessels are stenosed, and result in severe hypertension, particularly if the renal vessels are involved.

8.1.2 Phaeochromocytoma

Phaeochromocytoma is estimated to affect 2% of patients with NF1 [9]. Tumours may present in childhood, though this is rare. NF1-associated phaeochromocytoma may present in a less typical manner than in patients without NF1. Hypertension may not be detected and the high prevalence of anxiety and other neurobehavioural features in NF1 can also confound the identification of adrenergic symptoms. Similar to observations of phaeochromocytoma in other contexts, the adrenal medulla is the commonest site of origin and 12% of NF1-associated phaeochromocytomas are malignant when examined histologically. Bilateral tumours appear rare. Compared to sporadic phaeochromocytoma, NF1-associated lesions are on average smaller when detected, with less evidence of hypertension, but this may reflect early diagnosis following a higher index of suspicion, or incidental detection on imaging performed for other reasons [10]. No strong familial aggregation of phaeochromocytoma in NF1 is recognised, but co-occurrence of other neuroendocrine tumours, most commonly within the gastrointestinal tract, is a recurrent observation. Non-functional adrenal adenomas are also a common finding in patients with NF1, and demonstrate biallelic loss of function of NF1, though such lesions are not rare in the general population. Plasma metadrenaline assay is a core investigation in assessing for phaeochromocytoma, though elevated values may be observed in the absence of a secreting tumour in patients who are very anxious, or on medication that results in increased metadrenaline, such as monoamine oxidase inhibitors or sympathetomimetics, necessitating repeat testing.

8.1.3 Congenital Heart Disease in NF1

Ras-MAPK pathway functioning is critical to cardiac development, particularly of structures arising from the endocardial cushion. Where NF1 is dysregulated, Ras-MAPK-mediated endocardial-mesenchymal transition and proliferation are disrupted [11]. The most commonly identified lesions are therefore similar to those observed in other germline disorders of the Ras-MAPK pathway, particularly pulmonary stenosis, atrial septal defects and hypertrophic cardiomyopathy. Estimates for the overall prevalence of congenital heart disease in NF1 vary. 2.3% of patients with NF1 in the large early series of Lin et al [12] had a cardiac anomaly, and estimates consistently suggest that such findings are more common than the 0.5% prevalence observed in the general population. Much of this increased risk may be attributable to the congenital heart disease burden observed in patients with type I whole gene deletions [13], prompting the recommendation for specialist cardiological evaluation in these individuals in particular [14]. A low threshold for such investigations may be warranted in any patient with NF1, particularly if any clinical symptoms or signs are detected on routine history or examination. Complex congenital heart disease is uncommon in NF1, with only occasional reports of tetralogy of Fallot [12] and an absence of other complex defects that are relatively frequently observed in other congenital heart disease cohorts.

8.1.3.1 Pulmonary Stenosis

Pulmonary valve stenosis is present overall in 2% of patients with NF1, but the prevalence appears increased in certain families, particularly those with missense NF1 variants [15]. This is in keeping with the previous descriptions of 'Watson syndrome' or 'NF-Noonan syndrome', both of which can now confidently be attributed to pathogenic variants in *NF1* [15]. Pulmonary atresia or more complex congenital heart disease may also occur in such families. Pulmonary artery stenosis has also been recorded in patients with NF1.

8.1.3.2 Other Valvular Abnormalities

8% of 65 patients with NF1 studied by Incelik et al. [16] had mitral valve incompetence ($n = 5$), compared to population estimates of 1.2% [17]. Single patients in their cohort were found to have aortic regurgitation and tricuspid regurgitation, respectively. Aortic stenosis has also been reported [13]. Whether mitral valve abnormalities are associated with the joint hypermobility seen in a significant proportion of individuals with NF1 has yet to be established. In both the general population, and individuals with disorders of connective tissue, joint hypermobility commonly coexists with mitral valve prolapse [18].

8.1.3.3 Cardiac Septal Defects

The prevalence of atrial and ventricular septal defects appears increased in NF1, though definitive data are lacking, and the published literature may be subject to ascertainment bias. 3–4% of patients with NF1 studied in series have had secundum atrial septal defects identified [16, 19]. Unroofed coronary sinus, a rare cause of atrial septal defect, has also been reported in a single individual with NF1 [20]. Ventricular septal defects appear less common than atrial defects, with single patients reported in modestly sized NF1 cohorts, particularly those with whole gene deletion [13], suggesting a somewhat increased risk compared to the general population.

8.1.3.4 Hypertrophic Cardiomyopathy

Findings consistent with eccentric left ventricular hypertrophy have been reported in asymptomatic patients with NF1, namely increased left ventricular diastolic posterior wall thickness and intraventricular diastolic septal thickness [13]. The significance of these remains unclear, but arrhythmias or more severe degrees of myocardial hypertrophy are not known to be associated with NF1, and hence their presence should prompt consideration of an additional cause. Foetal onset of hypertrophic cardiomyopathy, as may be observed in Noonan syndrome, has only extremely rarely been reported in association with NF1 [21].

8.1.3.5 Sudden Cardiac Death

Whilst fatal arrhythmias have not been attributed to NF1, sudden cardiac death, including in childhood, is a recurrently reported rare complication. Cardiovascular causes are a major source of the excess childhood mortality observed in NF1. Kanter et al. [22] reported two unrelated patients with coronary artery occlusion likely to be due to NF1-associated vasculopathy. The pathogenesis of vasculopathy in NF1 is incompletely understood, but is a recognised manifestation throughout the vasculature (see discussion of moya-moya in Chap. 13). Another patient with whole gene deletion was reported to have died suddenly at 16 years of age of myocardial infarction, with multiple coronary artery aneursyms identified at post-mortem [23]. The prevalence of coronary artery disease in the general adult population may lead to underascertainment of NF1-associated arteriopathy in patients with other identifiable risk factors. Intramyocardial vasculopathy as the likely cause of sudden death was reported in a 33-year-old patient by Hamilton et al. [24]. Within the vessels, regions of intimal thickening with high cellularity were present, as were areas of fibrotic, hypocellular lipid-poor plaque formation.

8.1.3.6 Intracardiac Tumours

Intracardiac tumours are very rarely reported in NF1. Two of 16 patients with whole gene deletion in Nguyen et al's [13] series had such lesions identified echocardiographically, and only one patient in the 2322 of Lin et al's cohort [12] was known to have such a tumour.

8.2 Lymphatic Abnormalities

Diffuse or plexiform neurofibromatous tissue may involve or disrupt lymphatic structures, and result in lymphoedema of affected parts. Resections for neurofibroma, or surgical or radiotherapy treatment of malignancy may also be risk factors for the development of lymphoedema. Whether or not primary lymphatic dysplasia (as is occasionally recorded in other germline disorders of the Ras-MAPK pathway) may also occur in NF1 is unclear.

8.3 Gastrointestinal

Gastrointestinal neoplasia is common in NF1, but the proportion of patients estimated to be affected ranges widely from 2 to 25% [25]. Common lesions associated with NF1 throughout the body, including neurofibromas and malignant peripheral nerve sheath tumours (MPNST), may occur within the gastrointestinal tract. Hepatobiliary and/or pancreatic involvement by plexiform neurofibroma is well documented, particularly at the porta hepatis [26], but is rare. The incidence of gastrointestinal stromal tumours (GIST) and gut associated neuroendocrine tumours is greatly increased in NF1. The question of whether there is an increased risk of tumours more common in the general population, such as colorectal cancer, remains to be clarified (as discussed in Chap. 17).

Despite gastrointestinal tract neoplasia being relatively common, acute intestinal obstruction is a rare sequela of NF1. A systematic review identified intussusception (caused by GIST or neurofibroma), intrinsic obstruction by plexiform neurofibroma or stenosing colorectal carcinoma, and extrinsic obstruction caused by malignant GIST, plexiform neurofibroma or MPNST as recorded causes [27].

8.3.1 Gastrointestinal Stromal Tumours

GISTs arise in the gastrointestinal sub-mucosa, and are the commonest mesenchymal tumour in the GI tract, they are seen in up to 7% of patients with NF1 [28]. The natural history of these tumours diverges from that of sporadic GIST. At the molecular level, c-KIT, mutated in the large majority of sporadic GISTs, is not usually mutated in NF1-associated GIST, and inactivation of the wild-type NF1 allele appears crucial to the pathogenetic mechanism for these lesions, as is the case for other NF1-associated tumours. NF1-associated GISTs may behave in an indolent fashion, and surgery is not indicated for most lesions below 2 cm in diameter, though treatment options are more limited for advanced tumours as tyrosine kinase inhibition with agents such as imatinib, which can be effective adjuvant therapy for advanced c-KIT mutated GIST, may not be applicable. Regorafenib and sunitinib (other tyrosine kinase inhibitors) each have anecdotal evidence for efficacy in patients with NF1-associated GIST [29, 30].

An earlier age at diagnosis is seen than for non-NF1-associated GIST, and in contrast to sporadic GISTs, extragastric locations are more common. Multifocal GIST is associated with NF1, and this, in combination with 'quadruple negative' genotype (no c-KIT, PDGRFA, BRAF or SDH gene mutation identified), may be the presenting feature of hitherto unrecognised neurofibromatosis type I [31].

8.3.2 Neuroendocrine Tumours

Neuroendocrine cells exist throughout the GI tract, secreting gut regulatory hormones. Tumours arising from these cell lineages (neuroendocrine tumours, previously termed carcinoid tumours) affect a small percentage of people with NF1, and can present with consequences of hormone secretion, bleeding, local pressure effects (such as obstructive jaundice from an ampullary lesion [32]), or be identified incidentally on imaging. The most commonly secreted hormone in NF1-associated neuroendocrine tumours is somatostatin, and characteristic histological appearances include psammomatous calcification [33]. Whilst the duodenum and ampulla are the region in which these have been most frequently recognised [34], the prevalence of lesions elsewhere in the GI tract may be underestimated.

Rarely, neuroendocrine tumours can present with carcinoid syndrome, namely facial flushing, diarrhoea, right-sided heart lesions, facial telangiectasia or bronchoconstriction, but this is caused when functionally secreting tumour tissue drains via extrasplanchnic vessels, which usually only occurs in metastatic disease. The possibility of such a tumour should be borne in mind for patients with NF1 presenting with such symptoms.

8.3.2.1 Gangliocytic Paraganglioma

Gangliocytic paraganglioma, a subtype of neuroendocrine tumour, is a very rare complication of NF1, which may have a favourable prognosis. It is most commonly located in the duodenum (90%), expression of progesterone receptor and pancreatic polypeptide is usual [35] and metastasis beyond lymph nodes is rare. Such tumours accounted for only 3% of duodenal lesions identified in patients with NF1 reviewed by Relles et al. [33].

8.3.3 Gastrointestinal Neurofibromas, Adenomas, Other Polyps and Carcinomas

Especially in patients with a high load of neurofibromas elsewhere, neurofibromas may be seen anywhere in or around the gastrointestinal tract. These may cause local effects or bleeding, but may be most likely to be identified incidentally on radiological or endoscopic imaging. Malignant tumours and premalignant adenomatous polyps of the gastrointestinal tract have not been recognised to be more common in patients with NF1, but the relative prevalence of colorectal carcinoma in the general population has potential to mask any subtle association by a lack of ascertainment of all relevant cases, as discussed in Chap. 17. The association of NF1 with juvenile-like hamartomatous polyp formation has also been reported [36].

8.4 GI Motility in NF1: Abnormalities of Structure and Function of the Enteric Nervous System

Dysmotility of the gastrointestinal tract is a common finding in the general population, and therefore it is unsurprising that it also occurs in many patients with NF1. Constipation is the most commonly reported symptom, and first line management is as for patients in the general population. However, the increased risks of gastrointestinal neoplasia and specific causes of dysmotility in patients with NF1 need to be borne in mind and appropriate thresholds for prompt investigation instituted. Exclusion of coeliac disease is important as, whilst no definite association is recognised, coeliac disease may coexist in at least 1% of patients with NF1 and is treatable with a gluten free diet. Untreated coeliac disease may result in diarrhoea, anaemia and malaise and is an additional risk factor for small bowel malignancies such as lymphoma and adenocarcinoma.

Diffuse ganglioneuromatosis is a rare complication of NF1, also seen in Cowden syndrome (due to loss of function *PTEN* mutations) and multiple endocrine neoplasia type 2B (due to *RET* mutations). Presenting symptoms are varied, according to the site and extent of affected tissue, but may include bleeding, abdominal pain or refractory constipation. Whilst any organ supplied by the enteric nervous system may be involved, ileum, colon and appendix are most frequently identified to be involved. Biopsy demonstrates increased numbers of ganglion cells, Schwann cells and nerve fibres. Mucosal oedema and ulceration may be seen in affected regions. Coexistent plexiform neurofibroma of the mesentery has been reported in a patient with small bowel ganglioneuromatosis [37].

The rarity of such observations suggests that, whilst NF1 and MEN2B (in which such findings are more classical [38]), may be considered related neurocristopathies, further genomic and other factors are likely to be important in whether individuals with each of these conditions develop such manifestations. Further work is needed to determine the mechanisms of development and function of the enteric nervous system.

8.4.1 Gastroparesis

Gastroparesis is a troublesome condition that has anecdotally been reported in patients with NF1. It is plausible that autonomic nervous system dysfunction may underlie this, as is postulated in gastroparesis associated with diabetes mellitus [39], but the published literature in this area is sparse. Diagnosis is based on the combination of excluding mechanical causes of delayed gastric emptying and demonstrating objectively slow gastric transit by gastric emptying scintigraphy. An instance of gastroparesis presenting as a paraneoplastic phenomenon in a patient with NF1 has also been reported [40].

8.4.2 Irritable Bowel Syndrome and Constipation

Irritable bowel syndrome (IBS) is extremely common in the general population, but adults with NF1 have an even higher prevalence of such symptoms, with an odds ratio of around 3 for IBS and functional constipation [41]. In children, a small systematic study identified statistically significantly larger rectal diameter [42], and 20% of patients had an extended colonic transit time. Despite this strong association, there are few studies looking at the efficacy of specific interventions in patients with coexisting IBS and NF1, hence clinical management of IBS symptoms is similar to management of these in the general population, with the caveat that malignant pathology should be excluded as far as is possible in this group of patients.

8.5 Urogenital Features of NF1

Plexiform and diffuse neurofibromas involving the genitalia are unusual. Plexiforms involving the bladder and lower ureters have been reported somewhat more frequently, with the majority identified in males in early series [43]. The function of the urinary and genital tracts may be affected by adjacent pelvic neurofibromas or involvement of the nerve plexus supplying them. Urogenital malignancy risk in NF1, aside from pelvic MPNST, is not known to be elevated.

8.5.1 NF1 in the Genital Tract

Genital hypertrophy is recorded in association with NF1, but this literature is largely limited to case reports [44, 45]. Precocious puberty (affecting up to one-third of those with optic pathway glioma [46], and much less common in other children with NF1) may accentuate this. The internal or external genitalia may also be affected by the presence of neurofibromatous tissue and localised overgrowth observed [47]. Anecdotally, males with NF1 may be at a higher risk for cryptorchidism, as is the case for Noonan syndrome and other disorders of the Ras-MAPK pathway, but this is not a particularly rare phenomenon in boys in the general population and standard orchidopexy procedures are likely to be effective. Neurofibroma within the gonads appears extremely rare, with individual reports only [48]. Extensive plexiform neurofibroma involving multiple pelvic organs is a rare presentation that can be particularly challenging to manage.

Physiological aspects of fertility are not usually affected in individuals with NF1 unless pituitary or other endocrine problems are present. Sexual dysfunction may be prevalent for many, frequently interlinked, reasons including body image [49], other psychological factors and concurrent physical or mental health issues.

8.5.2 NF1 in the Urinary Tract

Congenital renal tract anomalies appear rare in NF1 [1]. Hydronephrosis may develop due to pelviureteric junction obstruction or ureteric compression by retroperitoneal neurofibroma [50]. Whilst plexiform neurofibromas of the urinary tract are rare, the bladder is the pelvic organ most commonly directly infiltrated by neurofibromatous tissue [51], and symptoms may include dysuria, haematuria and recurrent urinary tract infection. MPNST of the urinary tract appears, correspondingly, extremely rare, but has been reported [52].

Lower urinary tract dysfunction in NF1 may be due to plexiform neurofibroma involving the bladder wall, spinal cord or cauda equina involvement or compression, or central nervous system problems [53]. Obstruction of the urethra, as for the rectum or vagina, may occur due to extrinsic compression by neurofibromata [54]. Data regarding the prevalence of enuresis are not available, but, in keeping with the developmental delay observed in many children with NF1, it appears more prevalent than in the general paediatric population. A strong association of enuresis with attention deficit hyperactivity disorder has been shown in population cohorts [55], in keeping with anecdotal observations in NF1, though a recent systematic review [56] concluded that further studies of this are required.

8.6 Pulmonary

Intrathoracic neurofibromas are the most common manifestation of NF1 within the chest, and can pose dilemmas in management, with significant risk of malignant transformation and a lack of symptoms until an advanced stage. The majority appear to occur in the posterior mediastinum adjacent to the pleura, but intercostal nerve involvement or endobronchial lesions are occasionally seen [57]. Neurofibromatosis-associated diffuse lung disease (NFDLD), like NF1-associated pulmonary hypertension, may cause significant morbidity and mortality.

8.6.1 Neurofibromatosis Type I-Associated Diffuse Lung Disease

NFDLD is characterised by apical cystic or bullous change, and basal fibrosis witnessed by ground glass and reticulate appearances on imaging [58]. The cystic changes can increase the risk of pneumothorax and, where more widespread emphysematous or fibrotic changes are present, chronic respiratory failure.

8.6.2 NF1-Associated Pulmonary Arterial Hypertension

Pulmonary arterial hypertension in NF1 is infrequent but may be associated with a poor prognosis. Where present, it usually, but not exclusively, occurs in the setting of interstitial lung disease, and age at presentation is older than for other subtypes of pulmonary hypertension [59]. The response of patients with PH-NF1 to pharmaceutical therapies for pulmonary hypertension is not known, and early consideration of transplantation has been suggested [59], with the caveat of taking into account the increased malignancy risk that may apply to patients with NF1 receiving immunosuppressant medication. The observation of NF1 patients with pre-capillary pulmonary hypertension (who have no evidence of interstitial lung disease) suggests that PH-NF1 may be a manifestation of NF1-associated vasculopathy [60]. As for other forms of NF1-associated vasculopathy, the molecular and cellular mechanisms underlying this remain incompletely understood.

8.7 Haematological

The principal haematological association with NF1 is juvenile myelomonocytic leukaemia (JMML). JMML is, as discussed in Chap. 17, a rare myeloproliferative disorder characterised by Ras-MAPK pathway dysfunction, with 90% having an identifiable mutation in *NRAS*, *KRAS*, *PTPN11*, *NF1* or *CBL* [61]. Across JMML, driver mutations in *NRAS*, *KRAS* and *PTPN11* are usually somatic, whilst *NF1* and *CBL* often exhibit biallelic mutation, with the first 'hit' being in the germline. Whilst spontaneous remission may occur in 15% of JMML, patients with NF1 are likely to have progressive disease for which haematopoietic stem cell transplantation is required. The exact risk of JMML in NF1 is difficult to quantify, but recent Finnish cohort data suggests that this may be lower than previously thought, as no leukaemias were identified in 8376 person years of individuals with NF1 up to the age of 20 [62]. An association between juvenile xanthogranuloma (JXG) and JMML has long been recognised: it appears that NF1-associated JMML is seen almost exclusively in patients with JXG, though the risk for any individual patient with such lesions of developing JMML is only modest. Clinical surveillance with awareness of potential presenting symptoms of JMML is therefore required, and regular blood monitoring may also be considered [63]. The association of other haematological malignancies in NF1 is less conclusive, as discussed in Chap. 17, but the observation that 8/4939 children with ALL enrolled in the AIEOP-BFM ALL 2000 trial were known to have NF1 is compatible with a modest increase in risk [64] .

8.8 Glomus Tumours

Glomus tumours are very small mesenchymal lesions (only a few millimetres in diameter) that originate from the glomus body, a thermoregulatory shunt often located in the nail bed of the distal phalanx in fingers and toes. In the past, glomus tumours were often not diagnosed or misdiagnosed in NF1 patients, since it was thought that the pain was caused by an upstream neurofibroma affecting the nerve. The classical triad of glomus tumour symptoms include pain, localised tenderness and cold intolerance. Until 2009, only a few NF1 cases with glomus tumours were described and it was not clear if such lesions were part of the NF1 spectrum. In 2009, Brems and colleagues described 11 NF1 patients with glomus tumours, of which 5 presented with multifocal lesions [65]. The mean age was 40 years with a female predominance. Biallelic *NF1* inactivation was detected in the alpha-smooth muscle actin positive cells of the glomus tumour, resulting in over activation of the Ras-MAPK pathway after stimulation. Mitotic recombination of chromosome arm 17q has been detected in 22% of molecularly characterised NF1-associated glomus tumours [66]. To date, about 50 NF1-associated glomus tumour cases have been described in the literature [67, 68], but it has been estimated that glomus tumours may affect up to 5% of adult NF1 patients [69]. Glomus tumours can be clinically diagnosed with physical examination (e.g. pin-point pain) and a single question about the occurrence of pain in a digit during cold weather. The nail and pulp of the affected digit is often normal, MRI may demonstrate the lesions [69]. Surgical removal of symptomatic glomus tumours under local anaesthesia with or without sedation is the only effective treatment and may be curative. In general, the recurrence risk is low; however, when the bone is affected curettage is advised and the recurrence risk might be higher. Glomus tumours are almost always benign histologically.

References

1. Leppavirta J, Kallionpaa RA, Uusitalo E, Vahlberg T, Poyhonen M, Peltonen J, et al. Congenital anomalies in neurofibromatosis 1: a retrospective register-based total population study. Orphanet J Rare Dis. 2018;13(1):5.
2. Terry AR, Jordan JT, Schwamm L, Plotkin SR. Increased risk of cerebrovascular disease among patients with neurofibromatosis type 1: population-based approach. Stroke. 2016;47(1): 60–5.
3. Koss M, Scott RM, Irons MB, Smith ER, Ullrich NJ. Moyamoya syndrome associated with neurofibromatosis type 1: perioperative and long-term outcome after surgical revascularization. J Neurosurg Pediatr. 2013;11(4):417–25.
4. Dubov T, Toledano-Alhadef H, Chernin G, Constantini S, Cleper R, Ben-Shachar S. High prevalence of elevated blood pressure among children with neurofibromatosis type 1. Pediatr Nephrol. 2016;31(1):131–6.
5. Ferner RE, Huson SM, Evans DGR. Neurofibromatoses in clinical practice. London: Springer; 2011. p. 1–46.
6. Roberts K, Fan B, Brightwell R. Spontaneous accessory renal artery aneurysm rupture in a patient with neurofibromatosis type 1: a case report. Vasc Endovasc Surg. 2019;53(2): 150–3.
7. Bartline PB, McKellar SH, Kinikini DV. Resection of a large innominate vein aneurysm in a patient with neurofibromatosis type 1. Ann Vasc Surg. 2016;30:157.e1–5.
8. Warejko JK, Schueler M, Vivante A, Tan W, Daga A, Lawson JA, et al. Whole exome sequencing reveals a monogenic cause of disease in approximately 43% of 35 families with midaortic syndrome. Hypertension. 2018;71(4):691–9.
9. Ferner RE, Huson SM, Thomas N, Moss C, Willshaw H, Evans DG, et al. Guidelines for the diagnosis and management of individuals with neurofibromatosis 1. J Med Genet. 2007;44(2):81–8.
10. Shinall MC, Solorzano CC. Pheochromocytoma in neurofibromatosis type 1: when should it be suspected? Endocr Pract. 2014;20(8):792–6.
11. Lakkis MM, Epstein JA. Neurofibromin modulation of Ras activity is required for normal endocardial-mesenchymal transformation in the developing heart. Development. 1998;125(22):4359–67.
12. Lin AE, Birch PH, Korf BR, Tenconi R, Niimura M, Poyhonen M, et al. Cardiovascular malformations and other cardiovascular abnormalities in neurofibromatosis 1. Am J Med Genet. 2000;95(2):108–17.
13. Nguyen R, Mir TS, Kluwe L, Jett K, Kentsch M, Mueller G, et al. Cardiac characterization of 16 patients with large NF1 gene deletions. Clin Genet. 2013;84(4):344–9.
14. Miller DT, Freedenberg D, Schorry E, Ullrich NJ, Viskochil D, Korf BR, et al. Health supervision for children with neurofibromatosis type 1. Pediatrics. 2019;143(5):e20190660.
15. Ben-Shachar S, Constantini S, Hallevi H, Sach EK, Upadhyaya M, Evans GD, et al. Increased rate of missense/in-frame mutations in individuals with NF1-related pulmonary stenosis: a novel genotype-phenotype correlation. Eur J Hum Genet. 2013;21(5):535–9.
16. Incecik F, Herguner OM, Alinc Erdem S, Altunbasak S. Neurofibromatosis type 1 and cardiac manifestations. Turk Kardiyol Dern Ars. 2015;43(8):714–6.
17. Nalliah CJ, Mahajan R, Elliott AD, Haqqani H, Lau DH, Vohra JK, et al. Mitral valve prolapse and sudden cardiac death: a systematic review and meta-analysis. Heart. 2019;105(2):144–51.
18. Malfait F, Wenstrup R, De Paepe A. Classic Ehlers-Danlos syndrome. In: Adam MP, Ardinger HH, Pagon RA, Wallace SE, LJH B, Stephens K, et al., editors. GeneReviews((R)). Seattle: University of Washington; 1993.
19. Tedesco MA, Di Salvo G, Natale F, Pergola V, Calabrese E, Grassia C, et al. The heart in neurofibromatosis type 1: an echocardiographic study. Am Heart J. 2002;143(5):883–8.
20. Bender LP, Meyer MR, Rosa RF, Rosa RC, Trevisan P, Zen PR. Unroofed coronary sinus in a patient with neurofibromatosis type 1. Rev Paul Pediatr. 2013;31(4):546–9.

21. Ritter A, Cuddapah S, Degenhardt K, Kasperski S, Johnson MP, O'Connor MJ, et al. Fetal cardiomyopathy in neurofibromatosis type I: novel phenotype and review of the literature. Am J Med Genet A. 2019;179(6):1042–6.
22. Kanter RJ, Graham M, Fairbrother D, Smith SV. Sudden cardiac death in young children with neurofibromatosis type 1. J Pediatr. 2006;149(5):718–20.
23. Ruggieri M, D'Arrigo G, Abbate M, Distefano A, Upadhyaya M. Multiple coronary artery aneurysms in a child with neurofibromatosis type 1. Eur J Pediatr. 2000;159(7): 477–80.
24. Hamilton SJ, Allard MF, Friedman JM. Cardiac findings in an individual with neurofibromatosis 1 and sudden death. Am J Med Genet. 2001;100(2):95–9.
25. Bakker JR, Haber MM, Garcia FU. Gastrointestinal neurofibromatosis: an unusual cause of gastric outlet obstruction. Am Surg. 2005;71(2):100–5.
26. Yepuri N, Naous R, Richards C, Kittur D, Jain A, Dhir M. Nonoperative management may be a viable approach to plexiform neurofibroma of the porta hepatis in patients with neurofibromatosis-1. HPB Surg. 2018;2018:7814763.
27. Trilling B, Faucheron JL. Intestinal obstruction in von Recklinghausen's disease. Color Dis. 2014;16(10):762–8.
28. Miettinen M, Fetsch JF, Sobin LH, Lasota J. Gastrointestinal stromal tumors in patients with neurofibromatosis 1: a clinicopathologic and molecular genetic study of 45 cases. Am J Surg Pathol. 2006;30(1):90–6.
29. Fujimi A, Nagamachi Y, Yamauchi N, Tamura F, Kimura T, Miyajima N, et al. Gastrointestinal stromal tumor in a patient with neurofibromatosis type 1 that was successfully treated with regorafenib. Intern Med. 2019;58:1865.
30. Kalender M, Sevinc A, Tutar E, Sirikci A, Camci C. Effect of sunitinib on metastatic gastrointestinal stromal tumor in patients with neurofibromatosis type 1: a case report. World J Gastroenterol. 2007;13(18):2629–32.
31. Gasparotto D, Rossi S, Polano M, Tamborini E, Lorenzetto E, Sbaraglia M, et al. Quadruple-negative GIST is a sentinel for unrecognized neurofibromatosis type 1 syndrome. Clin Cancer Res. 2017;23(1):273–82.
32. Thavaraputta S, Graham S, Rivas Mejia AM, Lado-Abeal J. Duodenal somatostatinoma presenting as obstructive jaundice with the coexistence of a gastrointestinal stromal tumour in neurofibromatosis type 1: a case with review of the literature. BMJ Case Rep. 2019;12(1). https://doi.org/10.1136/bcr-2018-226702.
33. Relles D, Baek J, Witkiewicz A, Yeo CJ. Periampullary and duodenal neoplasms in neurofibromatosis type 1: two cases and an updated 20-year review of the literature yielding 76 cases. J Gastrointest Surg. 2010;14(6):1052–61.
34. Noe M, Pea A, Luchini C, Felsenstein M, Barbi S, Bhaijee F, et al. Whole-exome sequencing of duodenal neuroendocrine tumors in patients with neurofibromatosis type 1. Mod Pathol. 2018;31(10):1532–8.
35. Okubo Y, Yoshioka E, Suzuki M, Washimi K, Kawachi K, Kameda Y, et al. Diagnosis, pathological findings, and clinical management of gangliocytic paraganglioma: a systematic review. Front Oncol. 2018;8:291.
36. Ravegnini G, Quero G, Sammarini G, Giustiniani MC, Castri F, Pomponi MG, et al. Gastrointestinal juvenile-like (inflammatory/hyperplastic) mucosal polyps in neurofibromatosis type 1 with no concurrent genetic or clinical evidence of other syndromes. Virchows Arch. 2019;474(2):259–64.
37. Thway K, Fisher C. Diffuse ganglioneuromatosis in small intestine associated with neurofibromatosis type 1. Ann Diagn Pathol. 2009;13(1):50–4.
38. Gfroerer S, Theilen TM, Fiegel H, Harter PN, Mittelbronn M, Rolle U. Identification of intestinal ganglioneuromatosis leads to early diagnosis of MEN2B: role of rectal biopsy. J Pediatr Surg. 2017;52(7):1161–5.
39. Krishnasamy S, Abell TL. Diabetic Gastroparesis: principles and current trends in management. Diabetes Ther. 2018;9(Suppl 1):1–42.

40. Bernardis V, Sorrentino D, Snidero D, Avellini C, Paduano R, Beltrami CA, et al. Intestinal leiomyosarcoma and gastroparesis associated with von Recklinghausen's disease. Digestion. 1999;60(1):82–5.
41. Ejerskov C, Krogh K, Ostergaard JR, Fassov JL, Haagerup A. Constipation in adults with neurofibromatosis type 1. Orphanet J Rare Dis. 2017;12(1):139.
42. Pedersen CE, Krogh K, Siggaard C, Joensson IM, Haagerup A. Constipation in children with neurofibromatosis type 1. J Pediatr Gastroenterol Nutr. 2013;56(2):229–32.
43. Deniz E, Shimkus GJ, Weller CG. Pelvic neurofibromatosis: localized von Recklinghausen's disease of the bladder. J Urol. 1966;96(6):906–9.
44. Darcy C, Ullrich NJ. A 15-month-old girl presenting with clitoromegaly and a chest mass. Semin Pediatr Neurol. 2018;26:128–31.
45. Kousseff BG, Hoover DL. Penile neurofibromas. Am J Med Genet. 1999;87(1):1–5.
46. Cambiaso P, Galassi S, Palmiero M, Mastronuzzi A, Del Bufalo F, Capolino R, et al. Growth hormone excess in children with neurofibromatosis type-1 and optic glioma. Am J Med Genet A. 2017;173(9):2353–8.
47. Pascual-Castroviejo I, Lopez-Pereira P, Savasta S, Lopez-Gutierrez JC, Lago CM, Cisternino M. Neurofibromatosis type 1 with external genitalia involvement presentation of 4 patients. J Pediatr Surg. 2008;43(11):1998–2003.
48. Protopapas A, Sotiropoulou M, Haidopoulos D, Athanasiou S, Loutradis D, Antsaklis A. Ovarian neurofibroma: a rare visceral occurrence of type 1 neurofibromatosis and an unusual cause of chronic pelvic pain. J Minim Invasive Gynecol. 2011;18(4):520–4.
49. Smith KB, Wang DL, Plotkin SR, Park ER. Appearance concerns among women with neurofibromatosis: examining sexual/bodily and social self-consciousness. Psychooncology. 2013;22(12):2711–9.
50. Yilmaz K, Dusunsel R, Dursun I, Coskun A, Erten S, Kucukaydin M, et al. Neurofibromas of the bladder in a child with neurofibromatosis type 1 causing chronic renal disease. Ren Fail. 2013;35(7):1005–7.
51. Ure I, Gurocak S, Gonul II, Sozen S, Deniz N. Neurofibromatosis type 1 with bladder involvement. Case Rep Urol. 2013;2013:145076.
52. O'Brien J, Aherne S, Buckley O, Daly P, Torreggiani WC. Malignant peripheral nerve sheath tumour of the bladder associated with neurofibromatosis I. Can Urol Assoc J. 2008;2(6):637–8.
53. Bouty A, Dobremez E, Harper L, Harambat J, Bouteiller C, Zaghet B, et al. Bladder dysfunction in children with neurofibromatosis type I: report of four cases and review of the literature. Urol Int. 2018;100(3):339–45.
54. Subasinghe D, Keppetiyagama CT, De Silva C, Perera ND, Samarasekera DN. Neurofibroma invading into urinary bladder presenting with symptoms of obstructed defecation and a large perineal hernia. BMC Surg. 2014;14:21.
55. Shreeram S, He JP, Kalaydjian A, Brothers S, Merikangas KR. Prevalence of enuresis and its association with attention-deficit/hyperactivity disorder among U.S. children: results from a nationally representative study. J Am Acad Child Adolesc Psychiatry. 2009;48(1):35–41.
56. Niemczyk J, Wagner C, von Gontard A. Incontinence in autism spectrum disorder: a systematic review. Eur Child Adolesc Psychiatry. 2018;27(12):1523–37.
57. Boland JM, Colby TV, Folpe AL. Intrathoracic peripheral nerve sheath tumors-a clinicopathological study of 75 cases. Hum Pathol. 2015;46(3):419–25.
58. Alves Junior SF, Zanetti G, Alves de Melo AS, Souza AS Jr, Souza LS, de Souza Portes Meirelles G, et al. Neurofibromatosis type 1: state-of-the-art review with emphasis on pulmonary involvement. Respir Med. 2019;149:9–15.
59. Jutant EM, Girerd B, Jais X, Savale L, O'Connell C, Perros F, et al. Pulmonary hypertension associated with neurofibromatosis type 1. Eur Respir Rev. 2018;27(149). https://doi.org/10.1183/16000617.0053-2018.
60. Rodrigues D, Oliveira H, Andrade C, Carvalho L, Guimaraes S, Moura CS, et al. Interstitial lung disease and pre-capillary pulmonary hypertension in neurofibromatosis type 1. Respir Med Case Rep. 2018;24:8–11.

61. Niemeyer CM, Flotho C. Juvenile myelomonocytic leukemia: who's the driver at the wheel? Blood. 2019;133(10):1060–70.
62. Peltonen S, Kallionpaa RA, Rantanen M, Uusitalo E, Lahteenmaki PM, Poyhonen M, et al. Pediatric malignancies in neurofibromatosis type 1: a population-based cohort study. Int J Cancer. 2019;145:2926.
63. Paulus S, Koronowska S, Folster-Holst R. Association between juvenile myelomonocytic leukemia, juvenile xanthogranulomas and neurofibromatosis type 1: case report and review of the literature. Pediatr Dermatol. 2017;34(2):114–8.
64. Schutte P, Moricke A, Zimmermann M, Bleckmann K, Reismuller B, Attarbaschi A, et al. Preexisting conditions in pediatric ALL patients: spectrum, frequency and clinical impact. Eur J Med Genet. 2016;59(3):143–51.
65. Brems H, Park C, Maertens O, Pemov A, Messiaen L, Upadhyaya M, et al. Glomus tumors in neurofibromatosis type 1: genetic, functional, and clinical evidence of a novel association. Cancer Res. 2009;69(18):7393–401.
66. Stewart DR, Pemov A, Van Loo P, Beert E, Brems H, Sciot R, et al. Mitotic recombination of chromosome arm 17q as a cause of loss of heterozygosity of NF1 in neurofibromatosis type 1-associated glomus tumors. Genes Chromosomes Cancer. 2012;51(5):429–37.
67. Kumar MG, Emnett RJ, Bayliss SJ, Gutmann DH. Glomus tumors in individuals with neurofibromatosis type 1. J Am Acad Dermatol. 2014;71(1):44–8.
68. Harrison B, Moore AM, Calfee R, Sammer DM. The association between glomus tumors and neurofibromatosis. J Hand Surg Am. 2013;38(8):1571–4.
69. Stewart DR, Sloan JL, Yao L, Mannes AJ, Moshyedi A, Lee CC, et al. Diagnosis, management, and complications of glomus tumours of the digits in neurofibromatosis type 1. J Med Genet. 2010;47(8):525–32.

Genomics of Peripheral Nerve Sheath Tumors Associated with Neurofibromatosis Type 1

9

Eduard Serra, Bernat Gel, Juana Fernández-Rodríguez, and Conxi Lázaro

Contents

Genomics and bioinformatics disciplines suffered a great revolution after the consecution of the sequencing of the human genome and as a consequence molecular analysis changed of scale. Neurofibromatosis field has made use of these new technological capabilities but there is a lack of a comprehensive review on how

E. Serra (✉) · B. Gel
Hereditary Cancer Group, The Institute for Health Science Research Germans Trias i Pujol (IGTP), CIBERONC, Can Ruti Campus, Barcelona, Spain
e-mail: eserra@igtp.cat; bgel@igtp.cat

J. Fernández-Rodríguez · C. Lázaro
Hereditary Cancer Program, Catalan Institute of Oncology (ICO-IDIBELL-CIBERONC), L'Hospitalet de Llobregat, Barcelona, Spain
e-mail: jfernandez@idibell.cat

G. Tadini et al. (eds.), *Multidisciplinary Approach to Neurofibromatosis Type 1*,
https://doi.org/10.1007/978-3-319-92450-2_9

genomics impacted in the field and in particular to the knowledge gained on Neurofibromatosis type 1 (NF1) associated tumors. We divided this chapter into two parts: first we introduce the different tumors of the peripheral nervous system (PNS) associated with NF1, and second, we provide a summary on the contribution of genomics to the understanding of the molecular pathogenesis of these tumors. The second part is based only in a selection of works with the intention to provide a general view rather than an exhaustive collection of all the research produced in the field.

9.1 NF1-Associated Peripheral Nerve Sheath Tumors

One of the major clinical complications of NF1 patients is the development of different tumor types that arise in nervous and non-nervous tissues, both in childhood and adulthood. The PNS is particularly affected, with the development of different benign and malignant tumor types, like multiple cutaneous neurofibromas (cNFs), plexiform neurofibromas (pNFs), atypical neurofibromas (aNFs), and malignant peripheral nerve sheath tumors (MPNSTs).

9.1.1 Cutaneous Neurofibromas

Cutaneous neurofibromas (cNFs) are benign tumors that originate in the peripheral nervous system that resides in the skin, forming discrete and well-circumscribed non-encapsulated nodules. Other discrete neurofibromas can arise in the subcutaneous tissue (subcutaneous) or in deeper parts of the body. Discrete neurofibromas differentiate from other neurofibromas, like diffuse neurofibromas (ill-defined firm plaques) or plexiform neurofibromas (involving multiple nerve fascicles and growing along large nerves) [1].

cNFs normally appear during puberty and are present in more than 95% of Neurofibromatosis Type 1 patients [2]. Their number increases along life, although it is greatly variable depending on the NF1 patient, ranging from tens to thousands [3, 4]. The volume also increases with time, although the growth rate varies among individuals, depends on the location in the body, and could be different even among cNFs of a single patient [5]. cNFs can adopt different forms according to its growth stage, and there have been different attempts to classify them [2]. They may be itchy or painful, but most are asymptomatic. Although cNFs do not progress to malignancy and rarely are associated with clinical complications, they may have a great impact on the quality of life of NF1 patients due to the disfigurement, dysesthesia, and the psychological impact of the perceived disease visibility [6].

Neurofibromas are composed by different cell types, mainly Schwann cells (SCs) and fibroblasts, but also perineurial cells, infiltrating immune cells, axons, and others that are embedded in an abundant collagen-rich extracellular matrix [7, 8]. The classic histological appearance of a cNF is that of a hypocellular tumor with abundant mucoid stroma, floating strands of collagen, and scarce cells [1]. The exact identity of the cell that originates cNFs and the contribution of the tumor microenvironment to its formation are active research lines in the field (see below).

Neurofibromas are caused by the somatic inactivation of the *NF1* gene [9–11]. Of the different cell types composing cNFs only Schwann cells bear a double inactivation of the *NF1* gene [12, 13]. The ability to isolate pure populations of *NF1*(−/−) Schwann cells and analyze their genetic material has demonstrated that the majority of somatic *NF1* inactivation in cNFs are due to point mutations [13, 14]. Since somatic *NF1* mutations and neurofibroma-genesis are causally linked, genes controlling DNA repair mechanisms could be good candidate modifiers of the number of cNFs developed [13, 15, 16]. Furthermore, it has been reported that in a significant percentage of cNFs (~25%) somatic inactivation is evidenced by Loss of Heterozygosity (LOH) [10, 17–19]. Different works attempted to characterize the mechanisms underlying LOH in cNFs [16, 20]. The most frequent mechanism causing LOH in cNFs is homologous recombination, which is observed in about 60% of LOH-bearing cNFs [19] and which does not alter the number of *NF1* gene copies but reduces to homozygosity the constitutional *NF1* mutation [15]. These mitotic recombination events are generated by a single crossover located between the centromere and the *NF1* gene, resulting in isodisomy of almost all 17q arm. LOH due to the loss of the *NF1* gene accounts for about the remaining 40% of cNFs with LOH, with deletions ranging in size from 80 kb to 8 Mb within 17q [15]. Patients bearing constitutional *NF1* microdeletions do not exhibit LOH as a second hit [20].

Although double inactivation of the *NF1* gene is found in SCs, the specific identity of the cell type receiving this somatic inactivation and from which a neurofibroma is developed has not been fully characterized. In addition, it is not known whether this cell type is the same in cNFs and pNFs, although two recently generated mouse models in which *NF1* was ablated in cells expressing either Hoxb7 [21] or Prss56 [22] in the developing mouse, both generated cNF and pNF tumors. What it is known is that when selectively culturing Schwann cells from both types of neurofibromas, the somatic *NF1* mutation is restricted to this cell type and it is not observed in other cell types within neurofibromas, like endoneurial fibroblasts [12–14, 23]. Thus, we might not know the exact identity of the cell receiving the second *NF1* hit, but we know that it has the capacity to differentiate into Schwann cells. Studies with genetically modified mouse models for plexiform neurofibromas point to a SC precursor [24, 25]. There are a high number of cutaneous and plexiform neurofibromas that exhibit LOH due to homologous recombination [15, 18, 19]. One consequence of this molecular evidence is that the cell that receives the second *NF1* hit must be actively dividing, since homologous recombination needs cell division in order to operate.

As stated above, the number of cNFs developed in NF1 patients is highly variable, ranging from tens to thousands of tumors in a single patient. Different studies were developed to clarify the heritability of NF1 traits, the proportion of phenotypic variance that is explained by genetic variance. These studies identified the existence of a strong genetic component beyond the *NF1* gene influencing the variable number of cNFs developed that seem to follow a polygenic model [26, 27]. The role of the constitutional *NF1* mutation in this variation is still not clear. It has been observed that patients bearing the same germline mutation, even affected patients from the same family, can exhibit a very different number of cNFs [28]. However, different studies also suggested a potential role of the *NF1* germline mutation on cNF number [27, 29]. Two types of constitutional *NF1* mutations have clearly been found to influence neurofibroma number: Type-1 micro deletions (1.4 Mb deletions with breakpoints located within *NF1*-REPs a and c) seem to be associated with the early onset of a large number of cNFs [30, 31] and the c.2970-2972 delAAT mutation has been identified in patients with an absence of cNFs or any other clinically suspected neurofibroma type (plexiform or subcutaneous) [32, 33]. However, these two types of mutation only account for a small percentage of NF1 patients. There are currently no effective cNF therapies beyond surgery.

9.1.2 Plexiform Neurofibromas

Plexiform neurofibromas (pNFs) are big neurofibroma lesions that grow along large nerves, expanding and altering their form and adopting a rope-like appearance. In other cases, when multiple nerves are involved, it resembles "a bag of worms." A pNF may be intraneural or can spill out beyond the epineurium, diffusely infiltrating adjacent soft tissue. When peritumoral massive growth is present, the tumors are denominated massive soft tissue neurofibromas [1, 34]. A pNF may be visible or may lie internally. Terminology based on magnetic resonance imaging (MRI) characterizes pNFs as superficial or deep, invasive or displacing, and fascicular-nodular or diffuse [35]. Different classifications try to respond to clinical management needs, especially concerning their different risk of malignant progression.

pNFs are mainly developed in the context of NF1 and are thought to be congenital [36]. They are identified in around 30% of NF1 individuals by physical examination [3] and in around 50% if MRI is used [37]. pNFs exhibit highest growth rates mainly during early childhood [38]. This tumor type constitutes a major source of morbidity [36] and in some cases undergoes malignant transformation [39] progressing towards a malignant peripheral nerve sheath tumor (MPNST) [40].

pNFs have the same cellular composition as cNFs, although the identity of the cell originating them could be different. Each pNF arises from an independent biallelic inactivation of the *NF1* gene [41]. Thus, like cNFs [15] different pNFs arising in the same individual bear different somatic *NF1* mutations [42]. Besides the involvement of chromosome 17 in the inactivation of the *NF1* locus [43, 44], no other recurrent gross genomic alterations or recurrent point mutations have been identified in pNFs [42, 45]. Also, like cNFs, only pNF-derived Schwann cells are *NF1*(−/−) [23, 45]. In an analysis of intra pNF heterogeneity, in general pNFs were quite homogeneous both histologically and also at a molecular level. Despite this general homogeneity, certain heterogeneity regarding cell density and percentage of *NF1*(-/-) cells was identified [45].

In a recent genotype-phenotype study [46] constitutional missense mutations affecting one of five consecutive NF1 codons-Leu844, Cys845, Ala846, Leu847, and Gly848-located in the cysteine-serine-rich domain (CSRD) of neurofibromin were found to be positively associated with the presence of a major superficial plexiform neurofibromas and symptomatic spinal neurofibromas.

Surgery is still the only standard treatment for pNF. However, complete resection is difficult in many instances since they can acquire a large size and can be located in parts of the body difficult to operate. The MEK inhibitor (MEKi) Selumetinib has been used in children with inoperable pNFs showing tumor volume decrease (greater than 20% of the volume) in about 70% of the cases [47]. Further clinical trials using MEKis are ongoing.

9.1.3 Atypical Neurofibromas

Atypical neurofibromas (aNFs) have been defined as distinct and slowly growing nodular lesions that may or may not be associated with a pNF [43], exhibiting one or more histological atypical features but not fulfilling the criteria to be classified as an MPNST (they lack brisk mitotic activity or necrosis, for instance). Since not all neurofibromas exhibiting atypical features are the same, there has been an attempt to establish clear criteria to stratify them [48]. These criteria distinguish between cellular neurofibromas (neurofibromas with increased cellularity as the only atypical feature), neurofibromas with cytologic atypia (cytological atypia as the only atypical feature), and neurofibromas with multiple histological atypical features (cytologic atypia, rare mitoses, fascicular growth pattern, and increased cellularity). This latter group was named atypical neurofibromatous neoplasms with uncertain biological potential (ANNUBP) [48] and falls within the description used by other groups that studied aNFs [43].

aNFs in general, and ANNUBP in particular, are considered precursor lesions of MPNSTs based on clinical and pathological evidences of progression and on their genomic structure when compared to pNFs and MPNSTs [43, 49]. However, not all aNFs will end up forming an MPNST and currently we do not have the knowledge to predict which aNF will become malignant, what complicates their clinical management. aNFs are often already present in childhood. Under clinical examination they are frequently positive on 18-Fluorodeoxyglucose-Positron Emission Tomography (FDG-PET) scan [50]. Twenty-five percent of NF1 patients developing aNFs exhibit more than one aNF, being at greater risk of MPNST development [51]. Growth of distinct nodular lesions, pain, and FDG-PET avidity should raise concern for the presence of an aNF and, although complete resection may prevent the development of MPNSTs, some complicated locations together with an uncertain risk of transformation may complicate its clinical management [51, 52].

In addition to the biallelic *NF1* inactivation, the recurrent loss of the *CDKN2A/B* locus at 9p21.3 has been identified in aNFs [43, 45, 53]. Besides the pNF-aNF-MPNST progression, other ways of MPNST genesis might exist, since not all MPNSTs exhibit the loss of the *CDKN2A/B* locus [54, 55].

9.1.4 Malignant Peripheral Nerve Sheath Tumors

MPNSTs are rare malignancies with a peripheral nerve sheath origin. MPNSTs account for 3–10% of all soft tissue sarcomas and are a highly aggressive histological subtype. Approximately half of MPNSTs develop in patients with neurofibromatosis type 1 (NF1), while the other half develop sporadically [39, 56]. The incidence in the general population is of 1 per 100,000 [39] and the lifetime risk of an NF1 individual to develop an MPNST is at least of 10% [39, 57].

In NF1, MPNSTs commonly arise within a pre-existing pNF or aNF [40] and have a very bad prognostic due to its aggressiveness and metastatic potential, constituting the leading cause of morbidity and mortality in young and adults with NF1 [39, 57, 58]. Histologically, there is marked pleomorphism, mitosis, and invasion of adjacent tissues. The presence of a high tumor burden in NF1 patients can greatly difficult MPNST diagnose. FDG-PET scan is used to differentiate benign lesions from malignant tumors [50]. Patients with a *NF1* microdeletion as the constitutional *NF1* mutation have an increased risk for MPNST development [59, 60] and should have an adequate clinical surveillance.

MPNSTs exhibit biallelic inactivation of *NF1* [61]. A recent work [62] showed that a somatic *NF1* mutation was shared by an MPNST, the surrounding original pNF and its metastasis, linking in this way the cell originating pNFs and MPNSTs. In addition to *NF1* inactivation, a hallmark of MPNSTs is their normally hyperploid, highly rearranged, and complex genome [63, 64]. Recurrence in losses and gains of specific genomic regions containing cancer-associated genes have been reported and summarized [55, 65, 66] (see below).

Like many soft tissue sarcomas, complete resection with wide margins is essential in MPNST therapy, followed by radiation and/or chemotherapy [56, 67]. The 5-year survival rate after MPNST diagnosis in a NF1 patient is 20–50%, a much worse scenario than in sporadic cases and with a much earlier onset. Treatment failure is often associated with bone and lung metastases [39]. Standard sarcoma chemotherapy regimens are indicated for the treatment of MPNSTs, although its clinical benefit is limited. Several altered intracellular signal transduction cascades and deregulated tyrosine kinase receptors have been identified in MPNST and MPNST cell lines, posing the possibility of personalized targeted therapeutics (reviewed in [25, 65, 68, 69]). Different clinical trials assessed the activity of compounds like sorafenib or rapamycin analogs in patients with MPNSTs are ongoing [69]. In general, no objective responses have been observed when using single drug treatments.

Pre-clinical tumor models for MPNSTs have been developed to help testing the effectiveness of different types of therapeutic approaches. Subcutaneous and orthotopic xenograft of NF1-associated MPNST models have been generated from established cell lines, directly engrafting the human MPNSTs subcutaneously or orthotopically in the sciatic nerve. Patient-derived orthotopic xenograft (PDOX) models resemble primary tumors both histologically and genomically, and can mimic their metastatic capacity [70]. In addition, genetically engineered mouse models (GEMMs) carrying concomitant mutations in *Nf1* and *Tp53*, *Pten* or *Cdkn2a* develop MPNSTs and have been used to test different therapeutic approximations There exist also mixed models using allografts from GEMM (reviewed in [26]). Using these pre-clinical models, different treatment assays have been performed for MPNSTs, including the use of MEK inhibitors; mTOR inhibitors; a combination of MEK and mTOR inhibition; mTOR and HSP90 inhibition; mTOR and HDAC; AURKA; Wnt/ß-catenin signaling inhibition; BET bromodomain inhibitors alone or in combination with MEKi (reviewed in [25, 68, 69]).

9.2 Molecular Pathogenesis by Genomic Analysis

To review the contribution of genomics to the understanding of the molecular pathogenesis of NF1-associated PNS tumors, we performed a selection of works according to several criteria: we centered the analysis in human tumors, preferentially in the context of NF1 and that used technology based on microarrays and next generation sequencing (NGS) methodologies. The selection of works is mainly summarized in Table 9.1, in which information on the published work, the type of analysis, the type of samples used, and (when available) the data repository are provided. The works were grouped by areas: genome structure, data on single nucleotide variants (SNV) obtained by NGS, transcriptome, and epigenome; and there are works that impact in more than one area. There exist multitude of other works in the field that were not reviewed according to the established selection criteria (works on mouse models or other types of models, works using other types of technology like comparative genomic hybridization (CGH) or other cytogenetic techniques, etc.) that with no doubt equally contributed to the knowledge we have on the molecular pathogenesis of NF1 PNS tumors.

9.2.1 Genomic Structure

The molecular karyotype of neurofibromas and MPNSTs has been explored using tools such as array comparative genomic hybridization (aCGH), SNP-array, NGS-based approaches, or even methylation arrays.

Different works that used either aCGH or SNP-array to characterize the genomes of cNFs and pNFs (Table 9.1) arrived to the same conclusion: the genomic structure of cNF and pNF is identical, being an almost completely normal 2n genome. Only the long arm of chromosome 17 could be found recurrently altered as a result of somatic inactivation of the *NF1* gene, being affected by deletions or homologous recombination events generating loss of heterozygosity (LOH). The most extensive LOH study in cNFs ($N = 518$ from 113 NF1 patients) reported that 25% of cNFs exhibit LOH as a result of *NF1* somatic inactivation [19]. For pNFs, the percentage of somatic *NF1* inactivation by LOH mechanisms is higher, of about 50% [42, 45, 71].

aNFs have a similar genomic structure as pNFs. The only additional recurrent alteration identified in aNFs is the loss of the 9p arm and specifically the 9p21.3

Table 9.1 Genomic resources for NF1-associated peripheral nervous system tumors

	Work	Type of analysis	Type of material analyzed	Data repository
Genome structure	Cancer Genome Atlas Research Network (2017) Cell 171: 950–965.e28. DOI: 10.1016/j.cell.2017.10.014	SNP-array Affymetrix SNP 6.0	MPNSTs and other soft tissue sarcomas	NCI Genomic Data Commons—URL: https://portal.gdc.cancer.gov/projects/TCGA-SARC
	Adamowicz M et al. (2006) Genes Chromosomes Cancer 45(9): 829–8. DOI:10.1002/gcc.20343	aCGH 5p chromosome BAC-based	10 MPNSTs	
	Beert E et al. (2011) Genes Chromosomes Cancer, 50 (12) 1021–1032. DOI:10.1002/gcc.20921	aCGH Agilent 244K	Subcutaneous neurofibromas, plexiform neurofibromas, atypical neurofibromas, MPNSTs	ArrayExpress—Accession: E-MEXP-3052—URL: https://www.ebi.ac.uk/arrayexpress/experiments/E-MEXP-3052/
	Brekke HR et al. (2010) J Clin Onc 28:1573–1582. DOI:10.1200/JCO.2009.24.8989	Microarray slide with 3,568 BAC/PAC clones from the Norwegian Microarray Consortium	20 MPNSTs	
	Carrio M et al. (2018) Hum Mutat 39:1112–1125. DOI:10.1002/humu.23552	SNP-array Illumina HumanOmni-Express v1	Multiple parts of 6PNF, 2ANF	Synapse—Accession: syn7231973—URL: https://www.synapse.org/#!Synapse:syn7231973
	Castellsagué J et al. (2015) EMBO Mol Med 7(5):608-27. DOI: 10.15252/emmm.201404430	SNP-array Illumina Human 660W-Quad/Illumina HumanOmni-Express v1	Primary MPNSTs; ortho-xenografted MPNSTs	
	Ferrer M et al.(2018) Scientific Data 5:180106. DOI: 10.1038/sdata.2018.106	SNP-array Illumina HumanOmni2.5M + Exome array	17 primary and immortalized pNF-derived Schwann cells	Synapse—Accession: syn4940963—URL: http://www.synapse.org/pnfCellCulture
	Garcia-Linares C et al. (2010) Hum Mut 32:78–90. DOI:10.1002/humu.21387	SNP-array Illumina 370-Quad/Illumina Human660W-Quad	19 Cutaneous neurofibromas	
	Gosline S et al. (2017) Scientific Data 4:170045. DOI:10.1038/sdata.2017.45	SNP-array Illumina HumanOmni2.5–8	40 Cutaneous neurofibromas	Synapse—Accession: syn4984604—URL: http://www.synapse.org/cutaneousNF

	Hirbe A et al. (2015) Clin Canc Res 21 (18) 42014211. DOI: 10.1158/1078-0432.CCR-14-3049	WES NimbleGen libraries (Roche)/Illumina HiSeq 2000	PNF-MPNST-Metastasis progression	
	Kresse SH et al. (2008) Mol Cancer 7:48. DOI: 10.1186/1476-4598-7-48	BAC- and PAC-based array	7 high-grade MPNST	ArrayExpress—Accession: E-MEXP-869—URL: https://www.ebi.ac.uk/arrayexpress/experiments/E-MEXP-869/
	Lee W et al. (2014) Nat Genet 46(11): 1227–32. DOI:10.1038/ng.3095	SNP-array Affymetrix SNP 6.0	15 MPNST	dbGaP—Accession: phs000792.v1.p1—URL: https://www.ncbi.nlm.nih.gov/projects/gap/cgi-bin/study.cgi?study_id=phs000792.v1.p1
	Mantripragada K et al. (2008) Clin Cancer Res 14(4):1015–24. DOI:10.1158/1078-0432.CCR-07-1305	aCGH Custom PCR-based high resolution (57 genes)	35 MPNSTs, 16 plexiform, and 8 dermal neurofibromas	
	Mantripragada K et al. (2009) Genes Chrom & Cancer 48:897–907. DOI:10.1002/gcc.20695	Whole genome 32K BAC microarrays	24 MPNSTs and three neurofibroma samples	GEO—Accession: GSE16041—URL: https://www.ncbi.nlm.nih.gov/geo/query/acc.cgi?acc=GSE16041
	Pasmant E et al. (2011) J Natl Cancer Inst 103(22):1713-22. DOI: 10.1093/jnci/djr416	aCGH Agilent Human Genome 244K	22 PNFs	GEO—Accession: GSE24328—URL: https://www.ncbi.nlm.nih.gov/geo/query/acc.cgi?acc=GSE24328
	Pemov A et al. (2017) Oncogene 36(22):3168–3177. DOI:10.1038/onc.2016.464	SNP-array Illumina HumanOmni2.5–8	Short Schwann cell cultures from 23 PNFs	dbGaP—Accession: phs001403.v1.p1—URL: https://www.ncbi.nlm.nih.gov/projects/gap/cgi-bin/study.cgi?study_id=phs001403.v1.p1
	Röhrich M et al. (2016) Acta Neuropathologica, 131(6), 877–887. DOI:10.1007/s00401-016-1540-6	Methylation array Illumina Infinium HumanMethylation450K	34 MPNSTs, 33 neurofibromas, 6 ANFs	
	Sohier P et al. (2017) Genes Chromosomes Cancer 56:421–426. DOI 10.1002/gcc.22446	aCGH Agilent Human Genome 244K	8 MPNSTs, 1PNF, 7cNFs	GEO—Accession: GSE92647—URL: https://www.ncbi.nlm.nih.gov/geo/query/acc.cgi?acc=GSE92647

(continued)

Table 9.1 (continued)

	Work	Type of analysis	Type of material analyzed	Data repository
	Spurlock G et al. (2010) J Can Res Clin Oncol 136:1869–1880. DOI: 10.1007/s00432-010-0846-3	aCGH Agilent Human Genome 244K	PNF-MPNST progression	
	Upadhyaya M et al. (2012) Hum Mut 33:763–776. DOI:10.1002/humu.22044	SNP-array Affymetrix SNP 6.0	15 MPNSTs, 5PNFs	
	Yang J et al. (2011) Clin Canc Res 17:7563–7573. DOI10.1158/1078-0432.CCR-11-1707	aCGH Agilent Human Genome 44K	51MPNST (25 formalin-fixed paraffin-embedded) (26 fresh-frozen tumor samples)	GEO—Accession: GSE33881—URL: https://www.ncbi.nlm.nih.gov/geo/query/acc.cgi?acc=GSE33881
	Yu J et al. (2011) Clin Canc Res 17:1924–34. DOI:10.1158/1078-0432.CCR-10-1551	aCGH Affymetrix Genechip Mapping 500K	38 MPNSTs	
	Zhang M et al. (2014) Nat Genet 46:1170–1172. DOI:10.1038/ng.3116	WGS and WES/Illumina	8 MPNSTs (5 NF1-associated)	EGA—Accession: EGAS00001000974—URL: https://www.ebi.ac.uk/ega/studies/EGAS00001000974
SNVs data from NGS	Cancer Genome Atlas Research Network (2017) Cell 171:950–965.e28. DOI: 10.1016/j.cell.2017.10.014	WES Nimblegen SeqCap EZ Human Exome v3.0/Illumina HiSeq 2000	MPNSTs and other soft tissue sarcomas	NCI Genomic Data Commons—URL: https://portal.gdc.cancer.gov/projects/TCGA-SARC

	Brohl A et al. (2017) Sci Rep 7: 14992. DOI:10.1038/s41598-017-15183-1	WES NimbleGen SeqCap EZ Human Exome v2.0/Illumina HiScan	12 MPNSTs (10 NF1-associated); 7 tumors from TCGA data	
	Carrio M et al. (2018) Hum Mutat 39:1112–1125. DOI:10.1002/humu.23552	WES Agilent SureSelect Human All Exon/Illumina HiSeq	Multiple parts of 6PNF, 2ANF	Synapse—Accession: syn7231973—URL: https://www.synapse.org/#!Synapse:syn7231973
	Castellsagué J et al. (2015) EMBO Mol Med 7(5):608–27. DOI:10.15252/emmm.201404430	WES Agilent SureSelect Human AllExon/Illumina HiSeq 2000	Primary MPNSTs; ortho-xenografted MPNSTs	
	Ferrer M et al. (2018) Scientific Data 5:180106. DOI: 10.1038/sdata.2018.106	WES Agilent SureSelect Human All Exon v6/Illumina HiSeq2500	11 primary and immortalized pNF-derived Schwann cells	Synapse—Accession: syn4940963—URL: http://www.synapse.org/pnfCellCulture
	Gosline S et al. (2017) Scientific Data 4:170045. DOI:10.1038/sdata.2017.45	WGS NEBNext DNA Library Prep/Illumina HiSeqX	Cutaneous neurofibromas	Synapse—Accession: syn4984604—URL: http://www.synapse.org/cutaneousNF
	Hirbe A et al. (2015) Clin Canc Res 21 (18) 42014211. DOI: 10.1158/1078-0432.CCR-14-3049	WES Nimblegen SeqCap EZ Human Exome v3.0/Illumina HiSeq 2000	PNF-MPNST-Metastasis progression	
	Lee W et al. (2014) Nat Genet 46 (11): 1227–32. DOI:10.1038/ng.3095	WES Agilent SureSelect Human All Exon v4/Illumina HiSeq2500	15 MPNSTs	dbGaP—Accession: phs000792.v1.p1—URL: https://www.ncbi.nlm.nih.gov/projects/gap/cgi-bin/study.cgi?study_id=phs000792.v1.p1
	Lee W et al. (2014) Nat Genet 46 (11): 1227–32. DOI:10.1038/ng.3095	NGS panel MSK-IMPACT	37 MPNSTs	dbGaP—Accession: phs000792.v1.p1—URL: https://www.ncbi.nlm.nih.gov/projects/gap/cgi-bin/study.cgi?study_id=phs000792.v1.p1

(continued)

Table 9.1 (continued)

	Work	Type of analysis	Type of material analyzed	Data repository
	Pemov A et al. (2017) Oncogene 36(22):3168–3177. DOI:10.1038/onc.2016.464	WES Illumina TruSeq V1:32 and v2:30/Illumina HiSeq2500	Plexiform neurofibroma-derived Schwann cell cultures	dbGaP—Accession: phs001403.v1.p1—URL: https://www.ncbi.nlm.nih.gov/projects/gap/cgi-bin/study.cgi?study_id=phs001403.v1.p1
	Sohier P et al. (2017) Genes Chromosomes Cancer 56:421–426. DOI 10.1002/gcc.22446	WES	8 MPNSTs, 1PNF, 7cNFs	
	Zhang M et al. (2014) Nat Genet 46:1170–1172. DOI:10.1038/ng.3116	WGS, WES, and custom panel/Illumina HiSeq2500	50 MPNSTs (39 NF1-associated) (5 WGS, 3 WES and 42 custom panel)	EGA—Accession: EGAS00001000974—URL: https://www.ebi.ac.uk/ega/studies/EGAS00001000974
Transcrip-tome	Cancer Genome Atlas Research Network (2017) Cell 171:950–965.e28. DOI: 10.1016/j.cell.2017.10.014	RNA-Seq Illumina mRNA TruSeq/Illumina HiSeq 2000	MPNSTs and other soft tissue sarcomas	NCI Genomic Data Commons—URL: https://portal.gdc.cancer.gov/projects/TCGA-SARC
	Castellsagué J et al. (2015) EMBO Mol Med 7(5):608–27. DOI:10.15252/emmm.201404430	Expression array Affymetrix Human Gene 1.0 ST arrays	Primary MPNSTs; ortho-xenografted MPNSTs	GEO—Accession: GSE60082—URL: https://www.ncbi.nlm.nih.gov/geo/query/acc.cgi?acc=GSE60082
	Ferrer M et al. (2018) Scientific Data 5:180106. DOI: 10.1038/sdata.2018.106	RNA-Seq/Illumina HiSeq2500	18 primary and immortalized pNF-derived Schwann cells	Synapse—Accession: syn4940963—URL: http://www.synapse.org/pnfCellCulture
	Gosline S et al. (2017) Scientific Data 4:170045. DOI:10.1038/sdata.2017.45	RNA-Seq NEBNext mRNA Library Prep/Illumina HiSeq2500	Cutaneous neurofibromas	Synapse—Accession: syn4984604—URL: http://www.synapse.org/cutaneousNF
	Jouhilahti E-M (2012) PhD Thesis. ISBN 978-951-29-5135-2	Expression array Illumina HumanHT-12 V3.0	Neurofibroma-derived Schwann cell cultures NF1(+/−) and (−/−)	GEO—Accession: GSE32029—URL: https://www.ncbi.nlm.nih.gov/geo/query/acc.cgi?acc=GSE32029
	Karube K et al.(2006) J Clin Pathol 59:160–165. DOI: 10.1136/jcp.2004.023598	Expression array Takara Bio Cancer Chips version 4.0 of 886 genes	9 MPNSTs, 4 neurofibromas	

	Kolberg M et al. (2015) Mol Oncol 9(6):1129–39. DOI: 10.1016/j.molonc.2015.02.005	Expression array Human GenomeSurvey Microarray V2.0	8 neurofibromas; 30 MPNSTs (17 NF1 and 13 sporadic)	GEO—Accession: GSE66743—URL: https://www.ncbi.nlm.nih.gov/geo/query/acc.cgi?acc=GSE66743
	Lee W et al. (2014) Nat Genet 46(11): 1227–32. DOI:10.1038/ng.3095	RNA-Seq/Illumina2500	16 MPNSTs	dbGaP—Accession: phs000792.v1.p1—URL: https://www.ncbi.nlm.nih.gov/projects/gap/cgi-bin/study.cgi?study_id=phs000792.v1.p1
	Lévy P et al. (2007) Clin Cancer Res 13:398–407. DOI:10.1158/1078-0432.CCR-06-0182	Expression array Agilent 22K Human 1A	14 plexiform neurofibromas and 10 MPNSTs	ArrayExpress—Accession: E-TABM-69—URL: https://www.ebi.ac.uk/arrayexpress/experiments/E-TABM-69/
	Miller S et al. (2006) Can Res 66:2584–2591. DOI:10.1158/0008-5472.CAN-05-3330	Expression array Affymetrix GeneChips HU133A and HU133B	8 MPNST cell lines, NHSCs (and data from Watson et al. 2004)	
	Miller S et al. (2009) EMBO Mol Med 1:236–248. DOI 10.1002/emmm.200900027	Expression array Affymetrix GeneChips HU133 Plus 2.0	NHSC (10), dNFSC (11), pNFSC (11), MPNST cell lines (13), dNF (13), pNF (13), MPNST (6)	GEO—Accession: GSE14038—URL: https://www.ncbi.nlm.nih.gov/geo/query/acc.cgi?acc=GSE14038
	Nagayama S et al. (2002) Cancer Research 62:5859–5866. PMID:12384549	Expression array Own cDNA microarrays	4 MPNSTs	
	Pemov A et al. (2017) Oncogene 36(22):3168–3177. DOI:10.1038/onc.2016.464	RNA-Seq/Illumina	Short Schwann cell cultures from 23 PNFs	
	Subramanian S et al. (2010) The Journal of Pathology, 220(1), 58–70. DOI:10.1002/path.2633	Expression array Stanford cDNA microarrays	20 MPNSTs, 37 neurofibromas	

(continued)

Table 9.1 (continued)

	Work	Type of analysis	Type of material analyzed	Data repository
	Thomas L et al. (2015) Human Genomics 9:3. DOI:10.1186/s40246-015-0025-3	Expression array Affymetrix Human Exon 1.0 ST	8 MPNSTs, 7 PNFs (tumors related to Upadhyaya M et al. (2012))	
	Watson MA et al. (2004) 14:297–303. PMID:15446585	Expression array Affymetrix U95Av2 GeneChip	45 MPNSTs (25 NF1-associated)	
Epigenome	Cancer Genome Atlas Research Network (2017) Cell 171:950–965.e28. DOI:10.1016/j.cell.2017.10.014	miRNA-Seq mirVana miRNA Isolation/Illumina	MPNSTs and other soft tissue sarcomas	NCI Genomic Data Commons—URL: https://portal.gdc.cancer.gov/projects/TCGA-SARC
	Cancer Genome Atlas Research Network (2017) Cell 171:950–965.e28. DOI:10.1016/j.cell.2017.10.014	Methylation array Illumina Infinium HumanMethylation450K	MPNSTs and other soft tissue sarcomas	NCI Genomic Data Commons—URL: https://portal.gdc.cancer.gov/projects/TCGA-SARC
	De Raedt et al. (2014) Nature. DOI:10.1038/nature13561	ChIP-seq BRD4, H3K27Me3, H3K27Ac/Illumina HiSeq 2000	90-8TL cell line	GEO—Accession: GSE62499—URL: https://www.ncbi.nlm.nih.gov/geo/query/acc.cgi?acc=GSE62499
	Feber A et al. (2011) Genome Res 21(4): 515–24. DOI:10.1101/gr.109678.110	MeDIPseq/Illumina	10 MPNSTs, 10 NFs, 6 NHSCs (pooled)	GEO—Accession: GSE21714—URL: https://www.ncbi.nlm.nih.gov/geo/query/acc.cgi?acc=GSE21714
	Gong M et al. (2012) Neuro Oncol 14:1007–1017. DOI:10.1093/neuonc/nos124	LC Sciences (custom μParaflo array)	3 MPNSTs (1 NF1-related), 4 neurofibromas	

	Itani S et al. (2012) J Cancer Res Clin Oncol 138:1501–1509. DOI:10.1007/s00432-012-1223-1	TaqMan MicroRNA Assays Human PanelEarly Access Kit (Applied Biosystems)-157 miRNAs	6 MPNSTs, 6 NFs	
	Presneau N et al. (2012) Brit J Cancer 108(4):964–72. DOI:10.1038/bjc.2012.518	Agilent Human miRNA Microarray V2	10 neurofibromas, 10 MPNSTs (NF1 patients).	
	Röhrich M et al.(2016) Acta Neuropathologica, 131(6):877–887. DOI:10.1007/s00401-016-1540-6	Methylation array Illumina Infinium HumanMethylation450K		
	Subramanian S et al. (2010) The Journal of Pathology, 220(1):58–70. DOI:10.1002/path.2633	Stanford microRNA microarrays	20 MPNSTs, 37 neurofibromas	

WES Whole exome sequencing, *WGS* Whole genome sequencing, *aCGH* Array comparative genomic hybridization, *SNP-array* Single nucleotide polymorphism array band comprising the *CDKN2A/B* locus [43]. Other copy number changes were observed in some aNFs but they were far less frequent and occurred in a lower percentage of cells [43]. No additional genomic alterations besides those involving the *NF1* and *CDKN2A/B* inactivation were identified in another work that assessed tumor heterogeneity by analyzing different parts of two aNFs [45].

A different picture is the genomic composition of MPNSTs. The genome of malignant tumors is complicated to study due to the presence of non-tumor infiltrating cells (stroma) and the genomic heterogeneity of tumor cells. In addition, an important and still not resolved problem when assessing somatic copy number alterations (SCNAs) within hyperploid genomes (like those of MPNSTs) is inherent to the assay performed. Analyzing the genome structure by comparing the same amount of DNA from a 2n control tissue with the DNA from a hyperploid tumor generates a bias towards overestimating genomic losses and underestimating genomic gains. This bias needs to be taken into consideration when reaching conclusions on the copy number status of a particular genomic region. MPNSTs bear highly rearranged hyperploid genomes, in a clear contrast with pNFs [44, 64] and aNFs [43]. Many of the chromosomal alterations involve large chromosomal regions, at arm level or involving whole chromosomes, commonly present in the context of triploid or tetraploid genomes (see Table 9.1 for references).

9.2.2 Recurrently Altered Genomic Regions

Only a systematic bioinformatic integrative analysis of SCNA profiles of MPNSTs identified in independent works could assure a reliable list of recurrently altered chromosome regions. Looking for specific MPNST drivers within these regions represent a difficult task, even if a candidate gene approach within selected altered regions is applied. Nevertheless, the lack of recurrent point mutations in MPNSTs (see below) highlights the importance of analyzing their genomic structure to understand MPNST biology. Despite the absence of an integrative analysis, there are enough evidences to highlight at least some of these genomic regions and name some of the genes contained within them that have been associated with MPNST biology. Copy number gains have been recurrently identified at 5p (*TRIO, NKD2, IRX2*), 7p (*TWIST1, EGFR*), 7q (*HGF, MET*), 8q (*MYC*), 12q (*ERBB3, CDK4*), and 17q12-ter (*ERBB2, SOX9, BIRC5, TOP2A*). In addition copy number losses at 1p (*TP73*), 9p(9p21.3) (*CDKN2A/B*), 10q (*PTEN*), 11q(*EED*), 17p-17q11.2 (*TP53, NF1, SUZ12*) have also been recurrently reported [43, 44, 53, 63, 64, 72–79]. Many of these identified altered chromosomal regions are consistent with studies performed previous to the use of NGS and array techniques.

9.2.3 Mutational Landscape

Although mutation frequencies are highly dependent on the NGS analysis performed (platform used, type of assay, enrichment methodology, depth of coverage, etc.) and the type of bioinformatic analysis and parameters applied, certain generalities can be observed regarding the mutational landscape of NF1 PNS tumors. Considering only small somatic mutations (non-synonymous point mutations and small insertions/deletions) the analysis by exome sequencing of 23 pNFs [42] identified a median of 1 mutation with a range of 0–8 mutations per tumor. This result is consistent with the low number of mutations identified in other exome sequencing studies of pNFs and aNFs [45] or pNF-derived SCs [80] and similar to the very low mutation frequency and absence of recurrence identified in 40 cNFs after whole genome analysis [81]. In three independent analysis of MPNST exomes ($N = 70$ MPNSTs) the averaged median was of 55 mutations per MPNST, in a range of 7–472 mutations [66, 82, 83] also consistent with the low mutation frequency exhibited in general by soft tissue sarcomas [84].

In addition to exome and genome sequencing results, other works have supported the lack of activating mutations contributing to MPNST formation. A work checked in 5 MPNST cell lines the presence of 238 common mutations in 19 frequently activated oncogenes using mass spectroscopy-based analysis [85]. These authors did not identify activating mutations in any oncogene in these cell lines. Other works confirmed a minor role of mutations in other members of the Ras/MAPK pathway in MPNSTs [86].

A summary of the genomic structure and mutational landscape of NF1-associated PNS tumors would be the low frequency of point mutations in benign and malignant tumors, the necessary loss of *NF1* in cNFs and pNFs affecting chromosome 17q, the additional recurrent loss of *CDKN2A/B* in genomic alterations in aNFs, and the highly altered hyperploid genomes of MPNSTs together with the functional loss of the PRC2 complex. The combination of the resulting somatic copy number alteration in the altered genomes of MPNSTs seems to play an important role in its progression and viability.

9.2.3.1 *NF1, CDKN2A/B, TP53,* and *PRC2*: A Core Signature of Altered Tumor Suppressor Genes

Different works identified the loss of individual tumor suppressor genes (TSGs) in the biology of MPNSTs. The work by Lee et al. [55] consistently confirmed the implication of these TSGs and established the recurrent inactivation of a group of them (*NF1, CDKN2A/B, TP53,* and *PRC2*) defining a core signature in MPNSTs that has been consolidated by other works [66, 83]. The inactivation of this group of TSGs is more frequent by copy number alterations than by point mutations.

9.2.3.2 NF1

As already mentioned in this chapter, the loss of *NF1* is the key event driving cNF and pNF genesis. Although MPNST requires additional molecular events, NF1-associated MPNSTs invariably show the complete inactivation of *NF1*. This inactivation has been identified either by the detection of point mutations or by LOH analysis [55, 61, 86].

9.2.3.3 CDKN2A/B

The *CDKN2A/B locus* is a complex genomic region encoding both p19 (*ARF*) and p16 (*INK4A*) and p15 (*INK4B*) (respectively). These proteins are key regulators of the MDM2/p53 and CDK4/6/Rb pathways, important in regulating cell proliferation and cell viability. The loss of *CDKN2A/B* has been identified in aNFs (not in pNFs) although inactivation is never produced by point mutations [43, 45, 53]. Loss of the *CDKN2A/B* locus is also one of the most frequent alterations identified in MPNSTs, occurring in up to 70–80% in some studies [43, 44, 49, 54, 55, 64, 66, 77, 79, 87].

9.2.3.4 TP53

The presence of *TP53* mutations is specific of MPNSTs (not present in cNFs, pNFs, or aNFs) although there is certain discrepancy regarding their importance and extent. Different works identified *TP53* mutations in MPNSTs [88]. A work [89] assessed the mutation frequency of *TP53* in 145 consecutives clinically diagnosed MPNST cases collected over 36 years. Eighty-eight cases were histologically confirmed as MPNSTs, 30% of them were from NF1 patients ($N = 26$, 30%). *TP53* mutations were detected in 17 (24%) of 72 evaluable tumors, of which 36% were from NF1 patients. The authors concluded that *TP53* mutations are relatively rare in MPNSTs, compared to other cancers. However, these frequencies agree with other sarcomas [84]. Other authors also have suggested the relative role of *TP53* in MPNST tumorigenesis [66]. A work [62] discussed whether haploinsufficiency of *TP53* is sufficient for MPNST development, although other mechanisms of p53 inactivation beyond genetic alteration could also play a role [90].

9.2.3.5 Polycomb Repressive Complex 2 Components

Legius group [59] identified an elevated risk for MPNSTs in patients bearing constitutional *NF1* microdeletions. Since these microdeletions involve 13 genes in addition to *NF1*, the authors raised the possibility that a gene within the microdeletion region could contribute to the molecular pathogenesis of MPNSTs. One of these genes is *SUZ12*, a component of the polycomb repressive complex 2 (PRC2), involved in chromatin remodeling. The mutational analysis of 51 MPNSTs allowed the identification of mutations in *SUZ12* but also in EED, another PRC2 component [91]. Two additional groups further confirmed the high percentage of PRC2 inactivation by using SNP-array [55] and NGS analysis [55, 82] in a high number of MPNSTs. It has to be noted that second hit *NF1* deletions in cNFs and pNFs may also involve *SUZ12* [19, 45]. However, meanwhile cNF and pNFs SUZ12 deletions are in heterozygosity, not compromising PRC2 function, in the majority of MPNSTs mutations are in homozygosity or in more than one component of PRC2, completely ablating its function. Actually, a work [55] assessed the complete loss of trimethylation at lysine 27 of histone H3 (H3K27me3) by immunohistochemistry (IHC) validating its use in pathology.

9.2.4 MPNSTs Contain Highly Rearranged Stable Genomes

One of the questions to understand MPNST development is how the 2n genome of a pNF or aNF is transformed into the hyperploid and highly rearranged genome of an MPNST. Is it a progressive process due to a persistent genomic instability? Or it is rather produced by a catastrophic chromosomal event? There is still not sufficient data to properly evaluate this question but different observations made are worth mentioning. A main way to progress towards MPNST in the context of NF1 is starting from an aNF. Almost all aNFs have lost *NF1* and *CDKN2A/B* [43] and around 70% of MPNSTs also exhibit this double inactivation [43, 55, 77]. aNFs seem to have a high tendency to lose the *CDKN2A/B* locus since distinct independent deletions have been identified in different parts of the same aNF [45]. In this reported aNF, some areas bore one copy of the *CDKN2A/B* deleted, and in others the locus was homozygously deleted, correlating with a higher degree of histological atypical features [45]. Are aNF cells bearing *NF1* and *CDKN2A/B* inactivated at risk of genome instability? This is a possibility, since in [43] observed different percentages of triploid and tetraploid cells in 9/14 cytogenetically analyzed aNF-derived cells. However, on the other hand, the highly rearranged genome of MPNSTs seems to be stable. The molecular karyotype of patient-derived MPNST orthoxenografts (PDOXs) was found to be the same as their primary engrafted MPNST counterpart [70]. To establish a PDOX, a primary tumor has to be re-engrafted in different animals along several passages. In this process, a little part of the previous tumor is engrafted in the sciatic nerve of a new immunosuppressed animal and this is repeated several times, until the PDOX has a stable growth rate and can be cryopreserved for future experiments. Thus, considering the volume gained along all passages, the original tumor duplicates several times its original size. Castellsagué et al. [70] checked the structure of the genome of PDOX after at least six passages and found that their genome was more than 90% identical to the original primary tumor, denoting a high rate of genome stability. This result would be compatible with the hypothesis of a catastrophic event as the generator of the highly altered MPNST genome that subsequently would require genomic stability in order to progress as a tumor, although further experiments are required to reach a final conclusion.

9.2.5 Somatic *NF1* Mutation: Tracing the Cell of Origin in MPNST Progression

The cells originating an MPNST that developed in the context of a pre-existing pNF or aNF are descendants from the originating pNF and aNF cells. This has been demonstrated by showing that both the benign and the malignant tumor counterparts share the same *NF1* somatic inactivating alteration, evidencing the same clonal origin. Beert et al. [43] described a shared *NF1* deletion between an aNF and an intermediate MPNST. Hirbe et al. [62] described the presence of the same somatic *NF1* mutation shared by a histological progression of pNF, low grade MPNST, MPNST and even its metastasis. These findings were also supported by the work of Spurlock and colleagues [78] in which an LOH in the *NF1* region was shared by an MPNST and its surrounding pre-existing pNF, although the percentage of LOH in the pNF was low, but consistent with other works [45]. All together, these works demonstrate that MPNSTs have the same cellular origin as pNFs and aNFs.

9.2.6 Transcriptomics and Epigenomics

Different transcriptomic and epigenomic analysis have been performed of NF1-associated PNS tumors and their derived primary cells (Table 9.1). They were meant to identify genes and molecular pathways serving as biomarkers of tumor stage and/or therapeutic targets for treatment. Recently, different works have collected large data sets on the expression of cNFs and pNFs and derived cell lines [42, 80, 81] that constitute a valuable repository and will facilitate the differential expression analysis among NF1-associated PNS tumors.

Global transcriptome profiles of cNFs and pNFs seem to be very similar, so that an unsupervised cluster analysis cannot distinguish between both entities [92]. Interestingly, methylation profiles seem to provide higher specificity in this regard. The same type of analysis using methylome data was able to separate both tumor types [53]. The distinct methylation profiles of cNFs and pNFs could reflect differences in the epigenetic status of the cells originating them or differences in the proportion of cells composing them. In addition, methylome analysis clearly differentiated aNFs from other NFs and also from MPNSTs [53]. Expression analysis was also able to differentiate neurofibromas from MPNSTs [92]. When compared to normal human Schwann cells, MPNSTs exhibited a downregulation of Schwann cell differentiation markers (*SOX10, CNP, PMP22, NGFR*), whereas neural crest stem cell markers (*SOX9 and TWIST1*) were overexpressed [90, 92, 93].

The highly rearranged genomes of MPNSTs may complicate the expression analysis, since genomic alterations may have a great impact on gene expression, due to alterations of master transcriptional regulators or of specific gene copy number. For instance, transcriptome changes have been observed in MPNSTs that have lost PRC2 function, most times caused by the loss of one of its components. The lack of PRC2 function affects the activation of developmentally regulated master regulators and imprinted genes [55]. The loss of PRC2 has also an impact on chromatin and global epigenomic state [53, 91]. Other works analyzed the impact of SCNAs on the expression levels of genes contained in recurrently altered chromosomal regions in MPNSTs [74, 75, 77].

NF1 PNS tumors lack neurofibromin and consequently exhibit elevated levels of RAS/MAPK activity playing a central role in the cellular physiology of neurofibromas and MPNSTs. Other related signaling pathways, like the PI3K/AKT/mTOR pathway, have also been implicated in NF1-associated MPNST tumorigenesis (reviewed in [68]). Despite these well-characterized molecular mechanisms, several genomic studies tried to identify additional new signaling pathways present in neurofibromas or involved in the malignant transformation. For instance, Yang et al. [79] computed pathway enrichment scores from genes recurrently involved in SCNAs using Biocarta. This analysis resulted in 11 statistically significantly altered pathways, some consistent with known MPNST genetic alterations (*EGFR, CDKN2A*), and the IGF1R signaling pathway (a major cell survival pathway) playing a central role. Pathway analysis performed by Upadhyaya et al. [73], also taking information from genes altered by SCNAs, revealed the MPNST-specific amplification of seven Rho–GTPase pathway genes and several cytoskeletal remodeling/cell adhesion genes. Lévy et al. [94] identified Tenascin genes as potential players in pNF progression, as Thomas et al. [95] identified glutathione metabolism and Wnt signaling, the later consistent with previous works.

Feber et al. [96] generated a comprehensive analysis comparing the methylome of MPNSTs, benign neurofibromas, and normal Schwann cells. The authors found a complex pattern of epigenetic changes along progression towards MPNST, with predominant hypomethylation on satellite repeats in MPNSTs, although further work is necessary to assess the biological meaning of these methylation differences.

MicroRNAs (miRNAs) are non-coding single stranded RNAs 18–25 nucleotides long that suppress protein expression by binding to complementary sequences of messenger RNA (mRNA). The view on the role of miRNAs in NF1 tumorigenesis is still not well settled. The experimental data obtained so far indicate that a number of miRNAs may be involved in NF1 tumorigenesis, including miR-29c, miR-34a, miR-214, miR-10b, miR-204, and miR-21 [90, 97, 98]. The identification not only of differentially expressed microRNAs in tumors but also their target genes could provide a new insight into MPNST biology; however, there is still a lack of recurrence and consistency in the results obtained by the different works involving the study of miRNAs.

9.2.7 Genomic Information with Relevance in the Clinics

Drug discovery efforts for neurofibromas have been scarce, may be because benign tumors are not a main focus of attention for drug companies and research groups. A recent initiative has performed a high-throughput drug analysis for pNFs. Using a set of pNF-derived Schwann cell lines characterized at the genomic level by SNP-array analysis, RNA-seq, and whole exome sequencing, Ferrer et al. [80] carried out a dose response-based quantitative high-throughput screening by measuring the effect on cell viability of a collection of 1912 oncology-focused compounds. This work constitutes a valuable resource for future therapeutic tests for pNFs.

There exist more works on using the analysis of somatic copy number alterations or transcriptome analysis of MPNSTs to identify clinically relevant information either to identify biomarkers to help diagnosis or prognosis or to discover new targets for treatment. Nevertheless, the number of genomically analyzed MPNSTs to which clinical data has been correlated still needs to increase.

Regarding transcriptomics, Watson et al. [99] did not find any association between expression profiles and histological grade, tumor site, metastasis, recurrence, age, or patient survival. Using the transcriptome it was also difficult to differentiate between genes related to cell identity that could act as good biomarkers and genes constituting good therapeutic targets [92, 93]. Nevertheless, there exist successful examples combining human and mouse expression data that are now the basis of current clinical trials [47].

The genomic structure of MPNSTs has also been analyzed to obtain clinical useful information. Brekke et al. [77] identified the presence or absence of specific chromosomal arm level alterations (losses at 10q and Xq and gain of 16p) as a potential survival risk indicator. However, these correlations need to be further supported since not all alterations identified are among the most recurrently altered regions in MPNSTs. Yang et al. [79] characterized the genome status of 51 MPNSTs samples and identified several frequently gained or lost regions, containing several candidate genes. They correlated these genomic alterations with several clinical parameters such as tumor stage, tumor size, local recurrence, and metastasis. They were not able to associate individual alterations with patient survival, suggesting that multiple events might co-occur to affect survival. For instance, IGF1R copy number status was not correlated with survival. However, when patients were grouped according to the number of alterations in components of the IGF1R pathway (greater or lower of 10% altered pathway components) patients in the group with fewer alterations had a significantly better prognosis. Another similar work by Yu et al. [72] did not find clinical associations with the global degree of MPNST genome alterations. However, the authors associated the gain of 4 genomic regions located in chromosome 12 with poor patient survival. At the level of gene, CDK4 gain/amplification and increased FOXM1 protein expression were the most significant independent predictors for poor survival in MPNST patients. Upadhyaya et al. [73] did not identify any relationship between the grade of MPNSTs and the SCNA profile. Finally, Kolberg M et al. [74] aimed to identify clinically useful prognostic biomarkers by performing genome-wide RNA expression analysis followed by investigating upregulated genes at 17q. The authors used the combination of nuclear expression scores of three proteins to divide patients into risk groups with distinct survivals. In summary, the integration of genomic, molecular, and clinical data is a promising way to identify clinically relevant information for MPNSTs.

9.2.8 MPNST Genomics in the Context of Other Soft Tissue Sarcomas

Soft tissue sarcomas are relatively rare tumors that include up to 70 independent entities with different histopathological and molecular characteristics and prognosis [100].

According to their genomics, soft tissue sarcomas (STS) fall into two broad general groups: those with few genomic structural alterations and driven by specific translocations or activating mutations (one-third of all sarcomas) and those with complex karyotypes [84, 101]. MPNSTs fall in the group of soft tissue sarcomas with high levels of SCNAs and a low somatic point mutation burden, together with undifferentiated pleomorphic sarcomas (UPS), myxofibrosarcomas (MFS), and dedifferentiated liposarcomas (DDLPS). These karyotypically complex sarcomas can arise from a less aggressive form and progress towards malignancy, exhibiting then a much higher genomic complexity. Examples include the progression from atypical lipoma or well-differentiated liposarcoma to DDLPS or the progression from enchondroma to chondrosarcoma, together with the pNF-MPNST progression [101]. However, most high-grade karyotypically complex sarcomas present *de novo*, without antecedent lower-grade lesions. The epigenomic contribution in sarcomagenesis is also an active area of research [53].

If an unsupervised integrative cluster analysis is performed integrating DNA copy number, DNA methylation, and expression of mRNA and miRNA [84], MPNSTs still lie in its majority clustered together with UPS or MFS. However, if only gene and protein expression is considered, many MPNST cluster with synovial sarcoma (SS), a sarcoma with a simple genome, consistent with other reports [102]. It is interesting to note that genomic complexity is reflected in nuclear pleomorphism when analyzed by automated computation analysis of whole-slide digital pathology images [84].

The low number of point mutations makes difficult to identify mutation signatures in MPNSTs but the mutational signature associated with APOBEC was modestly elevated in MPNST compared to other sarcoma types, at similar levels as in DDLPS [84].

Considering data from TCGA [103] the oncogenic signaling pathways more frequently altered in MFS/UPS are RTK/Ras, cell cycle, and p53 signaling pathways, consistent with the genomic alterations that are found in MPNSTs. Sarcoma grading system and prediction capacity were improved by using a specific expression signature termed CINSARC (complexity index in sarcomas, composed of 67 genes related to mitosis and chromosome integrity) [104] although its validity in MPNSTs needs to be elucidated. NGS analyses of sarcomas have revealed the presence of many alterations that can be targeted using therapies that are already used in patients with other forms of cancer [105].

Our current state of knowledge on the NF1-associated PNS tumors still leaves many open questions. To which extent unpredictable factors like time of *NF1* inactivation and location of the originating cell influences the different types and morphologies of neurofibromas? Is the identity of the cell originating cNFs and pNFs the same? How a pNF with an almost unaltered genome can end up resulting in an MPNST with a highly altered and rearranged genome? Is there any biomarker for predicting aNF progression to MPNST? Can we formulate a defined molecular path (including genetics and epigenetics) from pNF up to MPNST and metastasis? How many ways of generating an MPNST exist? Are sporadic and NF1-associated MPNSTs sharing a molecular pathogenesis model? May be in the future genomic analysis can help elucidate these and other questions important for NF1 pathogenesis.

Acknowledgements We thank members of our labs for insightful discussions. We apologize to colleagues whose work could not be cited due to space limitation. The primary research in our laboratories for the topic of this review is supported by grants from: the Neurofibromatosis Therapeutic Acceleration Program (NTAP)- Johns Hopkins University School of Medicine. Its contents are solely the responsibility of the authors and do not necessarily represent the official views of the Johns Hopkins University School of Medicine; the Spanish Ministry of Science and Innovation, Carlos III Health Institute (ISCIII) (PI14/00577; PI16/00563, PI17/00524; PI19/00553, and CIBERONC) Plan Estatal de I. D. i 2013–16 and co-financed by the FEDER program—a way to build Europe—; the Government of Catalonia (2017SGR496) and CERCA Program/Generalitat de Catalunya; the Fundación PROYECTO NEUROFIBROMATOSIS, the Fundació La Marató de TV3; the NF Research Initiative -Boston Children's Hospital.

References

1. Stemmer-Rachamimov AO, Nielsen G. Pathologic and molecular diagnostic features of peripheral nerve sheath tumors in NF1. In: Upadhyaya M, Cooper D, editors. Neurofibromatosis type 1 molecular and cellular biology. Berlin: Springer; 2012. p. 429–43.
2. Ortonne N, Wolkenstein P, Blakeley JO, Korf B, Plotkin SR, Riccardi VM, et al. Cutaneous neurofibromas. Neurology. 2018;91(2 Supplement 1):S5–13.. [cited 2019 Feb 23]. Available from: http://www.ncbi.nlm.nih.gov/pubmed/29987130.
3. Huson SM, Harper PS, Compston DA. Von Recklinghausen neurofibromatosis. A clinical and population study in south-East Wales. Brain. 1988;111(Pt 6):1355–81.. [cited 2019 Feb 18]. Available from: http://www.ncbi.nlm.nih.gov/pubmed/3145091.
4. Duong TA, Bastuji-Garin S, Valeyrie-Allanore L, Sbidian E, Ferkal S, Wolkenstein P. Evolving pattern with age of cutaneous signs in neurofibromatosis type 1: a cross-sectional study of 728 patients. Dermatology. 2011;222(3):269–73. [cited 2019 Feb 18]. Available from: http://www.ncbi.nlm.nih.gov/pubmed/21540571.
5. Cannon A, Chen M-J, Li P, Boyd KP, Theos A, Redden DT, et al. Cutaneous neurofibromas in neurofibromatosis type I: a quantitative natural history study. Orphanet J Rare Dis. 2018;13(1):31. [cited 2019 Feb 17]. Available from: http://www.ncbi.nlm.nih.gov/pubmed/29415745.
6. Wolkenstein P, Zeller J, Revuz J, Ecosse E, Leplège A. Quality-of-life impairment in neurofibromatosis type 1: a cross-sectional study of 128 cases. Arch Dermatol. 2001;137(11):1421–5. [cited 2019 Feb 23]. Available from: http://www.ncbi.nlm.nih.gov/pubmed/11708944.
7. Krone W, Jirikowski G, Mühleck O, Kling H, Gall H. Cell culture studies on neurofibromatosis (von Recklinghausen). II. Occurrence of glial cells in primary cultures of peripheral neurofibromas. Hum Genet. 1983;63(3):247–51. [cited 2019 Feb 21]. Available from: http://www.ncbi.nlm.nih.gov/pubmed/6406358.
8. Peltonen J, Jaakkola S, Lebwohl M, Renvall S, Risteli L, Virtanen I, et al. Cellular differentiation and expression of matrix genes in type 1 neurofibromatosis. Lab Investig. 1988;59(6):760–71.. [cited 2019 Feb 23]. Available from: http://www.ncbi.nlm.nih.gov/pubmed/2462129.
9. Sawada S, Florell S, Purandare SM, Ota M, Stephens K, Viskochil D. Identification of NF1 mutations in both alleles of a dermal neurofibroma. Nat Genet. 1996;14(1):110–2.. [cited 2019 Feb 23]. Available from: http://www.nature.com/articles/ng0996-110.
10. Colman SD, Williams CA, Wallace MR. Benign neurofibromas in type 1 neurofibromatosis (NF1) show somatic deletions of the NF1 gene. Nat Genet. 1995;11(1):90–2.. [cited 2019 Feb 18]. Available from: http://www.nature.com/articles/ng0995-90.
11. Serra E, Puig S, Otero D, Gaona A, Kruyer H, Ars E, et al. Confirmation of a double-hit model for the NF1 gene in benign neurofibromas. Am J Hum Genet. 1997;61(3):512–9.. [cited 2019 Feb 23]. Available from: https://linkinghub.elsevier.com/retrieve/pii/S0002929707643146.
12. Serra E, Rosenbaum T, Winner U, Aledo R, Ars E, Estivill X, et al. Schwann cells harbor the somatic NF1 mutation in neurofibromas: evidence of two different Schwann cell subpopulations. Hum Mol Genet. 2000;9(20):3055–64.. [cited 2019 Feb 23]. Available from: http://www.ncbi.nlm.nih.gov/pubmed/11115850.
13. Maertens O, Brems H, Vandesompele J, De Raedt T, Heyns I, Rosenbaum T, et al. ComprehensiveNF1 screening on cultured Schwann cells from neurofibromas. Hum Mutat. 2006;27(10):1030–40. [cited 2019 Feb 23]. Available from: http://www.ncbi.nlm.nih.gov/pubmed/16941471.
14. Thomas L, Spurlock G, Eudall C, Thomas NS, Mort M, Hamby SE, et al. Exploring the somatic NF1 mutational spectrum associated with NF1 cutaneous neurofibromas. Eur J Hum Genet. 2012;20(4):411–9.. [cited 2019 Feb 23]. Available from: http://www.nature.com/articles/ejhg2011207.
15. Serra E, Rosenbaum T, Nadal M, Winner U, Ars E, Estivill X, et al. Mitotic recombination effects homozygosity for NF1 germline mutations in neurofibromas. Nat Genet. 2001;28(3):294–6.. [cited 2019 Feb 23]. Available from: http://www.ncbi.nlm.nih.gov/pubmed/11431704.

16. Serra E, Ars E, Ravella A, Sánchez A, Puig S, Rosenbaum T, et al. Somatic NF1 mutational spectrum in benign neurofibromas: mRNA splice defects are common among point mutations. Hum Genet. 2001;108(5):416–29.. [cited 2019 Feb 23]. Available from: http://www.ncbi.nlm.nih.gov/pubmed/11409870.
17. Serra E, Pros E, García C, López E, Gili MLL, Gómez C, et al. Tumor LOH analysis provides reliable linkage information for prenatal genetic testing of sporadic NFI patients. Genes Chromosom &amp. Cancer. 2007;46(9):820–7.. [cited 2019 Feb 23]. Available from: http://www.ncbi.nlm.nih.gov/pubmed/17563086.
18. Steinmann K, Kluwe L, Friedrich RE, Mautner V-F, Cooper DN, Kehrer-Sawatzki H. Mechanisms of loss of heterozygosity in neurofibromatosis type 1-associated plexiform neurofibromas. J Investig Dermatol. 2009;129(3):615–21. Mar [cited 2019 Feb 23]. Available from: https://linkinghub.elsevier.com/retrieve/pii/S0022202X15342500.
19. Garcia-Linares C, Fernández-Rodríguez J, Terribas E, Mercadé J, Pros E, Benito LL, et al. Dissecting loss of heterozygosity (LOH) in neurofibromatosis type 1-associated neurofibromas: importance of copy neutral LOH. Hum Mutat. 2011;32(1):78–90. [cited 2019 Feb 18]. Available from: http://www.ncbi.nlm.nih.gov/pubmed/21031597.
20. De Raedt T, Maertens O, Chmara M, Brems H, Heyns I, Sciot R, et al. Somatic loss of wild typeNF1 allele in neurofibromas: comparison ofNF1 microdeletion and non-microdeletion patients. Genes Chromosom Cancer. 2006;45(10):893–904.. [cited 2019 Feb 18]. Available from: http://www.ncbi.nlm.nih.gov/pubmed/16830335.
21. Chen Z, Mo J, Brosseau J-P, Shipman T, Wang Y, Liao C-P, et al. Spatiotemporal loss of *NF1* in Schwann cell lineage leads to different types of cutaneous neurofibroma susceptible to modification by the hippo pathway. Cancer Discov. 2019;9(1):114–29.. [cited 2019 Feb 17]. Available from: http://www.ncbi.nlm.nih.gov/pubmed/30348677.
22. Radomska KJ, Coulpier F, Gresset A, Schmitt A, Debbiche A, Lemoine S, et al. Cellular origin, tumor progression, and pathogenic mechanisms of cutaneous Neurofibromas revealed by mice with *Nf1* knockout in boundary cap cells. Cancer Discov. 2019;9(1):130–47. [cited 2019 Feb 23]. Available from: http://www.ncbi.nlm.nih.gov/pubmed/30348676.
23. Li H, Chang L-J, Neubauer DR, Muir DF, Wallace MR. Immortalization of human normal and NF1 neurofibroma Schwann cells. Lab Investig. 2016;96(10):1105–15.. [cited 2019 Feb 23]. Available from: http://www.ncbi.nlm.nih.gov/pubmed/27617404.
24. Jouhilahti EM. The roots of neurofibromas in neurofibromatosis type 1. A question of multipotency, differentiation and hiding. Turku: Turun Yliopisto University of Turku; 2012.
25. Ratner N, Miller SJ. A RASopathy gene commonly mutated in cancer: the neurofibromatosis type 1 tumour suppressor. Nat Rev Cancer. 2015;15(5):290–301. [cited 2019 Feb 23]. Available from: http://www.nature.com/articles/nrc3911.
26. Easton DF, Ponder MA, Huson SM, Ponder BA. An analysis of variation in expression of neurofibromatosis (NF) type 1 (NF1): evidence for modifying genes. Am J Hum Genet. 1993;53(2):305–13. [cited 2019 Feb 18]. Available from: http://www.ncbi.nlm.nih.gov/pubmed/8328449.
27. Sabbagh A, Pasmant E, Laurendeau I, Parfait B, Barbarot S, Guillot B, et al. Unravelling the genetic basis of variable clinical expression in neurofibromatosis 1. Hum Mol Genet. 2009;18(15):2768–78. [cited 2019 Feb 23]. Available from: http://www.ncbi.nlm.nih.gov/pubmed/19417008.
28. Ars E, Serra E, García J, Kruyer H, Gaona A, Lázaro C, et al. Mutations affecting mRNA splicing are the most common molecular defects in patients with neurofibromatosis type 1. Hum Mol Genet. 2000;9(2):237–47.. [cited 2019 Feb 17]. Available from: http://www.ncbi.nlm.nih.gov/pubmed/10607834.
29. Szudek J, Joe H, Friedman JM. Analysis of intrafamilial phenotypic variation in neurofibromatosis 1 (NF1). Genet Epidemiol. 2002;23(2):150–64.. [cited 2019 Feb 23]. Available from: http://www.ncbi.nlm.nih.gov/pubmed/12214308.
30. Kayes LM, Burke W, Riccardi VM, Bennett R, Ehrlich P, Rubenstein A, et al. Deletions spanning the neurofibromatosis 1 gene: identification and phenotype of five patients. Am J Hum

Genet. 1994;54(3):424–36. [cited 2019 Feb 21]; Available from: http://www.ncbi.nlm.nih.gov/pubmed/8116612.

31. Wu B-L, Austin MA, Schneider GH, Boles RG, Korf BR. Deletion of the entireNF1 gene detected by FISH: four deletion patients associated with severe manifestations. Am J Med Genet. 1995;59(4):528–35. [cited 2019 Feb 23]. Available from: http://www.ncbi.nlm.nih.gov/pubmed/8585580.
32. Upadhyaya M, Huson SM, Davies M, Thomas N, Chuzhanova N, Giovannini S, et al. An absence of cutaneous neurofibromas associated with a 3-bp inframe deletion in exon 17 of the NF1 gene (c.2970-2972 delAAT): evidence of a clinically significant NF1 genotype-phenotype correlation. Am J Hum Genet. 2007;80(1):140–51. [cited 2019 Feb 23]. Available from: http://www.ncbi.nlm.nih.gov/pubmed/17160901.
33. Koczkowska M, Callens T, Gomes A, Sharp A, Chen Y, Hicks AD, et al. Expanding the clinical phenotype of individuals with a 3-bp in-frame deletion of the NF1 gene (c.2970_2972del): an update of genotype–phenotype correlation. Genet Med. 2018;21(4):867–76. [cited 2019 Feb 21]; Available from: http://www.ncbi.nlm.nih.gov/pubmed/30190611.
34. Rodriguez FJ, Folpe AL, Giannini C, Perry A. Pathology of peripheral nerve sheath tumors: diagnostic overview and update on selected diagnostic problems. Acta Neuropathol. 2012;123(3):295–319.. [cited 2019 Feb 23]. Available from: http://www.ncbi.nlm.nih.gov/pubmed/22327363.
35. Mautner VF, Hartmann M, Kluwe L, Friedrich RE, Fünsterer C. MRI growth patterns of plexiform neurofibromas in patients with neurofibromatosis type 1. Neuroradiology. 2006;48(3):160–5.. [cited 2019 Feb 23]. Available from: http://www.ncbi.nlm.nih.gov/pubmed/16432718.
36. Korf BR. Plexiform neurofibromas. Am J Med Genet. 1999;89(1):31–7.. [cited 2019 Feb 21]. Available from: http://www.ncbi.nlm.nih.gov/pubmed/10469434.
37. Mautner V-F, Asuagbor FA, Dombi E, Fünsterer C, Kluwe L, Wenzel R, et al. Assessment of benign tumor burden by whole-body MRI in patients with neurofibromatosis 1. Neuro-Oncology. 2008;10(4):593–8. [cited 2019 Feb 23]. Available from: http://www.ncbi.nlm.nih.gov/pubmed/18559970.
38. Dombi E, Solomon J, Gillespie AJ, Fox E, Balis FM, Patronas N, et al. NF1 plexiform neurofibroma growth rate by volumetric MRI: relationship to age and body weight. Neurology. 2007;68(9):643–7.. [cited 2019 Feb 18]. Available from: http://www.ncbi.nlm.nih.gov/pubmed/17215493.
39. Evans DGR, Baser ME, McGaughran J, Sharif S, Howard E, Moran A. Malignant peripheral nerve sheath tumours in neurofibromatosis 1. J Med Genet. 2002;39(5):311–4.. [cited 2019 Feb 18]. Available from: http://www.ncbi.nlm.nih.gov/pubmed/12011145.
40. McCarron KF, Goldblum JR. Plexiform neurofibroma with and without associated malignant peripheral nerve sheath tumor: a clinicopathologic and immunohistochemical analysis of 54 cases. Mod Pathol. 1998;11(7):612–7. [cited 2019 Feb 23]. Available from: http://www.ncbi.nlm.nih.gov/pubmed/9688181.
41. Kluwe L, Friedrich RE, Mautner VF. Allelic loss of the NF1 gene in NF1-associated plexiform neurofibromas. Cancer Genet Cytogenet. 1999;113(1):65–9.. [cited 2019 Feb 21]. Available from: http://www.ncbi.nlm.nih.gov/pubmed/10459349.
42. Pemov A, Li H, Patidar R, Hansen NF, Sindiri S, Hartley SW, et al. The primacy of NF1 loss as the driver of tumorigenesis in neurofibromatosis type 1-associated plexiform neurofibromas. Oncogene. 2017;36(22):3168–77.. [cited 2019 Feb 23]. Available from: http://www.ncbi.nlm.nih.gov/pubmed/28068329.
43. Beert E, Brems H, Daniëls B, De Wever I, Van Calenbergh F, Schoenaers J, et al. Atypical neurofibromas in neurofibromatosis type 1 are premalignant tumors. Genes Chromosom Cancer. 2011;50(12):1021–32. [cited 2019 Feb 17]. Available from: http://www.ncbi.nlm.nih.gov/pubmed/21987445.
44. Mantripragada KK, Spurlock G, Kluwe L, Chuzhanova N, Ferner RE, Frayling IM, et al. High-resolution DNA copy number profiling of malignant peripheral nerve sheath tumors using targeted microarray-based comparative genomic hybridization. Clin Cancer Res.

2008;14(4):1015–24.. [cited 2019 Feb 23]. Available from: http://www.ncbi.nlm.nih.gov/pubmed/18281533.

45. Carrió M, Gel B, Terribas E, Zucchiatti AC, Moliné T, Rosas I, et al. Analysis of intratumor heterogeneity in neurofibromatosis type 1 plexiform neurofibromas and neurofibromas with atypical features: correlating histological and genomic findings. Hum Mutat. 2018;39(8):1112–25.. [cited 2019 Feb 17]. Available from: http://www.ncbi.nlm.nih.gov/pubmed/29774626.
46. Koczkowska M, Chen Y, Callens T, Gomes A, Sharp A, Johnson S, et al. Genotype-phenotype correlation in NF1: evidence for a more severe phenotype associated with missense mutations affecting NF1 codons 844–848. Am J Hum Genet. 2018;102(1):69–87.. [cited 2019 Feb 21]. Available from: http://www.ncbi.nlm.nih.gov/pubmed/29290338.
47. Dombi E, Baldwin A, Marcus LJ, Fisher MJ, Weiss B, Kim A, et al. Activity of Selumetinib in neurofibromatosis type 1–related plexiform neurofibromas. N Engl J Med. 2016;375(26):2550–60. [cited 2019 Feb 18]. Available from: http://www.ncbi.nlm.nih.gov/pubmed/28029918.
48. Miettinen MM, Antonescu CR, Fletcher CDM, Kim A, Lazar AJ, Quezado MM, et al. Histopathologic evaluation of atypical neurofibromatous tumors and their transformation into malignant peripheral nerve sheath tumor in patients with neurofibromatosis 1—a consensus overview. Hum Pathol. 2017;67:1–10. [cited 2019 Feb 23]. Available from: http://www.ncbi.nlm.nih.gov/pubmed/28551330.
49. Nielsen GP, Stemmer-Rachamimov AO, Ino Y, Moller MB, Rosenberg AE, Louis DN. Malignant transformation of neurofibromas in neurofibromatosis 1 is associated with CDKN2A/p16 inactivation. Am J Pathol. 1999;155(6):1879–84.. [cited 2019 Feb 23]. Available from: https://linkinghub.elsevier.com/retrieve/pii/S0002944010655071.
50. Ferner RE, Golding JF, Smith M, Calonje E, Jan W, Sanjayanathan V, et al. [18F]2-fluoro-2-deoxy-D-glucose positron emission tomography (FDG PET) as a diagnostic tool for neurofibromatosis 1 (NF1) associated malignant peripheral nerve sheath tumours (MPNSTs): a long-term clinical study. Ann Oncol. 2008;19(2):390–4. [cited 2019 Feb 18]. Available from: http://www.ncbi.nlm.nih.gov/pubmed/17932395.
51. Higham CS, Dombi E, Rogiers A, Bhaumik S, Pans S, Connor SEJ, et al. The characteristics of 76 atypical neurofibromas as precursors to neurofibromatosis 1 associated malignant peripheral nerve sheath tumors. Neuro-Oncology. 2018;20(6):818–25.. [cited 2019 Feb 18]. Available from: https://academic.oup.com/neuro-oncology/article/20/6/818/4835085.
52. Bernthal NM, Putnam A, Jones KB, Viskochil D, Randall RL. The effect of surgical margins on outcomes for low grade MPNSTs and atypical neurofibroma. J Surg Oncol. 2014;110(7):813–6.. Available from: http://www.ncbi.nlm.nih.gov/pubmed/25111615.
53. Röhrich M, Koelsche C, Schrimpf D, Capper D, Sahm F, Kratz A, et al. Methylation-based classification of benign and malignant peripheral nerve sheath tumors. Acta Neuropathol. 2016;131(6):877–87.. [cited 2019 Feb 23]. Available from: http://link.springer.com/10.1007/s00401-016-1540-6.
54. Kourea HP, Orlow I, Scheithauer BW, Cordon-Cardo C, Woodruff JM. Deletions of the INK4A gene occur in malignant peripheral nerve sheath tumors but not in neurofibromas. Am J Pathol. 1999;155(6):1855–60.. [cited 2019 Feb 21]. Available from: https://linkinghub.elsevier.com/retrieve/pii/S0002944010655046.
55. Lee W, Teckie S, Wiesner T, Ran L, Prieto Granada CN, Lin M, et al. PRC2 is recurrently inactivated through EED or SUZ12 loss in malignant peripheral nerve sheath tumors. Nat Genet. 2014;46(11):1227–32.. [cited 2019 Feb 17]. Available from: http://www.ncbi.nlm.nih.gov/pubmed/25240281.
56. Carli M, Ferrari A, Mattke A, Zanetti I, Casanova M, Bisogno G, et al. Pediatric malignant peripheral nerve sheath tumor: the Italian and German soft tissue sarcoma cooperative group. J Clin Oncol. 2005;23(33):8422–30.. [cited 2019 Feb 17]. Available from: http://www.ncbi.nlm.nih.gov/pubmed/16293873.
57. Uusitalo E, Rantanen M, Kallionpää RA, Pöyhönen M, Leppävirta J, Ylä-Outinen H, et al. Distinctive cancer associations in patients with neurofibromatosis type 1. J Clin Oncol.

2016;34(17):1978–86.. [cited 2019 Feb 23]. Available from: http://www.ncbi.nlm.nih.gov/pubmed/26926675.
58. Rasmussen SA, Yang Q, Friedman JM. Mortality in neurofibromatosis 1: an analysis using U.S. death certificates. Am J Hum Genet. 2001;68(5):1110–8.
59. De Raedt T, Brems H, Wolkenstein P, Vidaud D, Pilotti S, Perrone F, et al. Elevated risk for MPNST in NF1 microdeletion patients. Am J Hum Genet. 2003;72(5):1288–92.. [cited 2019 Feb 18]. Available from: http://linkinghub.elsevier.com/retrieve/pii/S0002929707606569.
60. Pasmant E, Sabbagh A, Spurlock G, Laurendeau I, Grillo E, Hamel M-J, et al. NF1 microdeletions in neurofibromatosis type 1: from genotype to phenotype. Hum Mutat. 2010;31(6):E1506–18. [cited 2019 Feb 23]. Available from: http://www.ncbi.nlm.nih.gov/pubmed/20513137.
61. Legius E, Marchuk DA, Collins FS, Glover TW. Somatic deletion of the neurofibromatosis type 1 gene in a neurofibrosarcoma supports a tumour suppressor gene hypothesis. Nat Genet. 1993;3(2):122–6.. [cited 2019 Feb 23]. Available from: http://www.nature.com/articles/ng0293-122
62. Hirbe AC, Dahiya S, Miller CA, Li T, Fulton RS, Zhang X, et al. Whole exome sequencing reveals the order of genetic changes during malignant transformation and metastasis in a single patient with NF1-plexiform Neurofibroma. Clin Cancer Res. 2015;21(18):4201–11.. [cited 2019 Feb 18]. Available from: http://clincancerres.aacrjournals.org/cgi/doi/10.1158/1078-0432.CCR-14-3049.
63. Kresse SH, Skårn M, Ohnstad HO, Namløs HM, Bjerkehagen B, Myklebost O, et al. DNA copy number changes in high-grade malignant peripheral nerve sheath tumors by array CGH. Mol Cancer. 2008;7(1):48.. [cited 2019 Feb 21]. Available from: http://molecular-cancer.biomedcentral.com/articles/10.1186/1476-4598-7-48.
64. Mantripragada KK, de Ståhl TD, Patridge C, Menzel U, Andersson R, Chuzhanova N, et al. Genome-wide high-resolution analysis of DNA copy number alterations in NF1-associated malignant peripheral nerve sheath tumors using 32K BAC array. Genes Chromosom Cancer. 2009;48(10):897–907.. [cited 2019 Feb 23]. Available from: http://www.ncbi.nlm.nih.gov/pubmed/19603524.
65. Brems H, Beert E, de Ravel T, Legius E. Mechanisms in the pathogenesis of malignant tumours in neurofibromatosis type 1. Lancet Oncol. 2009;10(5):508–15.. [cited 2019 Feb 17]. Available from: http://www.ncbi.nlm.nih.gov/pubmed/19410195.
66. Sohier P, Luscan A, Lloyd A, Ashelford K, Laurendeau I, Briand-Suleau A, et al. Confirmation of mutation landscape of NF1-associated malignant peripheral nerve sheath tumors. Genes Chromosomes Cancer. 2017;56(5):421–6. [cited 2019 Feb 23]. Available from: http://doi.wiley.com/10.1002/gcc.22446.
67. Moretti VM, Crawford EA, Staddon AP, Lackman RD, Ogilvie CM. Early outcomes for malignant peripheral nerve sheath tumor treated with chemotherapy. Am J Clin Oncol. 2011;34(4):417–21. [cited 2019 Feb 23]. Available from: https://insights.ovid.com/crossref?an=00000421-201108000-00014.
68. Katz D, Lazar A, Lev D. Malignant peripheral nerve sheath tumour (MPNST): the clinical implications of cellular signalling pathways. Expert Rev Mol Med. 2009;11:e30.. [cited 2019 Feb 21]. Available from: http://www.journals.cambridge.org/abstract_S1462399409001227.
69. Kim A, Pratilas CA. The promise of signal transduction in genetically driven sarcomas of the nerve. Exp Neurol. 2018;299(Pt B):317–25.. [cited 2019 Feb 21]. Available from: http://www.ncbi.nlm.nih.gov/pubmed/28859862.
70. Castellsagué J, Gel B, Fernández-Rodríguez J, Llatjós R, Blanco I, Benavente Y, et al. Comprehensive establishment and characterization of orthoxenograft mouse models of malignant peripheral nerve sheath tumors for personalized medicine. EMBO Mol Med. 2015;7(5):608–27. Available from: http://www.ncbi.nlm.nih.gov/pubmed/25810463/n; http://www.pubmedcentral.nih.gov/articlerender.fcgi?artid=PMC4492820.
71. Upadhyaya M, Spurlock G, Monem B, Thomas N, Friedrich RE, Kluwe L, et al. Germline and somatic NF1 gene mutations in plexiform neurofibromas. Hum Mutat. 2008;29(8):E103–11. [cited 2019 Feb 23]. Available from: http://www.ncbi.nlm.nih.gov/pubmed/18484666.

72. Yu J, Deshmukh H, Payton JE, Dunham C, Scheithauer BW, Tihan T, et al. Array-based comparative genomic hybridization identifies CDK4 and FOXM1 alterations as independent predictors of survival in malignant peripheral nerve sheath tumor. Clin Cancer Res. 2011;17(7):1924–34.. [cited 2019 Feb 23]. Available from: http://www.ncbi.nlm.nih.gov/pubmed/21325289.
73. Upadhyaya M, Spurlock G, Thomas L, Thomas NST, Richards M, Mautner V-F, et al. Microarray-based copy number analysis of neurofibromatosis type-1 (NF1)-associated malignant peripheral nerve sheath tumors reveals a role for Rho-GTPase pathway genes in NF1 tumorigenesis. Hum Mutat. 2012;33(4):763–76.. [cited 2019 Feb 23]. Available from: http://www.ncbi.nlm.nih.gov/pubmed/22331697.
74. Kolberg M, Høland M, Lind GE, Ågesen TH, Skotheim RI, Sundby Hall K, et al. Protein expression of BIRC5, TK1, and TOP2A in malignant peripheral nerve sheath tumours – a prognostic test after surgical resection. Mol Oncol. 2015;9(6):1129–39. [cited 2019 Feb 21]. Available from: http://www.ncbi.nlm.nih.gov/pubmed/25769404.
75. Adamowicz M, Radlwimmer B, Rieker RJ, Mertens D, Schwarzbach M, Schraml P, et al. Frequent amplifications and abundant expression of TRIO, NKD2, and IRX2 in soft tissue sarcomas. Genes Chromosom Cancer. 2006;45(9):829–38. [cited 2019 Feb 17]. Available from: http://www.ncbi.nlm.nih.gov/pubmed/16752383.
76. Karube K, Nabeshima K, Ishiguro M, Harada M, Iwasaki H. cDNA microarray analysis of cancer associated gene expression profiles in malignant peripheral nerve sheath tumours. J Clin Pathol. 2006;59(2):160–5. [cited 2019 Feb 21]. Available from: http://jcp.bmj.com/cgi/doi/10.1136/jcp.2004.023598.
77. Brekke HR, Ribeiro FR, Kolberg M, Agesen TH, Lind GE, Eknaes M, et al. Genomic changes in chromosomes 10, 16, and X in malignant peripheral nerve sheath tumors identify a high-risk patient group. J Clin Oncol. 2010;28(9):1573–82. [cited 2019 Feb 17]. Available from: http://ascopubs.org/doi/10.1200/JCO.2009.24.8989.
78. Spurlock G, Knight SJL, Thomas N, Kiehl T-R, Guha A, Upadhyaya M. Molecular evolution of a neurofibroma to malignant peripheral nerve sheath tumor (MPNST) in an NF1 patient: correlation between histopathological, clinical and molecular findings. J Cancer Res Clin Oncol. 2010;136(12):1869–80. [cited 2019 Feb 23]. Available from: http://www.ncbi.nlm.nih.gov/pubmed/20229272.
79. Yang J, Ylipaa A, Sun Y, Zheng H, Chen K, Nykter M, et al. Genomic and molecular characterization of malignant peripheral nerve sheath tumor identifies the IGF1R pathway as a primary target for treatment. Clin Cancer Res. 2011;17(24):7563–73. [cited 2019 Feb 23]. Available from: http://www.ncbi.nlm.nih.gov/pubmed/22042973.
80. Ferrer M, Gosline SJC, Stathis M, Zhang X, Guo X, Guha R, et al. Pharmacological and genomic profiling of neurofibromatosis type 1 plexiform neurofibroma-derived schwann cells. Sci Data. 2018;5:180106.. [cited 2019 Feb 18]. Available from: http://www.ncbi.nlm.nih.gov/pubmed/29893754.
81. Gosline SJC, Weinberg H, Knight P, Yu T, Guo X, Prasad N, et al. A high-throughput molecular data resource for cutaneous neurofibromas. Sci Data. 2017;4:170045.. [cited 2019 Feb 18]. Available from: http://www.nature.com/articles/sdata201745.
82. Zhang M, Wang Y, Jones S, Sausen M, McMahon K, Sharma R, et al. Somatic mutations of SUZ12 in malignant peripheral nerve sheath tumors. Nat Genet. 2014;46(11):1170–2.. [cited 2019 Feb 23]. Available from: http://www.ncbi.nlm.nih.gov/pubmed/25305755.
83. Brohl AS, Kahen E, Yoder SJ, Teer JK, Reed DR. The genomic landscape of malignant peripheral nerve sheath tumors: diverse drivers of Ras pathway activation. Sci Rep. 2017;7(1):14992.. [cited 2019 Feb 17]. Available from: http://www.nature.com/articles/s41598-017-15183-1.
84. Abeshouse A, Adebamowo C, Adebamowo SN, Akbani R, Akeredolu T, Ally A, et al. Comprehensive and integrated genomic characterization of adult soft tissue sarcomas. Cell. 2017;171(4):950–965.e28. [cited 2019 Feb 17]. Available from: http://www.ncbi.nlm.nih.gov/pubmed/29100075.

85. Sun D, Tainsky MA, Haddad R. Oncogene mutation survey in MPNST cell lines enhances the dominant role of hyperactive Ras in NF1 associated pro-survival and malignancy. Transl Oncogenomics. 2012;5:1–7. [cited 2019 Feb 23]. Available from: http://access.portico.org/stable?au=phw17ww43bd.
86. Bottillo I, Ahlquist T, Brekke H, Danielsen SA, van den Berg E, Mertens F, et al. Germline and somatic NF1 mutations in sporadic and NF1-associated malignant peripheral nerve sheath tumours. J Pathol. 2009;217(5):693–701. [cited 2019 Feb 17]. Available from: http://doi.wiley.com/10.1002/path.2494.
87. Pasmant E, Sabbagh A, Masliah-Planchon J, Ortonne N, Laurendeau I, Melin L, et al. Role of noncoding RNA ANRIL in genesis of plexiform neurofibromas in neurofibromatosis type 1. JNCI J Natl Cancer Inst. 2011;103(22):1713–22.. [cited 2019 Feb 23]. Available from: http://www.ncbi.nlm.nih.gov/pubmed/22034633.
88. Legius E, Dierick H, Wu R, Hall BK, Marynen P, Cassiman JJ, et al. TP53 mutations are frequent in malignant NF1 tumors. Genes Chromosomes Cancer. 1994;10(4):250–5. [cited 2019 Feb 23]. Available from: http://www.ncbi.nlm.nih.gov/pubmed/7522538.
89. Verdijk RM, den Bakker MA, Dubbink HJ, Hop WCJ, Dinjens WNM, Kros JM. *TP53* mutation analysis of malignant peripheral nerve sheath tumors. J Neuropathol Exp Neurol. 2010;69(1):16–26.. [cited 2019 Feb 23]. Available from: http://www.ncbi.nlm.nih.gov/pubmed/20010306.
90. Subramanian S, Thayanithy V, West RB, Lee C-H, Beck AH, Zhu S, et al. Genome-wide transcriptome analyses reveal p53 inactivation mediated loss of miR-34a expression in malignant peripheral nerve sheath tumours. J Pathol. 2010;220(1):58–70.. [cited 2019 Feb 23]. Available from: http://doi.wiley.com/10.1002/path.2633.
91. De Raedt T, Beert E, Pasmant E, Luscan A, Brems H, Ortonne N, et al. PRC2 loss amplifies Ras-driven transcription and confers sensitivity to BRD4-based therapies. Nature. 2014;514(7521):247–51. [cited 2019 Feb 18]. Available from: http://www.ncbi.nlm.nih.gov/pubmed/25119042.
92. Miller SJSJSJ, Jessen WJWJWJ, Mehta J, Hardiman A, Sites E, Kaiser S, et al. Integrative genomic analyses of neurofibromatosis tumours identify SOX9 as a biomarker and survival gene. EMBO Mol Med. 2009;1(4):236–48. [cited 2019 Feb 23]. Available from: http://www.ncbi.nlm.nih.gov/pubmed/20049725.
93. Miller SJ, Rangwala F, Williams J, Ackerman P, Kong S, Jegga AG, et al. Large-scale molecular comparison of human schwann cells to malignant peripheral nerve sheath tumor cell lines and tissues. Cancer Res. 2006;66(5):2584–91. [cited 2019 Feb 23]. Available from: http://cancerres.aacrjournals.org/lookup/doi/10.1158/0008-5472.CAN-05-3330.
94. Lévy P, Ripoche H, Laurendeau I, Lazar V, Ortonne N, Parfait B, et al. Microarray-based identification of *Tenascin C* and *Tenascin XB*, genes possibly involved in tumorigenesis associated with Neurofibromatosis type 1. Clin Cancer Res. 2007;13(2):398–407. [cited 2019 Feb 23]. Available from: http://www.ncbi.nlm.nih.gov/pubmed/17202312.
95. Thomas LE, Winston J, Rad E, Mort M, Dodd KM, Tee AR, et al. Evaluation of copy number variation and gene expression in neurofibromatosis type-1-associated malignant peripheral nerve sheath tumours. Hum Genomics. 2015;9(1):3. [cited 2019 Feb 23]. Available from: http://www.ncbi.nlm.nih.gov/pubmed/25884485.
96. Feber A, Wilson GA, Zhang L, Presneau N, Idowu B, Down TA, et al. Comparative methylome analysis of benign and malignant peripheral nerve sheath tumors. Genome Res. 2011;21(4):515–24. Available from: http://genome.cshlp.org/cgi/doi/10.1101/gr.109678.110.
97. Itani S, Kunisada T, Morimoto Y, Yoshida A, Sasaki T, Ito S, et al. MicroRNA-21 correlates with tumorigenesis in malignant peripheral nerve sheath tumor (MPNST) via programmed cell death protein 4 (PDCD4). J Cancer Res Clin Oncol. 2012;138(9):1501–9.. [cited 2019 Feb 19]. Available from: http://link.springer.com/10.1007/s00432-012-1223-1.
98. Presneau N, Eskandarpour M, Shemais T, Henderson S, Halai D, Tirabosco R, et al. MicroRNA profiling of peripheral nerve sheath tumours identifies miR-29c as a tumour suppressor gene involved in tumour progression. Br J Cancer. 2013;108(4):964–72.. [cited 2019 Feb 23]. Available from: http://www.ncbi.nlm.nih.gov/pubmed/23175151.

99. Watson MA, Perry A, Tihan T, Prayson RA, Guha A, Bridge J, et al. Gene expression profiling reveals unique molecular subtypes of neurofibromatosis type I-associated and sporadic malignant peripheral nerve sheath tumors. Brain Pathol. 2004;14(3):297–303. [cited 2019 Feb 23]. Available from: http://www.ncbi.nlm.nih.gov/pubmed/15446585.
100. Fletcher CDM. The evolving classification of soft tissue tumours - an update based on the new 2013 WHO classification. Histopathology. 2014;64(1):2–11.. [cited 2019 Feb 18]. Available from: http://www.ncbi.nlm.nih.gov/pubmed/24164390.
101. Taylor BS, Barretina J, Maki RG, Antonescu CR, Singer S, Ladanyi M. Advances in sarcoma genomics and new therapeutic targets. Nat Rev Cancer. 2011;11(8):541–57.. [cited 2019 Feb 23]. Available from: http://www.ncbi.nlm.nih.gov/pubmed/21753790.
102. Nagayama S, Katagiri T, Tsunoda T, Hosaka T, Nakashima Y, Araki N, et al. Genome-wide analysis of gene expression in synovial sarcomas using a cDNA microarray. Cancer Res. 2002;62(20):5859–66. [cited 2019 Feb 23]. Available from: http://www.ncbi.nlm.nih.gov/pubmed/12384549.
103. Sanchez-Vega F, Mina M, Armenia J, Chatila WK, Luna A, La KC, et al. Oncogenic signaling pathways in the cancer genome atlas. Cell. 2018;173(2):321–337.e10. [cited 2019 Feb 23]. Available from: http://www.ncbi.nlm.nih.gov/pubmed/29625050.
104. Chibon F, Lagarde P, Salas S, Pérot G, Brouste V, Tirode F, et al. Validated prediction of clinical outcome in sarcomas and multiple types of cancer on the basis of a gene expression signature related to genome complexity. Nat Med. 2010;16(7):781–7. [cited 2019 Feb 18]. Available from: http://www.ncbi.nlm.nih.gov/pubmed/20581836.
105. Dufresne A, Brahmi M, Karanian M, Blay J-Y. Using biology to guide the treatment of sarcomas and aggressive connective-tissue tumours. Nat Rev Clin Oncol. 2018;15(7):443–58.. [cited 2019 Feb 18]. Available from: http://www.nature.com/articles/s41571-018-0012-4.

Mechanotransduction and NF1 Loss—Partner in Crime: New Hints for Neurofibroma Genesis

10

Federica Chiara

Contents

10.1 Introduction

Neurofibromas are complex benign nerve sheath tumors, whose morbidity is mainly due to accumulation of fibrotic tissue in which NF1$^{-/-}$ Schwann cells (SCs) undergo uncontrolled proliferation, thus compressing nerves, organs, and blood vessels. Plexiform neurofibromas (PNs) are a subset of neurofibromas for which there are few options of treatment, and complete surgical removal is often not feasible due to PN location, infiltration, and size. PNs can progress to highly malignant sarcomas termed MPNSTs (malignant peripheral nerve sheath tumors), which are almost invariably lethal [1].

Neurofibromin (NF1), the product of the *NF1* gene, is a Ras-GAP controlling the GTPase activity of the p21Ras proto-oncogene. NF1 heterozygous cells display hyperactivation of Ras, which further increases when loss of heterozygosity (LOH) occurs at the NF1 locus [2]. Thus, activation of Ras/Raf/ERK signaling in SCs is sufficient to make them more susceptible to proliferative signals provided by a NF1$^{+/-}$ niche [3]. Nonetheless, the physiological response to Ras hyperactivation is cell-cycle arrest and/or senescence rather than transformation. Ras-mediated

F. Chiara (✉)
Department of Surgery, Oncology and Gastroenterology, University of Padova, Padova, Italy
e-mail: federica.chiara@unipd.it

G. Tadini et al. (eds.), *Multidisciplinary Approach to Neurofibromatosis Type 1*,
https://doi.org/10.1007/978-3-319-92450-2_10

transformation of SCs probably relies on a stepwise process that integrates circuits of amplification signals from the local environment [4, 5].

The current view is that the tumorigenic proliferation of NF1 heterozygous SCs depends on an inflammatory milieu triggering a robust burst of mitogenic signals from both collagen-secreting fibroblasts and pericytes in which $NF1^{+/-}$ mast cells ($MCsNF1^{+/-}$) could play a pivotal role [6]. $MCsNF1^{+/-}$ are present in large amount in neurofibroma microenvironment and have a central role in sustaining chronic inflammation, cell proliferation, and extracellular matrix (ECM) deposition leading to fibrotic tissue deposition [7]. However, this model does not clarify the molecular networks required for providing SCs with the tumorigenic properties they have in PNs, such as the ability of growing in the absence of basal membrane binding, a high proliferative potential, and a profound metabolic rewiring. To better understand the role of the $NF1^{+/-}$ niche in PN progression, we will put the scientific data collected in this research field in the wider conceptual framework emerging from the most recent studies in molecular oncology. Several lines of evidence mechanistically link fibrosis and cancer in the triad "wound healing/chronic fibrosis/cancer" (WHFC) inspired by the old concept that "tumor is a wound that does not heal." This view is based on the observation that the same cell types, as well as the same soluble and matrix elements that drive wound healing also fuel chronic fibrosis and tumor progression via distinct signaling pathways [8]. The final product of chronic fibrosis is an abnormal, fibrotic ECM, with specific settings of biochemical and biomechanical properties. The consequent dysregulation of mechanical homeostasis by new biomechanical forces generated by this anomalous ECM can drive tumor aggressiveness by inducing a mesenchymal-like switch in mutated cells so that they attain tumor-initiating or stem-like cell properties [9]. Thus, while genetic modifications in tumor cells unquestionably initiate tumor growth, a dynamically evolving ECM might determine its progression by modulating the behavior of both "initiated cells" and cancer-associated stromal cells [10]. In this scenario, PNs may arise from the primary event of NF1 loss in SCs that become more sensitive both to mitogenic stimuli of growth factors provided by chronic inflammation and to the ECM-derived mechanical stress, potently committing cells to transformation through a complex orchestration of changes in the genomic landscape of SCs cells. Importantly, high mechanical stress in solid tumors can impede drug delivery and may drive tumor progression toward malignancy. Therefore, a better understanding of these processes might provide hints for the design of novel anti-neoplastic drugs and strategies.

10.2 The Dark Side of Tissue Repair: Fibrosis

Fibrosis is defined as the excessive accumulation of fibrous connective tissue (components of the ECM such as collagen and fibronectin) in and around inflamed or damaged tissue, which can lead to permanent scarring and organ malfunction [11]. In physiological conditions ECM is a complex network of macromolecules that assemble into three-dimensional supramolecular structures [12, 13]. This molecular meshwork maintains the hydration and pH of the local microenvironment and regulates the availability of growth factors and cytokines, thus controlling growth, survival, motility, and differentiation of cells by tuning the ligation to specific cell receptors [14–16]. After tissue injury, inflammation prompts a reparative response called wound healing (WH) through the potent activation of macrophages and mast cells (MCs) [17, 18]. WH substitutes damaged cells with a collagen-enriched ECM, thus creating a scar endowed with strong, elastic fibers aligned in a parallel fashion (immature ECM) whose contraction permits the closure of the wound. Repetitive or persistent injurious stimuli determine chronic fibrosis, thus prolonging inflammation and indefinitely triggering an aberrant WH that leads to the formation of mature fibrotic ECM known as a scar. Under these dyshomeostatic conditions, the equilibrium between the population of M2 type macrophages that promote fibrosis (and are pro-neoplastic in the tumor microenvironment) and M1 type macrophages that drive the inflammatory response and are anti-fibrotic (and tumor suppressive in a neoplastic mass) is unbalanced, with M2 macrophages prevailing [19, 20]. Recent data indicate that also MCs are involved in all phases of WH/fibrotic cascade. MCs are chemoattracted by anaphylatoxins C3a and C5a of the complement system. Depending on the WH stage, MCs produce and secrete both tissue plasminogen activator (tPA) in its free and enzymatically active form and plasminogen, key components of the plasminogen/fibrinolytic system involved in fibrin homeostasis (i.e., resorption of blood clots) and tissue remodeling [20–22]. This suggests that MCs cooperate with macrophages in this process. Once a clot is created, MCs avoid further fibrin accumulation by prolonging the bleeding time [23] and by secreting the tryptase–heparin complexes that degrade fibrinogen in order to avoid its excessive conversion into fibrin by thrombin [24]. Mouse MCs express the thrombin receptor Par-1 [22] that triggers the release of fibrinogen-destroying tryptase–heparin complexes when the local concentration of thrombin is unusually high. In support of these data, some pediatric mastocytosis patients who have an excess of hTryptase-β+/heparin+ MCs in their tissues have excessive bleeding of their skin and gastrointestinal tract [25, 26]. These findings suggest an explanation of the concurrent association of neurofibromatosis type I and ulcerative colitis [27] reported in still few but significant clinical cases, being mast cells implicated in the pathogenesis of both diseases [28]. MCs act as scavengers of cell debris and, in conjunction with macrophages, help to generate new tissue through growth factors secretion (proliferation phase). In addition, MCs secrete the serine protease chymase that promotes both secretion and activation of TGF-beta, the main factor triggering ECM deposition, in different cell types (ECM deposition phase) [29, 30].

Under the potent stimulation of TGF-beta and of growth factors such as platelet-derived growth factor (PDGF), which are secreted by both macrophages and mast cells, and of tensional forces exerted by the fibrotic ECM, fibroblasts proliferate and differentiate into myofibroblasts. This population of stromal cells displays a high capacity to synthesize ECM components that exert further tensile forces [31–33]. Therefore, myofibroblasts can promote the formation of large, rigid collagen bundles that mechanically strengthen and stiffen the tissue after their crosslinking by lysyl oxidases (LOX) enzymes and eventually contribute to wound closure.

Hyperproliferation of these stromal cells and of other cell types is a hallmark of aberrant wound healing sustained by chronic inflammation [34]. In experimental models of renal, pulmonary, and cardiac fibrosis, endothelial cells can switch to a mesenchymal phenotype, a process known as endothelial–mesenchymal transition (EndMT). It is possible to envision that also in PN microenvironment EndMT, together with epithelial–mesenchymal transition (EMT), can contribute to fibroblast accumulation, which in turn can generate mesenchymal cells that express the myofibroblast markers αSMA (smooth muscle protein A) and smooth muscle protein 22α. However, it is unclear whether functional myofibroblasts seen in fibrosis or cancer derive from epithelial or endothelial cells. Certainly, vascular endothelial cells have demonstrated considerable plasticity to generate other cell types during embryonic development and disease progression [35].

Among the signaling pathways that control transition to a mesenchymal phenotype, transforming growth factor-β (TGFβ) family signaling has a predominant role through the SMAD3/β-catenin axis. In response to TGFβ, SMAD3 induces expression and nuclear import of transcription factor MRTFs and cooperates with MRTFs to induce myofibroblast differentiation, partly by inducing the expression of SNAIL2 [36, 37]. In addition, β-catenin, which is released from cell-to-cell tight junctions, antagonizes the inhibitory effect of SMAD3 on the MRTF–SRF complex, which in turn increases αSMA expression. A variety of other cell types may be recruited and differentiated into myofibroblasts [38]. For instance, in injured liver, both portal fibroblasts and hepatic stellate cells can generate myofibroblasts, depending on the site and type of damage. In the nerve, both interstitial pericytes and fibroblasts are supposed to be a major source of myofibroblast recruitment [39].

With the intent to explain the hyperproliferative phenotype of SCs in neurofibromas, Parrinello et al. proposed that $NF1^{-/-}$ SCs possess a lower ability to bind and wrap axons due to decreased expression of Sema 4F, one of the molecules involved in this process. In their mouse model, $NF^{+/-}$ nerves present a subtle axonal segregation defect that becomes evident in bundles constituted by C-fiber axons (unmyelinated axons) or Remak bundles. Postnatally, Remark bundles show an increased number of unsorted axons, defined as unstable. According to this model, over time these defects result both in disruption of the bundles and in inadequate Schwann cell–axonal interactions, leading to neuropathy. As expected, axonal damage triggers the rapid de-differentiation of Schwann cells, which revert to a progenitor-like state and enter cell cycle. Concomitantly, an inflammatory response initiates, with recruitment of macrophages and masts cells, which clear myelin and axonal debris and elicit a robust cytokine and growth factor stimulation of the stromal cells. The authors state that, while in normal tissues there is the activation of molecular mechanisms that silence the WH process, a self-sustaining WH loop is established in NF1 neurons, once the inflammatory response is elicited. It has been speculated that this "chronic inflammatory loop" depends on a continuous process of SC dissociation, de-differentiation, and proliferation, together with infiltration of immune cells and ECM deposition [6, 40]. $NF^{+/-}$ MCs fuel this "chronic inflammation," as Ras hyperactivation prompts multiple gain-of-function effects. $NF^{+/-}$ MCs overexpress the c-Kit receptor, a key regulator of mast cell generation and bioactivity and therefore

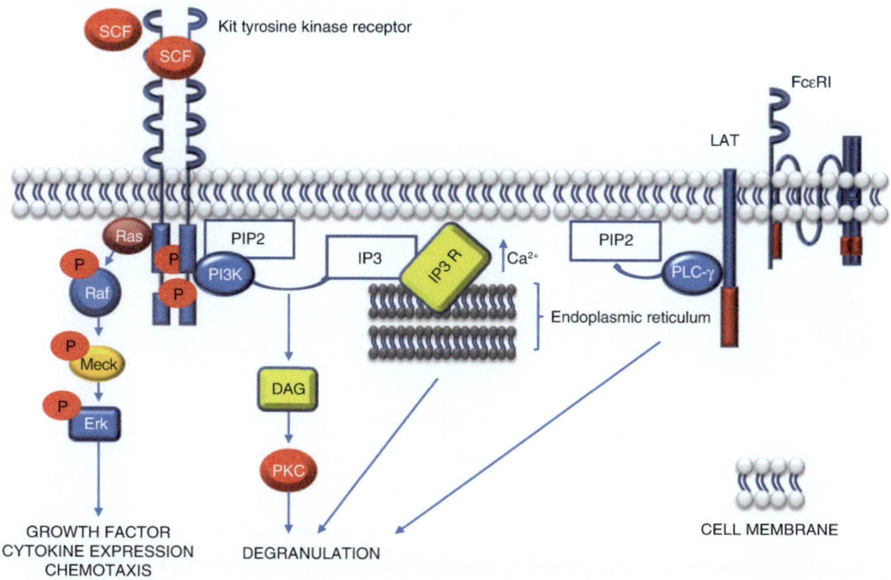

Fig. 10.1 Kit tyrosine kinase receptor activation is essential for mast cell growth, differentiation, and survival and for inducing mast cell migration/homing through chemotaxis. KIT catalytic activity and downstream signaling is initiated upon dimerization induced by binding of its specific ligand stem cell factor (SCF) or random collisions favored by receptor overexpression. The consensus of studies on mast cells suggests that downstream signaling generated by activated KIT alone is insufficient to induce degranulation but it cooperates with the high affinity for IgE receptor, FcεRI via PI3K signaling that ultimately elicits PKC activation. In addition, following aggregation with FcεRI, the adaptor molecule LAT (linker for activation of T cells) becomes phosphorylated in a LYN- and SYK (spleen tyrosine kinase)-dependent manner. This results in direct or indirect binding to LAT of the cytosolic adaptor molecules PLC-γ triggering degranulation. Kit receptor activation induces cytokine production and chemotaxis through Ras/Erk axis. *DAG* diacylglycerol, *IP3* inositol-1,4,5-trisphosphate, *PIP2* phosphatidylinositol-4,5-bisphosphate

the number of MCs recruited at the inflammatory site in a c-Kit-dependent way is higher in NF1 patients compared to healthy individual [7]. Moreover, c-Kit-dependent processes as cell proliferation, survival, migration, and degranulation *in vitro* and *in vivo* are increased, as Ras is an effector of the c-Kit receptor (Fig. 10.1), [29, 41]. Accordingly, knocking-down the c-kit gene in the hematopoietic differentiation lineage prevents tumorigenesis in a PN murine model [42]. Transplantation experiments have shown that these aberrant MCs critically sustain tumor microenvironment through trophic support. Notably, the amount of secreted, pro-inflammatory cytokines is increased in $NF^{+/-}$ MCs [43]. For instance, Yang et al. demonstrated that $NF1^{+/-}$ MCs secrete 2.5-fold higher levels of TGF-β than WT mast cells *in vitro* [42] (Fig. 10.2). These data increasingly support the idea that $NF1^{+/-}$ MCs are critical effectors in the paracrine induction of neurofibroma pathogenesis.

It is now well established that MCs correlate with NF1-associated PNs, and several evidences suggest that they take part in the process of neurofibromagenesis.

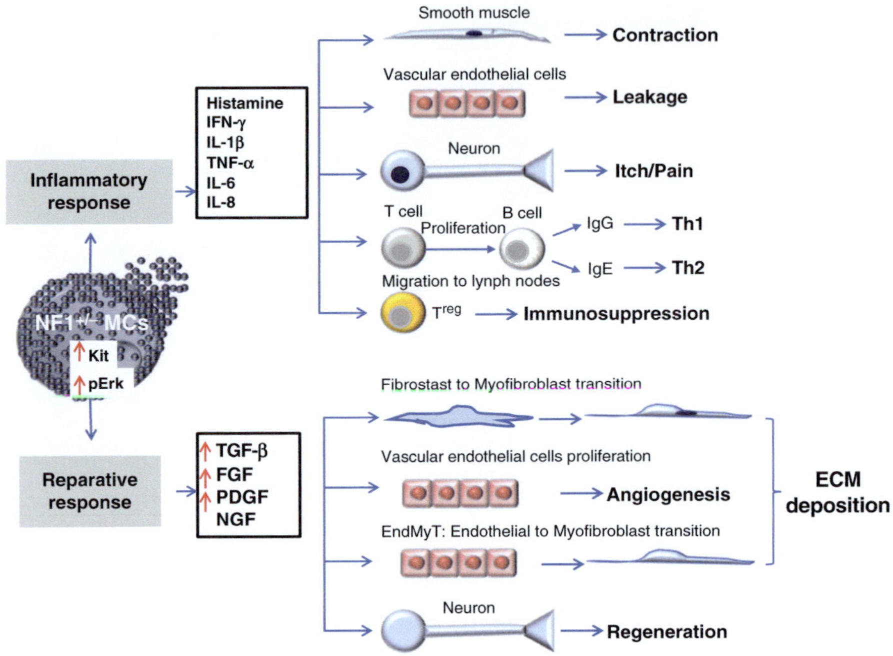

Fig. 10.2 Mast cells (MCs) during wound healing govern both inflammatory and reparative pathway. MCs secreted histamine acts through its various receptors to induce smooth muscle contraction or relaxation, enhanced permeability across vascular endothelial cells, and itching or pain by activating sensory neurons. Production of a wide range of cytokines and chemokines promotes adaptive immune responses (Th1 and Th2) and immunosuppression. The figure shows that in $NF1^{-/+}$ MCs both growth factors and cytokine secretion are increased under the control of an overactivated Kit tyrosine kinase receptor due to both increased ligand stimulation and random collisions

Tucker et al. examined the density and distribution of MCs within NF1-associated neurofibromas classified histologically as encapsulated or diffuse based on the presence or absence of the perineurium. They observed that mast cell density and distribution differentiate the two basic types of NF1-associated neurofibromas and correlated with the invasiveness behavior of PN [44]. Coherently, $NF1^{-/-}$ Schwann cells overexpress the ligand of tyrosine kinase receptor c-Kit, the stem cell factor (SCF), which is responsible for increased attraction of mast cells. Remarkably, Vincent Riccardi reported a successful therapy after a long treatment with Ketotifen, a potent MC stabilizer. He described amelioration of neurofibroma-associated itching, pain, and tenderness, and patients reported that there was a consistent improvement in a general sense of well-being, considering the decrease in the rates of appearance and growth of cutaneous neurofibromas [45]. This evident benefit is consistent with recent reports accounting for a functional cooperation between MCs and axons in pain control. The proximity between MCs and neurons potentiates critical molecular crosstalks that result in a synergistic contribution to the initiation and propagation of long-term changes in pain responses to chronic inflammation via intricate signal networks of neurotransmitters, cytokines, and adhesion molecules [46]. Sensory and autonomic (essentially sympathetic) nerves are present within the skin and influence a variety of physiological and pathological cutaneous functions. During inflammation or trauma, and particularly during WH, a significant increase in levels of neuromediators occurs [47]. This effect is MC dependent and plays an important regulatory role; however, further studies are needed to mechanistically elucidate this functional connection.

In light of these observations, a therapeutic strategy based on MC stabilizers could be an advisable choice to tackle several NF1-associated symptoms, such as persistent itching, hypertrophic scars, congenital melanocytic nevi, or autoimmune diseases, only citing few of them that might rely on MC deregulation [26]. Vincent Riccardi was the first to propose important connections between Nf1 loss and excessive WH [48]. Hence, knockout mice have shown fibroblast hyperplasia and increased collagen accumulation [49]. In 2007, Miyawaki et al. investigated whether wounds produced in the patients with NF1 produce keloid or hypertrophic scars. This study showed that the patients with NF-1 and PN form scars without keloid or hypertrophic changes, whereas those with a solitary neurofibroma after surgery had a higher risk to develop hypertrophic scars [50]. The following studies do not retrace the same path: Koivunen et al. found an equally effective epidermal WH between NF1 patients and healthy controls [49]. In addition, dermal WH appeared to function normally in NF1 patients based on retrospective and follow-up study of biopsy scars, suggesting that neurofibromin is not a crucial WH regulator. Given these different report data, more evidences are required to connect the etiology of PN and scar in a WH milieu.

Salgado et al. have functionally connected the Large/Giant Congenital Melanocytic Nevi, one of the NF1 hallmarks, with increased MC number and activity [51, 52]. In addition, histological analyses of fractures in mouse models that recapitulate features of the clinical pseudarthrosis of tibia (CPT) showed invasion by fibrous and highly proliferative tissue; mean amounts of fibrous tissue were increased upward of tenfold in fractures of $NF1^{-/-}$ mice compared to their wild type counterpart. In healed fractures, the increased proliferating, active ERK-positive cells were not osteoclasts but probably stromal cells, indicating that in CPT chronic inflammation stimulates their proliferation and that they seriously affect bone reconstitution in the fracture callus [53, 54]. CPT is also accompanied by proliferative disorders under inflammatory conditions in arteries and veins. Two reports [55, 56] describe thick-walled arteries and veins with a small lumen within the fibrotic tissue near the pseudarthrosis site. The proliferation rate of the periarteriolar tissue underneath the wound was increased and proliferative cells appeared positive for active ERK, suggesting that Nf1 loss, chronic fibrosis, and WH form a signaling system that alters tissue homeostasis independently of the kick-off stimulus. Yet, vasculopathies are frequent in NF1, as first observed by Vincent Riccardi, and vasculopathy is now well accepted as a NF1 hallmark [57–60]. Further work is required to mechanistically dissect and integrate these clinical and experimental observations. The most recent research on chronic fibrosis paves the way to reach this goal. Nancy Ratner's group published a computational analysis of the gene signature characteristics of the MC/SC network [61]. This work represents a step forward in understanding the major pathways involved in the interplay between these cell types and suggested a model by which decreased type-I interferon signaling plays a central role in neurofibroma growth.

In spite of their interest, these data need a note of caution. In fact, in other tumor models leukocyte subsets other than MCs do infiltrate, including both myeloid- and lymphoid-lineage cells that do not meet the classical definition of cells involved in an inflammatory immune response. For instance, in pancreatic carcinoma cellular immunity is greatly influenced by cytokines and chemokines that derive from tumor cells themselves (for example, IL-6, IL-1, IL-10, etc.) or by immune cells different from MCs (IL-4, IL-5, IL-13, IFN-γ, etc.), further enriching the complexity of the tumor microenvironment. The scenario is made more multifaceted by the discovery of new fibrogenic mesenchymal progenitor cells (MPCs) in the lungs of patients with idiopathic pulmonary fibrosis (IPF) suggesting the existence of fibrotic mechanisms that do not relate to inflammation [31, 62]. Taken together, these evidences suggest the possibility that molecular mechanisms alternative to MC-dependent inflammation might sustain fibrosis also in PNs. Therefore, while there are substantial evidences that early inflammation is a risk factor for PNs development, the molecular mechanisms accounting for the profound genomic changes should be placed in a progression model initiated by the biological changes triggered by the first genetic lesion, the LOH of the Nf1 gene, toward malignant transformation, under the biomechanical pressure elicited by fibrosis.

10.3 The Fibrotic Tissue as a Tumor Incubator: New Hints to Envision PN Development

Numerous clinical and pathological observations have established a clear relationship between inflammation, fibrosis, and cancer [8, 63]. A first observation highlighted that tumors are likened to wounds that fail to heal [64, 65]. In fact, tumor stroma exhibits some of the characteristics found in an unresolved wound [66] such as a "stiffened" microenvironment. In the present paragraph, we will report new findings dissecting the role of ECM stiffness on cancer development following a rational tread linking fibrosis and PN onset (Fig. 10.3).

Abnormal ECM deposition, remodeling, and posttranslational modifications of ECM components are today well-recognized incubators for cancer development. For instance, skin fibrosis associated with recessive dystrophic epidermolysis bullosa leads to highly metastatic skin carcinomas [67]; progressive lung scarring associated with IPF is a risk factor for lung cancer development [68]. In liver, persistent chronic inflammation has been associated with progressive hepatic fibrosis and the development of cirrhosis histologically characterized by destruction of liver tissue structure following a marked ECM accumulation. ECM stiffness is a prognostic factor of cirrhosis and correlates with hepatic adenocarcinoma onset [69]. Coherently, YAP transcription factor expression and activity, one of the hallmarks of the stiff ECM derived from the Hippo pathway, has been identified in fibrosis of the lung [70] and liver [71].

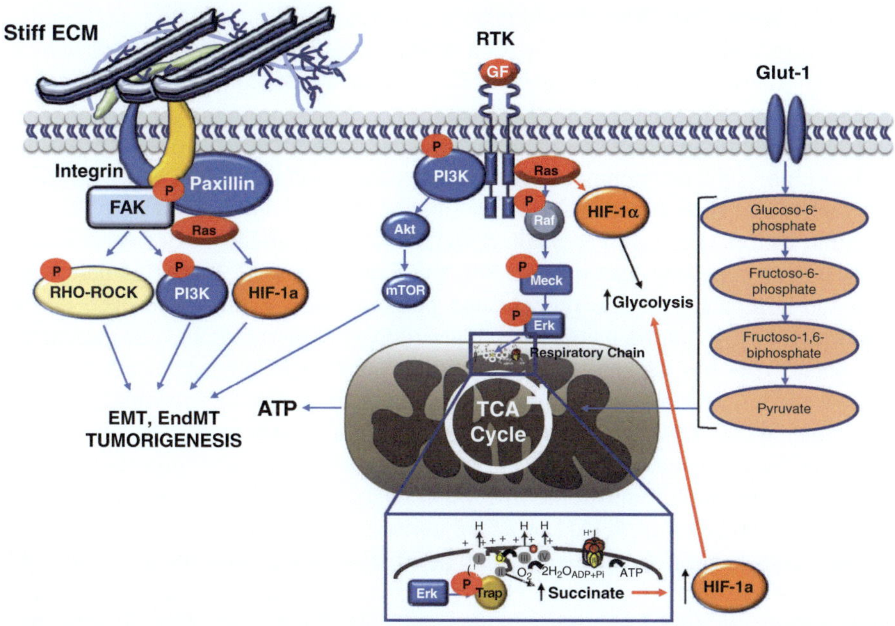

Fig. 10.3 Tumorigenesis is a complex program induced by the aberrant activation of different cellular processes. Both Extracellular matrix (ECM) stiffness and oncogenic activation of Ras GTPase represent two hits able to induce a radical change in the gene landscape of the cells. Cells bearing oncogenic mutations under ECM pressure respond with a profound gene expression renewal activating programs fundamental to orchestrate either the metabolic switch toward glycolysis or cell identity such as epithelial–mesenchymal transition (EMT) and endothelial–mesenchymal (End-MT) transition

Tissue measurement of the elastic modulus (stiffness) by atomic force microscopy (AFM) has confirmed the observation that local ECM of developing solid tumors is generally enriched of thick collagen fibers with respect to their normal counterparts. Although tumors are a gathering of stiff and compliant regions, tumors harboring the stiffest regions were overall the most aggressive [72]. In particular, patients with breast tumors containing the highest number of stiff regions within the stroma have the worst prognosis. Up to now, no study has been carried out to figure out whether ECM stiffness could represent a prognostic marker for growth or malignant transformation of PNs, despite the presence of a high number of stiff nodules in rapidly growing neurofibromas.

It is well known that a crucial event for cancer progression is the transition to a mesenchymal phenotype, forcing cells to undergo a global reprogramming toward the acquisition of structural and functional changes, including loss of cell polarity and tight cell–cell junctions. Very recent experimental studies provided the proof of concept that stiff ECM orchestrates a complex program for activation of a pro-wound repair state through continuous instructions to resident and invading immune and inflammatory cells and normal cell populations (i.e., pericytes, resident stem cells, fibroblasts) [31]. The physiological counterpart of this program is activated in cells during WH and is responsible for a gene expression rewiring in the sense of an epithelial–mesenchymal transition (EMT), initiated and controlled by signaling pathways that respond to extracellular cues.

EMT is a biological routine that plays essential roles during specific conditions, such as embryonic development. Its aberrant reactivation promotes cancer cell plasticity and fuels both tumor initiation and metastatic spread through a panel of transcription factors (EMT-TF) as Snail, SNAI226, ZEB1 and ZEB2, E47 (also known as TCF3), Krüppel-like factor 8 (KLF8), and Brachyury [73]. Emerging data highlight the complexity of the process and pinpoint aspects that have been poorly explored [74, 75]. Indeed, a high level of plasticity between epithelial and mesenchymal phenotypes has lately been proposed when cells displaying transient "hybrid" states were described [75]. This program is kept under control by a feedback process. An epithelial cell must be permissive to undergo a full EMT: the mesenchymal end-stage can be achieved when different regulatory networks are fundamentally disturbed; this probably requires the disruption of more than one molecular circuitry. Indeed, the activation of SNAI1 or ZEB2 transcription factors disturbs homeostasis in some tissues, but if the cell is not fully permissive, EMT is unable to occur. EMT in cells is often observed when the expression of an EMT transcription factor is combined with an additional acquired oncogenic activity. For instance, in pancreatic ductal adenocarcinoma (PDAC) concomitant activation of TWIST combined with a mutant K-Ras may set off EMT through different signaling cascades. The tumor progression model of the pancreatic adenocarcinoma indicates that ductal cells are first sensitized to EMT by K-Ras hyperactivation [76, 77]. The first evidence about a possible connection between Ras activation caused by neurofibromin loss and EMT dates back to 2010, when Arima et al. observed an increase in the mRNA and protein expression levels of EMT-related transcription factors in neurofibroma specimens and NF1-derived Schwann cells [78]. In 2012 Beak et al. identified neurofibromin as a key mediator of epicardial EMT and in the generation epicardial-derived cells (EPDCs). Mutant epicardial cells transitioned more readily to mesenchymal cells *in vitro* and *in vivo* and loss of Nf1 caused increased EPDC proliferation and resulted in more cardiac fibroblasts [79]. These data may explain the recurrence of cardiac hypertrophy, a phenotypic trait that is part of the spectrum of NF1-related diseases and in general of several other RASopathies, as Noonan Syndrome [80].

Although a mechanistic explanation functionally linking loss of neurofibromin and EMT has to be elucidated, inspired by PDAC model, it is possible to speculate that the double allelic mutation of *NF1* makes cells permissive to EMT, as it elicits Ras overactivation. Nonetheless, it has to be considered that loss of a RAS-GAP as neurofibromin compromises Ras inactivation only by hampering the Ras-associated GTPase function, whereas the oncogenic mutations of Ras keep it into a constitutive and growth factor independent activity and therefore have a wider impact on the enzyme and on the transduction pathway that stems from it. Hence, it is reasonable to envisage that $NF1^{-/-}$ cells need an additional stimulus that cooperates with deregulation of Ras signaling to drive the gene reprogramming required for EMT; such a stimulus could come from a stiff matrix.

Cells sense and convert exogenous forces into signaling pathways through a mechanism termed mechanotransduction. The best understood mechanotransduction mechanism is initiated through ECM-dependent integrin activation and clustering, resulting in vinculin activation that promotes focal adhesion assembly, focal adhesion kinase (FAK) and paxillin phosphorylation, subsequent Rho–ROCK-dependent actin remodeling, and reciprocal actomyosin-mediated cell contractility. ECM stiffness and elevated epithelial mechanosignaling enhance growth factor receptor-dependent PI3K signaling to foster malignant cell behavior. Meanwhile, tumor cells also generate high traction forces that disrupt cell–cell junctions, compromise tissue polarity, promote anchorage-independent survival, and enhance invasion through EMT [73].

A hallmark of EMT is the downregulation of E-cadherin to reinforce the destabilization of adherent's junctions. The EMT transitioning cells lose their association with epithelial cells and acquire an affinity for mesenchymal cells through homotypic N-cadherin interactions; these interactions are weaker than homotypic E-cadherin interactions and facilitate cell migration and invasion [74, 81]. EMT also activates the expression of neural cell adhesion molecule (NCAM), another adhesion molecule that interacts with N-cadherin to modulate the activity of RTKs that are associated with it [82]. NCAM interacts with the SRC family tyrosine kinase FYN to facilitate the assembly of focal adhesions, migration, and invasion. This is interesting in the NF1 perspective, as NCAM has been found in non-myelinating SCs from normal nerves and overexpressed by SCs from patients with chronic axonal neuropathies and Schwannomas. By contrast, its expression was lower in MPNST, probably because SC identity is lost in favor of dedifferentiated, highly invasive cells. Many of the pathological conditions described up to now express mesenchymal markers, as well as a stem-like molecular signature that has been associated with stiff ECM, to treatment resistance [83]. The therapeutic experience on PDAC clearly teaches that fibrotic tissue is a real barrier for several therapeutic molecules. The picture is made more complicated by the EMT that already has profoundly changed the gene expression pattern of the cells toward pluripotency and this is probably the reason why the trial with pirfenidone did not succeed on patients with NF1. Indeed, the Weaver group clearly showed that TGFβ- and other pro-fibrogenic growth factor inhibition is ineffective on PDAC since the thick and mature Collagen fibers are already formed and biomechanically control gene expression of both tumor and stromal cells [76]. However, new therapeutic strategies are under investigation, one of these has been suggested by Jian et al. [84]. The authors show that in PDAC tumors immunotherapy associated with Focal adhesion kinases (FAK inhibitor) could be a successful strategy.

One of the hallmarks of cancer development is rewiring of cellular metabolism [85]. It has long been postulated that cancer cells upregulate aerobic glycolysis in order to provide the building blocks necessary to rapidly proliferate [86]. Recently, the role of the mitochondri on as a biosynthetic "factory" for cancer cell proliferation has become more apparent [87], while accumulating evidences have shown a new interplay between biophysical forces and metabolism. According to this new model, Ras-dependent activation of PI3K/AKT signaling regulates the expression of glucose transporters, GLUT1 and GLUT4 [88], via hexokinase, thereby stimulating phosphofructokinase activity and increasing glucose uptake [89, 90], an action critical for enhanced aerobic glycolysis.

In parallel, matrix stiffness further potentiates this loop mediating PI3K activation of AKT via Fak kinase and Myc-dependent matrix stiffness-induced expression of miR18a, which inhibits PTEN expression and metabolism switch to glycolysis. In addition, both increased thickness and compromised vasculature change tumor microenvironment and trigger a poor outcome predictor: hypoxia [91]. Through activation of HIF-1, a potent oncogenic transcription factor, hypoxia acts to reinforce the Warburg effect, as HIF1α induces the expression of genes encoding glycolytic enzymes and glucose transporters. Metabolic reprogramming by Ras oncogene is carried out predominantly through the upregulation of hypoxia-inducible factor 1α (HIF1α), which forms the HIF transcription factor when bound to HIF1β and is well recognized for its ability to stimulate a glycolytic shift. Ras-induced concurrent activation of MAPK and PI3K effector pathways triggers the stimulation of mTOR activity and mTOR-mediated cap-dependent translation of HIF1α. RAS-dependent upregulation of HIF1α has been implicated in enhancing both the transport and the glycolytic capture of glucose, as well as its processing to biosynthetic intermediates. Oncogenic RAS increases the transcription of the glucose transporter GLUT1, thus providing cells the increased ability to take up glucose. The oncogene regulates also the expression of glycolytic enzymes, such as hexokinase, phosphofructokinase, and lactate dehydrogenase. Given this multiplicity of metabolic changes governed by oncogenic Ras, it is possible to envisage the participation of other Ras-targets other than HIF1α, still unknown.

A fascinating interplay between Ras activity, HIF 1α, and metabolic changes in NF1 has been very recently unrevealed by Andrea Rasola's group. They found that the lack of neurofibromin induces a glycolytic phenotype and decreased respiration in a Ras/ERK-dependent way [92]. The authors provide an interesting mechanistic model by which in the mitochondrial matrix a fraction of active ERK1/2 binds to and activates the mitochondrial chaperone TRAP1 that in turn inhibits succinate dehydrogenase (SDH), the respiratory complex II [93]. Consequently, the resulting increase in intracellular levels of the oncometabolite succinate inhibits the prolyl hydroxylases responsible for dispatching HIF-1α to the proteasome for degradation [94].

Altogether, these findings indicate the existence of a crosstalk among NF1 loss-dependent signaling, ECM stiffening, EMT, and metabolic interconnections, having a profound impact on tumor progression. Although additional studies are required to fully characterize the complexity of this signaling network, this new axis could represent a novel avenue to pursue in the search of the molecular cascades responsible for neurofibroma onset and development.

References

1. Gottfried ON, Viskochil DH, Couldwell WT. Neurofibromatosis type 1 and tumorigenesis: molecular mechanisms and therapeutic implications. Neurosurg Focus. 2010;28(1):E8.

2. Rubin JB, Gutmann DH. Neurofibromatosis type 1 – a model for nervous system tumour formation? Nat Rev Cancer. 2005;5(7):557–64.
3. Harrisingh MC, Perez-Nadales E, Parkinson DB, Malcolm DS, Mudge AW, Lloyd AC. The Ras/Raf/ERK signalling pathway drives Schwann cell dedifferentiation. EMBO J. 2004;23(15):3061–71.
4. Aragona M, Panciera T, Manfrin A, Giulitti S, Michielin F, Elvassore N, et al. A mechanical checkpoint controls multicellular growth through YAP/TAZ regulation by actin-processing factors. Cell. 2013;154(5):1047–59.
5. Levental KR, Yu H, Kass L, Lakins JN, Egeblad M, Erler JT, et al. Matrix crosslinking forces tumor progression by enhancing integrin signaling. Cell. 2009;139(5):891–906.
6. Parrinello S, Noon LA, Harrisingh MC, Wingfield Digby P, Rosenberg LH, Cremona CA, et al. NF1 loss disrupts Schwann cell-axonal interactions: a novel role for semaphorin 4F. Genes Dev. 2008;22(23):3335–48.
7. Staser K, Yang FC, Clapp DW. Mast cells and the neurofibroma microenvironment. Blood. 2010;116(2):157–64.
8. Yamauchi M, Barker TH, Gibbons DL, Kurie JM. The fibrotic tumor stroma. J Clin Investig. 2018;128(1):16–25.
9. Tschumperlin DJ, Ligresti G, Hilscher MB, Shah VH. Mechanosensing and fibrosis. J Clin Invest. 2018;128(1):74–84.
10. Kweh F, Zheng M, Kurenova E, Wallace M, Golubovskaya V, Cance WG. Neurofibromin physically interacts with the N-terminal domain of focal adhesion kinase. Mol Carcinog. 2009;48(11):1005–17.
11. Ueha S, Shand FH, Matsushima K. Cellular and molecular mechanisms of chronic inflammation-associated organ fibrosis. Front Immunol. 2012;3:71.
12. Frantz C, Stewart KM, Weaver VM. The extracellular matrix at a glance. J Cell Sci. 2010;123(Pt 24):4195–200.
13. Mouw JK, Ou G, Weaver VM. Extracellular matrix assembly: a multiscale deconstruction. Nat Rev Mol Cell Biol. 2014;15(12):771–85.
14. Bonnans C, Chou J, Werb Z. Remodelling the extracellular matrix in development and disease. Nat Rev Mol Cell Biol. 2014;15(12):786–801.
15. Mouw JK, Yui Y, Damiano L, Bainer RO, Lakins JN, Acerbi I, et al. Tissue mechanics modulate microRNA-dependent PTEN expression to regulate malignant progression. Nat Med. 2014;20(4):360–7.
16. Rubashkin MG, Ou G, Weaver VM. Deconstructing signaling in three dimensions. Biochemistry. 2014;53(13):2078–90.
17. Ehrlich HP. A snapshot of direct cell-cell communications in wound healing and scarring. Adv Wound Care. 2013;2(4):113–21.
18. Chen CZ, Peng YX, Wang ZB, Fish PV, Kaar JL, Koepsel RR, et al. The scar-in-a-jar: studying potential antifibrotic compounds from the epigenetic to extracellular level in a single well. Br J Pharmacol. 2009;158(5):1196–209.
19. Wynn TA, Ramalingam TR. Mechanisms of fibrosis: therapeutic translation for fibrotic disease. Nat Med. 2012;18(7):1028–40.
20. Mescher AL. Macrophages and fibroblasts during inflammation and tissue repair in models of organ regeneration. Regeneration. 2017;4(2):39–53.
21. Stenton GR, Nohara O, Dery RE, Vliagoftis H, Gilchrist M, Johri A, et al. Proteinase-activated receptor (PAR)-1 and -2 agonists induce mediator release from mast cells by pathways distinct from PAR-1 and PAR-2. J Pharmacol Exp Ther. 2002;302(2):466–74.
22. Vliagoftis H. Thrombin induces mast cell adhesion to fibronectin: evidence for involvement of protease-activated receptor-1. J Immunol. 2002;169(8):4551–8.
23. Kauhanen P, Kovanen PT, Reunala T, Lassila R. Effects of skin mast cells on bleeding time and coagulation activation at the site of platelet plug formation. Thromb Haemost. 1998;79(4):843–7.
24. Prieto-Garcia A, Zheng D, Adachi R, Xing W, Lane WS, Chung K, et al. Mast cell restricted mouse and human tryptase. Heparin complexes hinder thrombin-induced coagulation of

plasma and the generation of fibrin by proteolytically destroying fibrinogen. J Biol Chem. 2012;287(11):7834–44.
25. Kettelhut BV, Metcalfe DD. Pediatric mastocytosis. J Invest Dermatol. 1991;96(3):15S–8S.
26. Wulff BC, Wilgus TA. Mast cell activity in the healing wound: more than meets the eye? Exp Dermatol. 2013;22(8):507–10.
27. Fukunaga S, Takedatsu H, Mitsuyama K, Torimura T. A rare case of ulcerative colitis with neurofibromatosis type 1. Kurume Med J. 2017;64:25–7.
28. Douaiher J, Succar J, Lancerotto L, Gurish MF, Orgill DP, Hamilton MJ, et al. Development of mast cells and importance of their tryptase and chymase serine proteases in inflammation and wound healing. Adv Immunol. 2014;122:211–52.
29. Gilfillan AM, Beaven MA. Regulation of mast cell responses in health and disease. Crit Rev Immunol. 2011;31(6):475–529.
30. Ribatti D, Crivellato E. Mast cells, angiogenesis, and tumour growth. Biochim Biophys Acta. 2012;1822(1):2–8.
31. Herrera J, Henke CA, Bitterman PB. Extracellular matrix as a driver of progressive fibrosis. J Clin Investig. 2018;128(1):45–53.
32. Chen H, Xu Y, Yang G, Zhang Q, Huang X, Yu L, et al. Mast cell chymase promotes hypertrophic scar fibroblast proliferation and collagen synthesis by activating TGF-beta1/Smads signaling pathway. Exp Ther Med. 2017;14(5):4438–42.
33. Gruber BL. Mast cells in the pathogenesis of fibrosis. Curr Rheumatol Rep. 2003;5(2): 147–53.
34. Oskeritzian CA. Mast cells and wound healing. Adv Wound Care. 2012;1(1):23–8.
35. Medici D, Kalluri R. Endothelial-mesenchymal transition and its contribution to the emergence of stem cell phenotype. Semin Cancer Biol. 2012;22(5–6):379–84.
36. Wang S, Meng XM, Ng YY, Ma FY, Zhou S, Zhang Y, et al. TGF-beta/Smad3 signalling regulates the transition of bone marrow-derived macrophages into myofibroblasts during tissue fibrosis. Oncotarget. 2016;7(8):8809–22.
37. Meng XM, Nikolic-Paterson DJ, Lan HY. TGF-beta: the master regulator of fibrosis. Nat Rev Nephrol. 2016;12(6):325–38.
38. Falke LL, Gholizadeh S, Goldschmeding R, Kok RJ, Nguyen TQ. Diverse origins of the myofibroblast-implications for kidney fibrosis. Nat Rev Nephrol. 2015;11(4):233–44.
39. Tomasek JJ, Gabbiani G, Hinz B, Chaponnier C, Brown RA. Myofibroblasts and mechanoregulation of connective tissue remodelling. Nat Rev Mol Cell Biol. 2002;3(5):349–63.
40. Staser K, Yang FC, Clapp DW. Plexiform neurofibroma genesis: questions of Nf1 gene dose and hyperactive mast cells. Curr Opin Hematol. 2010;17(4):287–93.
41. Khalaf WF, Yang FC, Chen S, White H, Bessler W, Ingram DA, et al. K-ras is critical for modulating multiple c-kit-mediated cellular functions in wild-type and Nf1+/− mast cells. J Immunol. 2007;178(4):2527–34.
42. Yang FC, Ingram DA, Chen S, Zhu Y, Yuan J, Li X, et al. Nf1-dependent tumors require a microenvironment containing Nf1+/−− and c-kit-dependent bone marrow. Cell. 2008;135(3):437–48.
43. Chernousov MA, Yu WM, Chen ZL, Carey DJ, Strickland S. Regulation of Schwann cell function by the extracellular matrix. Glia. 2008;56(14):1498–507.
44. Tucker T, Riccardi VM, Sutcliffe M, Vielkind J, Wechsler J, Wolkenstein P, et al. Different patterns of mast cells distinguish diffuse from encapsulated neurofibromas in patients with neurofibromatosis 1. J Histochem Cytochem. 2011;59(6):584–90.
45. Riccardi VM. Ketotifen suppression of NF1 neurofibroma growth over 30 years. Am J Med Genet A. 2015;167(7):1570–7.
46. Monk KR, Wu J, Williams JP, Finney BA, Fitzgerald ME, Filippi MD, et al. Mast cells can contribute to axon-glial dissociation and fibrosis in peripheral nerve. Neuron Glia Biol. 2007;3(3):233–44.
47. Suzuki R, Furuno T, Okamoto K, Teshima R, Nakanishi M. ATP plays a role in neurite stimulation with activated mast cells. J Neuroimmunol. 2007;192(1–2):49–56.

48. Riccardi VM. Histogenesis control genes and neurofibromatosis 1. Eur J Pediatr. 2000;159(7):475–6.
49. Koivunen J, Karvonen SL, Yla-Outinen H, Aaltonen V, Oikarinen A, Peltonen J. NF1 tumor suppressor in epidermal wound healing with special focus on wound healing in patients with type 1 neurofibromatosis. Arch Dermatol Res. 2005;296(12):547–54.
50. Miyawaki T, Billings B, Har-Shai Y, Agbenorku P, Kokuba E, Moreira-Gonzalez A, et al. Multicenter study of wound healing in neurofibromatosis and neurofibroma. J Craniofac Surg. 2007;18(5):1008–11.
51. Ball NJ, Kho GT. Melanocytic nevi are associated with neurofibromas in neurofibromatosis, type I, but not sporadic neurofibromas: a study of 226 cases. J Cutan Pathol. 2005;32(8):523–32.
52. Salgado CM, Silver RB, Bauer BS, Basu D, Schmitt L, Khakoo Y, et al. Skin of patients with large/giant congenital melanocytic nevi shows increased mast cells. Pediatr Dev Pathol. 2014;17(3):198–203.
53. El-Hoss J, Sullivan K, Cheng T, Yu NY, Bobyn JD, Peacock L, et al. A murine model of neurofibromatosis type 1 tibial pseudarthrosis featuring proliferative fibrous tissue and osteoclast-like cells. J Bone Miner Res. 2012;27(1):68–78.
54. El-Hoss J, Cheng T, Carpenter EC, Sullivan K, Deo N, Mikulec K, et al. A combination of rhBMP-2 (recombinant human bone morphogenetic protein-2) and MEK (MAP kinase/ERK kinase) inhibitor PD0325901 increases bone formation in a murine model of Neurofibromatosis type I pseudarthrosis. J Bone Joint Surg Am. 2014;96(14):e117.
55. Kuorilehto T, Kinnunen P, Nissinen M, Alanne M, Leskela HV, Lehenkari P, et al. Vasculopathy in two cases of NF1-related congenital pseudarthrosis. Pathol Res Pract. 2006;202(9):687–90.
56. Hermanns-Sachweh B, Senderek J, Alfer J, Klosterhalfen B, Buttner R, Fuzesi L, et al. Vascular changes in the periosteum of congenital pseudarthrosis of the tibia. Pathol Res Pract. 2005;201(4):305–12.
57. Riccardi VM. The vasculopathy of NF1 and histogenesis control genes. Clin Genet. 2000;58(5):345–7.
58. Kaas B, Huisman TA, Tekes A, Bergner A, Blakeley JO, Jordan LC. Spectrum and prevalence of vasculopathy in pediatric neurofibromatosis type 1. J Child Neurol. 2013;28(5):561–9.
59. Saif I, Seriki D, Moore R, Woywodt A. Midaortic syndrome in neurofibromatosis type 1 resulting in bilateral renal artery stenosis. Am J Kidney Dis. 2010;56(6):1197–201.
60. Falcone JL, Go MR, Baril DT, Oakley GJ, Makaroun MS, Chaer RA. Vascular wall invasion in neurofibromatosis-induced aortic rupture. Vasc Endovasc Surg. 2010;44(1):52–5.
61. Choi K, Komurov K, Fletcher JS, Jousma E, Cancelas JA, Wu J, et al. An inflammatory gene signature distinguishes neurofibroma Schwann cells and macrophages from cells in the normal peripheral nervous system. Sci Rep. 2017;7:43315.
62. Yang L, Herrera J, Gilbertsen A, Xia H, Smith K, Benyumov A, et al. IL-8 mediates idiopathic pulmonary fibrosis mesenchymal progenitor cell fibrogenicity. Am J Physiol Lung Cell Mol Physiol. 2018;314(1):L127–L36.
63. Rybinski B, Franco-Barraza J, Cukierman E. The wound healing, chronic fibrosis, and cancer progression triad. Physiol Genomics. 2014;46(7):223–44.
64. Dvorak HF. Tumors: wounds that do not heal. Similarities between tumor stroma generation and wound healing. N Engl J Med. 1986;315(26):1650–9.
65. Schafer M, Werner S. Cancer as an overhealing wound: an old hypothesis revisited. Nat Rev Mol Cell Biol. 2008;9(8):628–38.
66. Bissell MJ, Radisky D. Putting tumours in context. Nat Rev Cancer. 2001;1(1):46–54.
67. Guerra L, Odorisio T, Zambruno G, Castiglia D. Stromal microenvironment in type VII collagen-deficient skin: the ground for squamous cell carcinoma development. Matrix Biol. 2017;63:1–10.
68. Avdeev SN. Idiopatic pulmonary fibrosis: a new paradigm. Ter Arkh. 2017;89(1):112–22.
69. Friedman SL. Mechanisms of hepatic fibrogenesis. Gastroenterology. 2008;134(6):1655–69.
70. Liu F, Lagares D, Choi KM, Stopfer L, Marinkovic A, Vrbanac V, et al. Mechanosignaling through YAP and TAZ drives fibroblast activation and fibrosis. Am J Physiol Lung Cell Mol Physiol. 2015;308(4):L344–57.

71. Calvo F, Ege N, Grande-Garcia A, Hooper S, Jenkins RP, Chaudhry SI, et al. Mechanotransduction and YAP-dependent matrix remodelling is required for the generation and maintenance of cancer-associated fibroblasts. Nat Cell Biol. 2013;15(6):637–46.
72. Tung JC, Barnes JM, Desai SR, Sistrunk C, Conklin MW, Schedin P, et al. Tumor mechanics and metabolic dysfunction. Free Radic Biol Med. 2015;79:269–80.
73. Brabletz T, Kalluri R, Nieto MA, Weinberg RA. EMT in cancer. Nat Rev Cancer. 2018;18(2):128–34.
74. Tzanakakis G, Kavasi RM, Voudouri K, Berdiaki A, Spyridaki I, Tsatsakis A, et al. Role of the extracellular matrix in cancer-associated epithelial to mesenchymal transition phenomenon. Dev Dynamics. 2017;247(3):368–81.
75. Nieto MA, Huang RY, Jackson RA, Thiery JP. Emt: 2016. Cell. 2016;166(1):21–45.
76. Laklai H, Miroshnikova YA, Pickup MW, Collisson EA, Kim GE, Barrett AS, et al. Genotype tunes pancreatic ductal adenocarcinoma tissue tension to induce matricellular fibrosis and tumor progression. Nat Med. 2016;22(5):497–505.
77. Neesse A, Algul H, Tuveson DA, Gress TM. Stromal biology and therapy in pancreatic cancer: a changing paradigm. Gut. 2015;64(9):1476–84.
78. Arima Y, Hayashi H, Kamata K, Goto TM, Sasaki M, Kuramochi A, et al. Decreased expression of neurofibromin contributes to epithelial-mesenchymal transition in neurofibromatosis type 1. Exp Dermatol. 2010;19(8):e136–41.
79. Baek ST, Tallquist MD. Nf1 limits epicardial derivative expansion by regulating epithelial to mesenchymal transition and proliferation. Development. 2012;139(11):2040–9.
80. Calcagni G, Limongelli G, D'Ambrosio A, Gesualdo F, Digilio MC, Baban A, et al. Cardiac defects, morbidity and mortality in patients affected by RASopathies. CARNET study results. Int J Cardiol. 2017;245:92–8.
81. Northey JJ, Przybyla L, Weaver VM. Tissue force programs cell fate and tumor aggression. Cancer Discov. 2017;7(11):1224–37.
82. Stukel JM, Willits RK. Mechanotransduction of neural cells through cell-substrate interactions. Tissue Eng Part B Rev. 2016;22(3):173–82.
83. Sotiriou C, Neo SY, McShane LM, Korn EL, Long PM, Jazaeri A, et al. Breast cancer classification and prognosis based on gene expression profiles from a population-based study. Proc Natl Acad Sci U S A. 2003;100(18):10393–8.
84. Jiang H, Hegde S, Knolhoff BL, Zhu Y, Herndon JM, Meyer MA, et al. Targeting focal adhesion kinase renders pancreatic cancers responsive to checkpoint immunotherapy. Nat Med. 2016;22(8):851–60.
85. Hanahan D, Weinberg RA. Hallmarks of cancer: the next generation. Cell. 2011;144(5):646–74.
86. Warburg O. On respiratory impairment in cancer cells. Science. 1956;124(3215):269–70.
87. Ahn CS, Metallo CM. Mitochondria as biosynthetic factories for cancer proliferation. Cancer Metab. 2015;3(1):1.
88. Flier JS, Mueckler MM, Usher P, Lodish HF. Elevated levels of glucose transport and transporter messenger RNA are induced by ras or src oncogenes. Science. 1987;235(4795):1492–5.
89. Laplante M, Sabatini DM. mTOR signaling in growth control and disease. Cell. 2012;149(2):274–93.
90. Laplante M, Sabatini DM. mTOR Signaling. Cold Spring Harb Perspect Biol. 2012;4(2):a011593.
91. Vaupel P. Prognostic potential of the pre-therapeutic tumor oxygenation status. Adv Exp Med Biol. 2009;645:241–6.
92. Masgras I, Ciscato F, Brunati AM, Tibaldi E, Indraccolo S, Curtarello M, et al. Absence of neurofibromin induces an oncogenic metabolic switch via mitochondrial ERK-mediated phosphorylation of the chaperone TRAP1. Cell Rep. 2017;18(3):659–72.
93. Guzzo G, Sciacovelli M, Bernardi P, Rasola A. Inhibition of succinate dehydrogenase by the mitochondrial chaperone TRAP1 has anti-oxidant and anti-apoptotic effects on tumor cells. Oncotarget. 2014;5(23):11897–908.
94. Sciacovelli M, Guzzo G, Morello V, Frezza C, Zheng L, Nannini N, et al. The mitochondrial chaperone TRAP1 promotes neoplastic growth by inhibiting succinate dehydrogenase. Cell Metab. 2013;17(6):988–99.

Diagnosis and Management of Benign Nerve Sheath Tumors in NF1: Evolution from Plexiform to Atypical Neurofibroma and Novel Treatment Approaches

11

Andrea M. Gross, Eva Dombi, and Brigitte C. Widemann

Contents

11.1 Introduction

As a genetic tumor predisposition syndrome, one of the hallmark features of neurofibromatosis type 1 (NF1) is the development of both histologically benign and malignant tumors. The wide variety and heterogeneous presentations of the benign tumors in NF1 often provide both diagnostic and treatment challenges for patients and caregivers [1, 2]. Notably, three of the six NIH Consensus Criteria for the diagnosis of NF1 refer to the presence of benign or low grade tumors (neurofibromas, optic pathway gliomas, and Lisch nodules (iris hamartomas)) [3], which highlights their importance in this condition. In this chapter, we will discuss the presentation, diagnosis, and management options for these benign tumors, with a focus on neurofibromas (summary in Table 11.1).

A. M. Gross · E. Dombi · B. C. Widemann (✉)
National Cancer Institute, Pediatric Oncology Branch, Bethesda, MD, USA
e-mail: andrea.gross@nih.gov; dombie@mail.nih.gov; widemanb@mail.nih.gov

G. Tadini et al. (eds.), *Multidisciplinary Approach to Neurofibromatosis Type 1*,
https://doi.org/10.1007/978-3-319-92450-2_11

Table 11.1 Characteristics of neurofibromatosis type 1 (NF1) associated peripheral nerve sheath tumors: cutaneous neurofibromas (cNF), plexiform neurofibromas (pNF), atypical neurofibromas (aNF), and malignant peripheral nerve sheath tumors (MPNST). Table modified from Widemann et al [4]

Tumor type	NF1 cutaneous neurofibroma	NF1 plexiform neurofibroma	NF1 atypical neurofibroma	Malignant peripheral nerve sheath tumor
Lifetime incidence (%)	Up to 99	25–50	Unknown	8–15.8
Median age at diagnosis (years)	Adolescent–young adult	Young child	27 (range 7.6–60)	13–36
Development	Nerve	Nerve	pNF/nerve	pNF/aNF/nerve
Tumor genetics	Biallelic *NF1* loss	Biallelic *NF1* loss	+ loss *CDKN2A/B*	+ *Polycomb repressive complex: EED, SUZ12, p53, others*
Histopathology	Benign	Benign	Borderline: aNF and ANNUBP[a]	Malignant: Low[b] to high grade
Clinical findings/ symptoms	Discrete lesions in the dermis or epidermis; increase in size and number over time	Large slow growing tumor, pain, functional loss, disfigurement	Firm nodular tumor, faster growth than PN, pain, functional loss	Rapidly enlarging tumor, worsening pain, functional loss
Imaging	Photography, 3D photography, ultrasound	MRI (STIR), whole-body MRI	MRI with contrast and apparent diffusion coefficient, FDG-PET	MRI with contrast and apparent diffusion coefficient + CT chest/abdomen/ pelvis, FDG-PET
Treatment	Surgical removal or ablation (tumors may regrow) Clinical trials	Complete surgical resection many times not feasible Clinical trials: MEK inhibitor	Surgical resection if feasible with low morbidity (wide negative margins not required)	*High grade MPNST*: Complete surgical resection with wide negative margins As indicated: Radiation, chemotherapy *Low grade MPNST*: Complete surgical resection, wide negative margins not required

[a]ANNUBP: Atypical neurofibromatous neoplasms of uncertain biologic potential. Characteristic histologic features of atypical neurofibromas and ANNUBP are in the 2017 review by Miettinen et al. [60]

[b]Low grade MPNST has histologic features similar to ANNUBP

MRI Magnetic Resonance Imaging, *FDG-PET* fluorodeoxyglucose -positron emission tomography

11.2 Cutaneous Neurofibromas

Cutaneous neurofibromas (cNF), discrete lesions occurring in the skin (dermis or epidermis) [5], arise from neoplastic Schwann cells [6, 7] and contain other cells including mast cells, fibroblasts, perineural cells, and endothelial cells [1, 8–10].

The natural history of cNF is that they tend to increase both in size and number over time [11]. They are benign lesions which do not progress to malignancy and occur in up to 99% of adult patients with NF1 [11, 12]. While histologically benign, cNF can cause severe morbidity resulting from disfigurement and emotional distress [13]. Though cNF are less common in children and young adults, they still have an estimated prevalence of up to 40% in pre-pubertal children [14]. Retrospective reports suggest that cNF growth may increase in the setting of hormonal changes such as puberty and pregnancy [15]; however, this has yet to be validated in prospective studies.

Though cNF are highly prevalent, there is wide variability in the number and location of cNF between individual patients. There are a few very specific genotype–phenotype correlations for the development of cNF [5]. For example, some patients with NF1 microdeletions are more likely to develop cNF in childhood [16], and patients with a larger burden of pNF tend to have a larger number of cNF [17]. In contrast, patients with a specific *NF1* deletion in p.Met992del, or a missense mutation affecting p.Arg1809, rarely develop any cNF [18–21]. However, outside of these limited circumstances, it is not currently possible to predict which patients will develop cNF during their lifetime, and even parents and children with the same germline mutation may have significant differences in their cNF burden.

Treatment options for cNF are limited at this time, with destruction (e.g., laser or electrodessication) [11, 22] or surgical removal of tumors causing discomfort or disfigurement currently being the only standard treatment [23]. Some of the challenges in designing clinical trials for the treatment of these lesions have been the lack of validated measurement tools and varied classification systems for cNF. In 2018, Ortonne et al. proposed a unified classification system that accounts for both clinical variation in appearance (e.g., flat vs pedunculated lesions) and histologic variation (e.g., diffuse vs plexiform appearance) [5]. This system is currently being validated in a prospective clinical trial, and various different measurement techniques are being evaluated for their use in future clinical trials to treat these tumors. A recent summit on cNF has reviewed the current knowledge of cNF in NF1 and developed research priorities to achieve the goal of developing effective therapies for cNF [5, 24–27].

11.3 Plexiform Neurofibromas (pNF)

In contrast to cNF, pNF consist of a proliferation of cells within peripheral nerves and involve multiple nerve fascicles and branches [28]. These are histologically benign tumors with cell populations similar to cNF. A genomic analysis of pNF demonstrated that, similarly to cNF, biallelic NF1 loss is the pathogenic driver of pNF [29]. While histologically and genomically similar, the clinical behavior of cNF and pNF are strikingly different. In comparison to cNF, pNF are typically diagnosed at a young age and assumed to be congenital. The size of pNF frequently increase rapidly in childhood while significant progression is rare later in life. Finally, in contrast to cNF, pNF are at risk for transformation to malignant peripheral nerve sheath tumors (MPNSTs) [30, 31], aggressive sarcomas which cause severe morbidity and mortality in NF1.

11.3.1 Clinical Diagnosis of pNF

The clinical presentation and diagnosis of pNF depend on their location in the body. Some pNF have a very complex shape and occasionally grow to extreme size. Plexiform neurofibromas with a superficial component can be diagnosed early in life, usually by the observation of subtle asymmetry and enlargement of tissue, which can be rapidly progressive. Superficial components of pNF may also have a sponge-like texture and show hyperpigmentation and excess hair growth. Large areas of skin hyperpigmentation may be indicative of deeper pNF in that body region. Deep pNF may not be diagnosed until they result in clinical symptoms and can be very large by this time. Plexiform neurofibromas in the limbs can be associated with overgrowth of the extremity, which can be severe [28]. Figure 11.1 shows a rapidly progressive extremity neurofibroma.

Plexiform neurofibromas can develop in any peripheral nerve in the body and therefore the symptoms and morbidities they can cause vary widely across patients. Several studies have shown that the amount of pNF burden can correlate with the degree of symptoms, with larger pNF being associated with a higher risk of complications [32]. Importantly, these morbidities often develop at a young age [32, 33]. In a retrospective review of the National Cancer Institute (NCI) NF1 Natural History cohort, we found that among 41 patients with a median age of 8 years old, 36 (70%) had at least one neurofibroma-related morbidity at presentation [34]. These

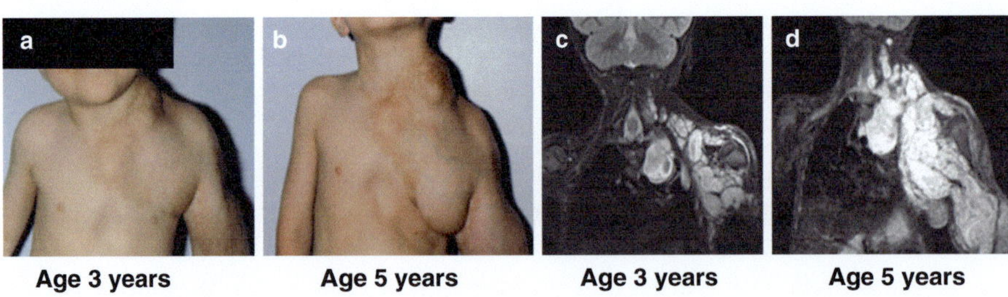

Fig. 11.1 Growth of a plexiform neurofibroma over time. Example of rapid plexiform neurofibroma growth based on photography (**a**, **b**) and coronal STIR MRI (**c**, **d**) in a young child: Substantial growth of a large left neck/chest/arm plexiform neurofibroma over the course of 2 years. There is hyperpigmentation overlying the plexiform neurofibroma and overgrowth of the affected left arm. This patient had minimal function and sensation in the affected arm

morbidities spanned a wide range including motor dysfunction, airway impairment, pain, visual impairment, and disfigurement. After an observation period of ≥7 years per patient, no patient with stable or growing pNF had spontaneous resolution of an associated morbidity. Rather, there was a significant increase in the number of morbidities per patient over time. Though small pNF were found to cause morbidity in some locations, such as orbital tumors, we found that larger pNF and faster pNF growth rate were associated with more motor dysfunction and pain, respectively. Though pNF are histologically benign, large pNF burden is not only associated with worsening morbidity, but also with an increased risk of mortality from NF1-related complications including malignant transformation [35].

11.3.2 Imaging of pNF

Imaging of pNF has greatly aided in the clinical characterization of these tumors. Earlier studies using either computerized tomography (CT) or X-ray imaging [36, 37] tended to underestimate the incidence of these tumors. Magnetic resonance imaging (MRI) can better distinguish pNF from surrounding tissue and has allowed for more accurate characterization and quantification of these tumors [38, 39]. Therefore, MRI has become the standard imaging approach for pNF and based on MRI imaging pNF occur in up to 50% of patients with NF1 [28, 40]. Typical pNF appear bright on T2 weighted imaging sequences and often exhibit the "central dot sign," areas of decreased signal intensity within clusters of grape like pNF components. MRI sequences do not require contrast agent administration when the purpose is to measure the size of the lesion [39, 41]. Plexiform neurofibromas can involve both deep and superficial tissue layers and contain diffuse or nodular/fascicular components. As a specific subset of pNF, superficial pNF are confined to skin and subcutaneous tissue and have a characteristic imaging appearance with diffuse rather than fascicular or nodular morphology [42]. Examples of the MRI appearance of different types of pNF are shown in Fig. 11.2. More recently whole-body MRI has become available to comprehensively evaluate total tumor burden in

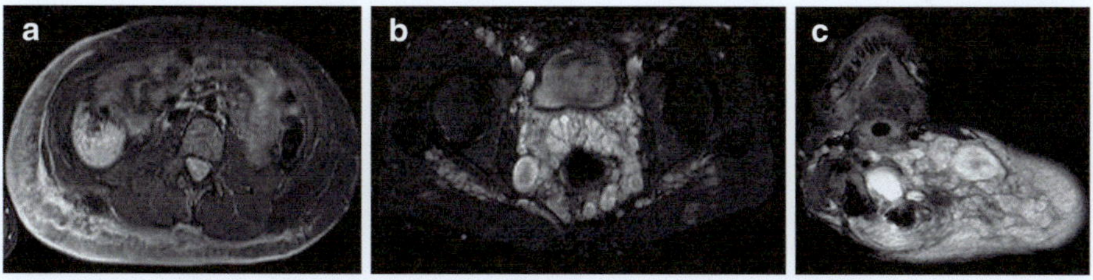

Fig. 11.2 Different locations and MRI appearances of pNF: (**a**) Superficial truncal plexiform neurofibroma confined the cutaneous and subcutaneous tissue. This neurofibroma does not have nodular or fascicular components; (**b**) Deep pelvic plexiform neurofibroma arising beneath the muscle fascia with nodular and fascicular components; and (**c**) Neck plexiform neurofibroma with superficial and deep involvement which has diffuse, nodular, and fascicular components

NF1, to characterize the natural history of NF1 and to detect tumors at risk for malignant transformation [43, 44].

MRI of pNF has also been critical to the understanding of the natural history of peripheral nerve sheath tumors and to the ability to accurately detect and measure pNF size in clinical trials. Early interventional clinical trials targeting pNF used tumor response criteria that are used for solid tumors and are based on one-dimensional (1-D) and two-dimensional (2-D) tumor measurements [45–48]. Given that pNF are frequently large, have a complex (non-spherical) shape, and a slow growth pattern, it was recognized that these methods have limited value in the assessment of treatment outcome for pNF. In order to reproducibly and sensitively quantify the size of these complex lesions and detect small changes in size over time, volumetric methods of assessing pNF burden were developed using MR imaging characteristics [41, 49, 50]. In the method developed at the NCI, non-contrast, short T1-Inversion Recovery (STIR-MR) images, on which pNF are bright lesions compared with normal surrounding tissue, were used to develop a program for automated image analysis [41]. This method has good reproducibility and inter-observer variability and is more sensitive in detecting small changes in pNF size compared to line measurements. This method has been used at the NCI, Pediatric Oncology Branch to evaluate the changes in pNF size over time on our NF1 natural history trial (NCT00924196) and to evaluate pNF volume on most ongoing multi-center clinical trials for children with NF1 and pNF [51]. Other volumetric MRI methods have been used and are in development [50, 52]. Recently, the method developed at the NCI, which has been used in most clinical trials, was compared to the volumetric method developed at Massachusetts General Hospital and demonstrated good agreement between the two methods [49].

11.3.3 Natural History of pNF Growth

Use of the semi-automated volumetric MRI analysis at the NCI has contributed to the understanding of the natural history of the growth of pNF [41]. Young children (age ≤8 years) appear to have the fastest pNF growth rate [53, 54] and there does not appear to be an acceleration in growth rate during puberty [55, 56]. In adults, pNF typically only have minimal growth. Spontaneous and small decreases in pNF volumes (median 3.4% decrease in tumor volume per year) have been described in one study [57]. Of note, this longitudinal study did not identify new pNF over time [57]. These findings speak against prior clinical observations that growth of pNF may be erratic [28] and also emphasize the need for the development of effective therapies targeting pNF for young patients when pNF grow most rapidly.

11.3.4 Atypical Neurofibromas (aNF)

In addition to characterizing the natural history of pNF growth, the NCI natural history study also allowed for identification and characterizing of distinct nodular lesions. These lesions were first identified on MRI studies performed to monitor the growth of pNF. Key characteristics included lesions with nodular character

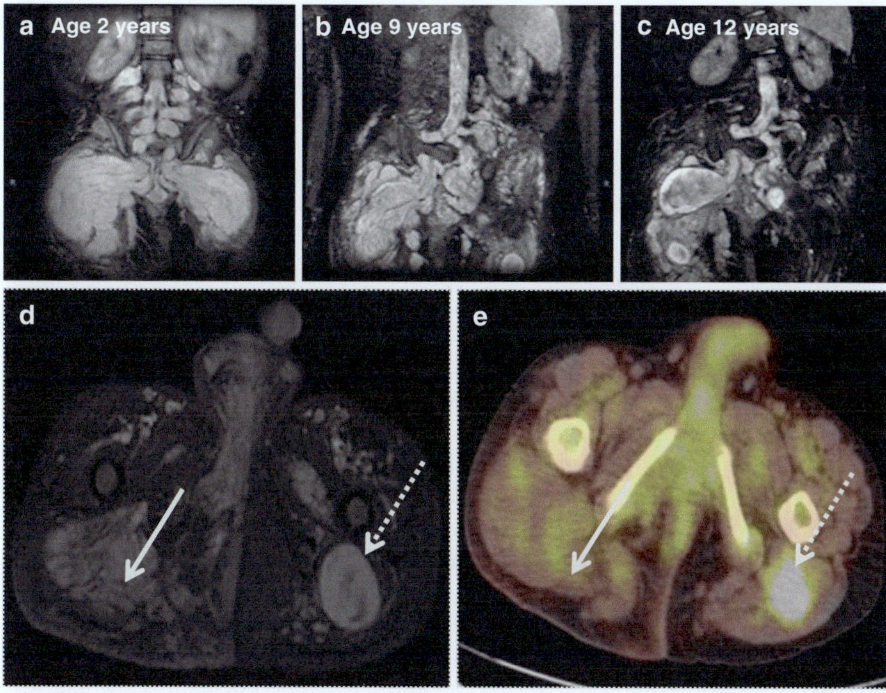

Fig. 11.3 Upper panel (**a–c**): Coronal STIR MRI documenting the development of a distinct nodular lesion within a plexiform neurofibroma (pNF) over the course of 10 years. This lesion was confirmed to be an atypical neurofibroma (aNF) by biopsy and pathology evaluation. Lower panel (**d**, **e**): Axial STIR MRI (**d**) and fluorodeoxyglucose (FDG) positron emission tomography (**e**) of a pelvic plexiform neurofibroma (solid arrow) and atypical neurofibroma (dashed arrow). In contrast to the plexiform neurofibroma, the atypical neurofibroma demonstrates FDG avidity

$\geq$3 cm in size, clearly standing out from surrounding pNF or development outside of a plexiform neurofibroma (Fig. 11.3). Volumetric MRI analysis of these lesions demonstrated more rapid growth compared to the adjacent pNF and evaluation with fluorodeoxyglucose positron emission tomography (FDG-PET) showed increased FDG uptake in these lesions compared to low uptake in the pNF. These findings together suggested a different biology of distinct nodular lesions compared to surrounding pNF and concern that these lesions may be transforming to malignancy. Biopsies of these lesions were performed and confirmed atypical neurofibromas (aNF) in many cases [58, 59]. Atypical neurofibromas are diagnosed based on pathologic characteristics including nuclear atypia, increased cellularity, and loss of neurofibroma architecture [60]. These lesions were first defined as precursor lesions for MPNST by Eric Legius and his team who described loss of *CDKN2A/B* in aNF and in MPNST but not subcutaneous and pNF [61]. Since then the importance of aNF as MPNST precursors has been confirmed. A retrospective review of patients with NF1 and aNF treated in Belgium, the UK, and at the NCI in the USA confirmed that most of these lesions are firm nodules on palpation, appear as distinct encapsulated lesions on MR imaging, and are at risk for malignant transformation [59]. This is of clinical relevance, as surgical resection of many aNF can be performed without causing substantial morbidity. In addition, compared to high grade MPNST, which requires surgical resection with wide negative margins for potential cure, resection of aNF with narrow margins appears adequate with small risk for recurrence [62, 63]. It thus appears that at least a subset of MPNST does not develop directly from pNF but from aNF, which arise within or outside of pNF. A recent consensus conference established criteria for pathologic characterization of aNF [60] and for their clinical management [64].

11.3.5 Treatment and Clinical Trials for pNF

Currently, there are no potentially curative treatment options for pNF other than surgery. Complete resection of pNF, however, is often not feasible due to the large size of the tumor, rich vascular supply, and invasion of the surrounding tissues. In addition, regrowth of pNF after surgery is common [65, 66], particularly in young patients with head and neck pNF [67].

NF1 tumors are characterized by activated RAS resulting in the initiation of a cascade of signaling events such as activation of Raf and MAPK that lead to increased cell proliferation [68, 69]. In addition, activation of the mTOR pathway has been identified in benign and malignant NF1 tumors [70–72], and the tumor microenvironment contributes to the pathogenesis of pNF [8]. Schwann cells have been shown to secrete kit ligand, which recruits mast cells and results in abnormal growth properties [73–75]. Blocking RAS activity signaling thus provides a rational approach towards the treatment of pNF.

Recently, the method developed at the NCI, which has been used in most clinical trials, was compared to the volumetric method developed at Massachusetts General Hospital and demonstrated good agreement between the two methods [49] (thalidomide [47] and tipifarnib phase I [48]). In recent clinical trials tumor progression is defined as an increase in tumor volume by ≥20% and response as a ≥20% decrease in pNF volume compared to baseline. In 2013, consensus recommendations for the imaging and response assessment of pNF in clinical trials were issued by an international working group, the Response Evaluation in Neurofibromatosis and Schwannotomosis (REiNS) collaboration, which aims to develop meaningful and standardized endpoints and outcome measures for clinical trials in patients with NF1, NF2 and schwannomatosis [76, 39], which concluded that volumetric tumor assessment is preferable to all other MRI analysis techniques. The main advantage of volumetric analysis is that it allows earlier detection of progression and thus limits duration of exposure to potentially toxic investigational agents.

A number of clinical trials targeting pNF have been completed and are reviewed by Gutmann and colleagues [77] including the farnesyltransferase inhibitor tipifarnib [78], the antifibrotic agent pirfenidone [79–81], the mTOR inhibitor sirolimus [82, 83], and the antiangiogenic and immune modulatory agent peginterferon alfa-2b [84, 85]. Most of these trials aimed to detect an improvement in progression free survival (PFS), and all volumetric response assessments were performed centrally at the NCI. The tipifarnib trial was the first to use volumetric MRI analysis to describe PFS. In the absence of control data and with an unknown natural history of NF1 pNF at the time the trial was initiated, this trial was designed as a randomized, double-blinded, placebo-controlled, flexible crossover trial. This design would offer each patient, either on the first or the second treatment phase, access to tipifarnib, provided disease progressed in the first phase. The median time to progression (TTP) of progressive pNF treated on the placebo group (29 patients) was 10.6 months. Tipifarnib did not result in a doubling of the TTP compared to the placebo arm. This has been the only placebo-controlled trial for pNF conducted to date and has provided valuable data on the natural history of progressive pNF. Three subsequent open label phase II trials (pirfenidone [86], sirolimus [87], and peginterferon alfa-2b [85]) used the tipifarnib trial placebo group to evaluate if the agent of interest would result in an increase in the TTP compared to the placebo control group. Compared to the tipifarnib placebo control group, only peginterferon alfa-2b achieved a doubling in the TTP [76]. Sirolimus achieved a statistically significant increase in the median TTP by 3.5 months [82]. Plexiform neurofibroma volume decreases by ≥20% in these trials were only observed in 4 of 82 (5%) patients treated with peginterferon alfa-2b [85]. In a recent phase II trial of the c-kit and PDGFR inhibitor imatinib conducted by Kent Robertson, pNF volume decrease ranging from 20 to 40% was observed in 6 of 23 response evaluable patients [52]. This trial used a different method of volumetric analysis and responses were limited to patients with very small pNF (≤20 mL). In contrast, most target pNF enrolled on NCI clinical trials had much larger volumes: Tipifarnib median pNF volume 364 mL (range 20.5–5573 mL); pirfenidone: median pNF volume 349 mL (range 12–5629 mL). Conducting trials with the goal of improving PFS is challenging, as these trials take substantial time to complete. A Department of Defense sponsored NF Clinical trials Consortium subsequently developed trials with response as the primary trial endpoint.

Until recently, most clinical trials targeting pNF focused on tumor measurement to assess the effect of a new agent, but did not incorporate patient reported or functional endpoints. One of the challenging aspects about designing clinical trials for pNF has been determining ways to reproducibly and sensitively detect change in pNF-related morbidity over time. Both patient reported outcome (PRO) and functional outcome measures are needed to measure the heterogeneous pNF-related symptoms. Several groups are tackling this challenge, including the REiNS collaboration which brings together clinicians, researchers, and patient advocates to develop meaningful clinical endpoints for pNF-related trials [88]. In addition, other groups are working to validate both functional and PRO measures in the NF1 population [89, 90], and several ongoing clinical trials including trials with MEK inhibitors are evaluating these measures in the setting of pNF directed medical therapies.

11.4 MEK Inhibition and Other Targeted Therapies for pNF

MEK inhibitors are targeted agents against the mitogen-activated protein kinase kinase (MEK), which is downstream of the hyperactivated RAS pathway in NF1-related neoplasms [91]. Prior to initiation of the first clinical trial with MEK inhibitors for pNF, MEK inhibition (PD0325901) was shown to abrogate myeloproliferative disease in a NF1 mouse model [92]. In a subsequent phase I trial (NCT01362803) of the MEK inhibitor selumetinib (AZD6244, ARRY-142886) in children with NF1 and inoperable pNF unprecedented shrinkage of pNF was observed with 17 of 24 (71%) of patients achieving a partial response (>20% shrinkage by volumetric MRI) [51]. The tumors in this study ranged widely in size, with a median volume of 1205 mL, and shrinkage was seen even in these larger tumors. Notably, even the patients who did not achieve a volumetric partial response appeared to have some benefit from treatment, with no patients experiencing disease progression after a median of 30 cycles (1 cycle = 28 days) on treatment. This contrasts starkly with the natural history of pNF, where the median time to progression is approximately 10 months [78], as well as with the results of previous clinical trials as detailed in the previous section. The maximum volumetric shrinkage seen in this study was minus 47% from baseline and this was achieved after approximately 18 months of therapy. Overall, selumetinib was well tolerated with the major side effects including development of an acneiform rash, gastrointestinal symptoms, and asymptomatic elevation in creatine kinase [51].

Though anecdotal improvements in pNF-related morbidities such as pain and disfigurement were reported in the phase I trial of selumetinib, these were not prospectively evaluated in that trial. The ongoing phase 2 study of selumetinib in pediatric patients with NF1 and inoperable pNF addresses this issue by incorporating extensive standardized functional and PRO measures (NCT01362803). Given the wide heterogeneity of the pNF-related morbidities in our population, a wide variety of measurements are being used and are tailored to each patient's pNF location and clinical presentation. For example, patients with a tumor impacting the airway undergo serial polysomnography, spirometry, and impulse oscillometry at the same time as each MRI restaging exam for the first year. Results of this study recapitulated the results seen in the phase I study with an overall response rate of 70%. In addition, statistically and clinically meaningful improvements in both pain and motor function were observed [93, 94]. An ongoing study for adults with inoperable pNF is evaluating similar functional and PRO measures as well as obtaining pre- and on-treatment tumor biopsies (NCT02407405).

Similarly, the MEK inhibitors trametinib and PD0325901 have shown activity in NF1-related pNF [95, 96], and there is an ongoing clinical trial of another MEK inhibitor, binimetinib (NCT03231306), which has the advantage of having a pediatric liquid formulation. Of note, the use of MEK inhibitors in NF1-related tumors has been confirmed in a study of low grade gliomas which showed evidence of activity [97, 98].

Other targeted therapies may also be useful for treating pNF in the future. For example, cabozantinib, a multi-receptor tyrosine kinase inhibitor, showed preliminary activity with 8 of 19 patients (42%) achieving a partial response in a study of adolescents and young adults with inoperable pNF (NCT02101736) [99].

11.4.1 Use of Preclinical Trials to Inform Clinical Trials Directed at pNF

Genetically engineered mouse models of NF1 and neurofibroma have become available to evaluate targeted agents in preclinical trials, with the goal to select the most active agents for clinical evaluation [74, 100–102]. One of the first agents in a neurofibroma model to demonstrate a consistent decrease in neurofibroma volumes was the MEK inhibitor (PD0325901) [68], and similar activity was observed with the MEK inhibitor selumetinib [51]. While these results were not available prior to the initiation of the selumetinib phase I trial for pNF, these findings validate the neurofibroma mouse model and support that preclinical studies may aid in the evaluation and selection of new agents for clinical trials.

11.5 Future Directions

The use of unique clinical trial endpoints, including volumetric MRI, functional and PRO measures, has allowed for exciting new research in the treatment of benign nerve sheath tumors in NF1. Though MEK inhibition has shown promising results, not all patients demonstrate a response, and some patients experience pNF regrowth after a dose reduction or discontinuation of selumetinib. While these new medical therapies may be able to decrease tumor volume, many pNF-related morbidities, such as vision loss, may not be reversible, and therefore the potential for preventing growth of pNF in young children may be a promising approach for future clinical trials. Importantly, preclinical studies utilizing validated mouse models of neurofibromas now offer the opportunity to discover potentially active agents. Several ongoing clinical trials are evaluating novel treatments for pNF. Future studies, including combination of targeted therapies and treatments for aNF, are in consideration.

References

1. Friedman J. Neurofibromatosis 1: clinical manifestations and diagnostic criteria. J Child Neurol. 2002;17:548–54.
2. Monroe CL, Dahiya S, Gutmann DH. Dissecting clinical heterogeneity in Neurofibromatosis type 1. Annu Rev Pathol. 2017;12:53–74.
3. National Institutes of Health Consensus Development Conference Statement: neurofibromatosis. Bethesda, MD., USA, July 13-15, 1987. Neurofibromatosis. 1988;1(3):172–8.
4. Widemann, B. C. and A. Italiano. Biology and Management of Undifferentiated Pleomorphic Sarcoma, Myxofibrosarcoma, and Malignant Peripheral Nerve Sheath Tumors: State of the Art and Perspectives. J Clin Oncol. 2018;36(2):160–167.
5. Ortonne N, et al. Cutaneous neurofibromas: Current clinical and pathologic issues. Neurology. 2018;91(2 Supplement 1):S5–S13.
6. Wu M, Wallace MR, Muir D. Tumorigenic properties of neurofibromin-deficient Schwann cells in culture and as syngrafts in Nf1 knockout mice. J Neurosci Res. 2005;82(3):357–67.
7. Rutkowski JL, et al. Genetic and cellular defects contributing to benign tumor formation in neurofibromatosis type 1. Hum Mol Genet. 2000;9(7):1059–66.

8. Le LQ, Parada LF. Tumor microenvironment and neurofibromatosis type I: connecting the GAPs. Oncogene. 2007;26(32):4609–16.
9. Munchhof AM, et al. Neurofibroma-associated growth factors activate a distinct signaling network to alter the function of neurofibromin-deficient endothelial cells. Hum Mol Genet. 2006;15(11):1858–69.
10. Yang FC, et al. Neurofibromin-deficient Schwann cells secrete a potent migratory stimulus for Nf1+/− mast cells. J Clin Invest. 2003;112(12):1851–61.
11. Cannon A, et al. Cutaneous neurofibromas in Neurofibromatosis type I: a quantitative natural history study. Orphanet J Rare Dis. 2018;13(1):31.
12. Ferner RE, et al. Guidelines for the diagnosis and management of individuals with neurofibromatosis 1. J Med Genet. 2007;44(2):81–8.
13. Page PZ, et al. Impact of neurofibromatosis 1 on quality of life: a cross-sectional study of 176 American cases. Am J Med Genet A. 2006;140(18):1893–8.
14. Boulanger JM, Larbrisseau A. Neurofibromatosis type 1 in a pediatric population: Ste-Justine's experience. Can J Neurol Sci. 2005;32(2):225–31.
15. Dugoff L, Sujansky E. Neurofibromatosis type 1 and pregnancy. Am J Med Genet. 1996;66(1):7–10.
16. Leppig KA, et al. Familial neurofibromatosis 1 microdeletions: cosegregation with distinct facial phenotype and early onset of cutaneous neurofibromata. Am J Med Genet. 1997;73(2):197–204.
17. Jett K, et al. Quantitative associations of scalp and body subcutaneous neurofibromas with internal plexiform tumors in neurofibromatosis 1. Am J Med Genet A. 2015;167(7):1518–24.
18. Pinna V, et al. p.Arg1809Cys substitution in neurofibromin is associated with a distinctive NF1 phenotype without neurofibromas. Eur J Hum Genet. 2015;23(8):1068–71.
19. Quintans B, et al. Neurofibromatosis without neurofibromas: confirmation of a genotype-phenotype correlation and implications for genetic testing. Case Rep Neurol. 2011;3:86–90.
20. Santoro C, et al. Arg(1809) substitution in neurofibromin: further evidence of a genotype-phenotype correlation in neurofibromatosis type 1. Eur J Hum Genet. 2015;23(11):1460–1.
21. Upadhyaya M, et al. An absence of cutaneous neurofibromas associated with a 3-bp inframe deletion in exon 17 of the NF1 gene (c.2970-2972 delAAT): evidence of a clinically significant NF1 genotype-phenotype correlation. Am J Hum Genet. 2007;80(1):140–51.
22. Elwakil TF, Samy NA, Elbasiouny MS. Non-excision treatment of multiple cutaneous neurofibromas by laser photocoagulation. Lasers Med Sci. 2008;23(3):301–6.
23. Williams VC, et al. Neurofibromatosis type 1 revisited. Pediatrics. 2009;123(1):124–33.
24. Blakeley JO, et al. Creating a comprehensive research strategy for cutaneous neurofibromas. Neurology. 2018;91(2 Supplement 1):S1–4.
25. Brosseau JP, et al. The biology of cutaneous neurofibromas: Consensus recommendations for setting research priorities. Neurology. 2018;91(2 Supplement 1):S14–20.
26. Verma SK, et al. Considerations for development of therapies for cutaneous neurofibroma. Neurology. 2018;91(2 Supplement 1):S21–30.
27. Cannon A, et al. Clinical trial design for cutaneous neurofibromas. Neurology. 2018;91(2 Supplement 1):S31–7.
28. Korf BR. Plexiform neurofibromas. Am J Med Genet. 1999;89(1):31–7.
29. Pemov A, et al. The primacy of NF1 loss as the driver of tumorigenesis in neurofibromatosis type 1-associated plexiform neurofibromas. Oncogene. 2017;36(22):3168–77.
30. Evans DG, et al. Malignant peripheral nerve sheath tumours in neurofibromatosis 1. J Med Genet. 2002;39(5):311–4.
31. Ferner RE, Gutmann DH. International consensus statement on malignant peripheral nerve sheath tumors in neurofibromatosis. Cancer Res. 2002;62(5):1573–7.
32. Nguyen R, et al. Plexiform neurofibromas in children with neurofibromatosis type 1: Frequency and associated clinical deficits. Journal of Pediatrics. 2011;159:652–655.e2.
33. Cnossen MH, et al. A prospective 10 year follow up study of patients with neurofibromatosis type 1. Arch Dis Child. 1998;78(5):408–12.
34. Gross AM, et al. Association of plexiform neurofibroma volume changes and development of clinical morbidities in neurofibromatosis 1. Neuro-Oncology. 2018;20(12):1643–51.

35. Prada CE, et al. Pediatric plexiform neurofibromas: impact on morbidity and mortality in neurofibromatosis type 1. J Pediatr. 2012;160(3):461–7.
36. Schorry EK, et al. Thoracic tumors in children with neurofibromatosis-1. Am J Med Genet. 1997;74(5):533–7.
37. Tonsgard JH, et al. CT imaging in adults with neurofibromatosis-1: frequent asymptomatic plexiform lesions. Neurology. 1998;50(6):1755–60.
38. Plotkin SR, et al. Quantitative assessment of whole-body tumor burden in adult patients with neurofibromatosis. PLoS One. 2012;7(4):e35711.
39. Dombi E, et al. Recommendations for imaging tumor response in neurofibromatosis clinical trials. Neurology. 2013;81:S33–40.
40. Mautner VF, et al. Assessment of benign tumor burden by whole-body MRI in patients with neurofibromatosis 1. Neuro-Oncology. 2008;10(4):593–8.
41. Solomon J, et al. Automated detection and volume measurement of plexiform neurofibromas in neurofibromatosis 1 using magnetic resonance imaging. Comput Med Imaging Graph. 2004;28(5):257–65.
42. Mautner VF, et al. MRI growth patterns of plexiform neurofibromas in patients with neurofibromatosis type 1. Neuroradiology. 2006;48(3):160–5.
43. Cai W, et al. Tumor burden in patients with neurofibromatosis types 1 and 2 and schwannomatosis: determination on whole-body MR images. Radiology. 2009;250(3):665–73.
44. Ahlawat S, et al. Current whole-body MRI applications in the neurofibromatoses: NF1, NF2, and schwannomatosis. Neurology. 2016;87(7 Suppl 1):S31–9.
45. Gupta A, et al. Phase I study of thalidomide for the treatment of plexiform neurofibroma in neurofibromatosis 1. Neurology. 2003;60:130–2.
46. Widemann BC, et al. Phase 1 trial and pharmacokinetic study of the farnesyl transferase inhibitor tipifarnib in children and adolescents with refractory leukemias: a report from the Children's Oncology Group. Pediatr Blood Cancer. 2011;56(2):226–33.
47. Estey E, et al. Therapeutic response in phase I trials of antineoplastic agents. Cancer Treat Rep. 1986;70(9):1105–15.
48. Therasse P, et al. New guidelines to evaluate the response to treatment in solid tumors. J Natl Cancer Inst. 2000;92(3):205–16.
49. Cai W, et al. Volumetric MRI analysis of plexiform neurofibromas in neurofibromatosis type 1: comparison of two methods. Acad Radiol. 2018;25(2):144–52.
50. Poussaint TY, et al. Interobserver reproducibility of volumetric MR imaging measurements of plexiform neurofibromas. AJR Am J Roentgenol. 2003;180(2):419–23.
51. Dombi E, et al. Activity of selumetinib in neurofibromatosis type 1-related plexiform neurofibromas. N Engl J Med. 2016;375(26):2550–60.
52. Robertson KA, et al. Imatinib mesylate for plexiform neurofibromas in patients with neurofibromatosis type 1: a phase 2 trial. Lancet Oncol. 2012;13(12):1218–24.
53. Dombi E, et al. NF1 plexiform neurofibroma growth rate by volumetric MRI: relationship to age and body weight. Neurology. 2007;68(9):643–7.
54. Korf B. Natrual history of plexiform neurofibormas in NF1. New Orleans: Children's Tumor Foundation; 2012.
55. Akshintala S, et al. Longitudinal evaluation of peripheral nerve sheath tumors in neurofibromatosis type 1: Growth analysis of plexiform neurofibromas and distinct nodular lesions. Neuro Oncol; 2020.
56. Dagalakis U, et al. Puberty and plexiform neurofibroma tumor growth in patients with neurofibromatosis type I. J Pediatr. 2013;164(3):620–4.
57. Nguyen R, et al. Growth dynamics of plexiform neurofibromas: a retrospective cohort study of 201 patients with neurofibromatosis 1. Orphanet J Rare Dis. 2012;7:75.
58. Meany H, et al. 18-fluorodeoxyglucose-positron emission tomography (FDG-PET) evaluation of nodular lesions in patients with Neurofibromatosis type 1 and plexiform neurofibromas (PN) or malignant peripheral nerve sheath tumors (MPNST). Pediatr Blood Cancer. 2013;60(1):59–64.
59. Higham CS, et al. The characteristics of 76 atypical neurofibromas as precursors to neurofibromatosis 1 associated malignant peripheral nerve sheath tumors. Neuro-Oncology. 2018;20(6):818–25.

60. Miettinen MM, et al. Histopathologic evaluation of atypical neurofibromatous tumors and their transformation into malignant peripheral nerve sheath tumor in patients with neurofibromatosis 1-a consensus overview. Hum Pathol. 2017;67:1–10.
61. Beert E, et al. Atypical neurofibromas in neurofibromatosis type 1 are premalignant tumors. Genes Chromosomes Cancer. 2011;50(12):1021–32.
62. Bernthal NM, et al. The effect of surgical margins on outcomes for low grade MPNSTs and atypical neurofibroma. J Surg Oncol. 2014;110(7):813–6.
63. Higham C, et al. Atypical neurofibromas in NF1: Clinical, imaging and pathology characteristics. Austin: Children's Tumor Foundation; 2016.
64. Reilly KM, et al. Neurofibromatosis Type 1-Associated MPNST State of the Science: Outlining a Research Agenda for the Future. J Natl Cancer Inst. 2017;109(8):djx124.
65. Canavese F, Krajbich JI. Resection of plexiform neurofibromas in children with neurofibromatosis type 1. J Pediatr Orthop. 2011;31(3):303–11.
66. Needle MN, et al. Prognostic signs in the surgical management of plexiform neurofibroma: the Children's Hospital of Philadelphia experience, 1974-1994. J Pediatr. 1997;131(5):678–82.
67. Needle MN, et al. Prognostic signs in the surgical management of neurofibroma : the Children's Hospital of Philadelphia experience, 1974-1994. J Pediatr. 1997;131:678–82.
68. Jessen WJ, et al. MEK inhibition exhibits efficacy in human and mouse neurofibromatosis tumors. J Clin Invest. 2013;123(1):340–7.
69. Weiss B, Bollag G, Shannon K. Hyperactive Ras as a therapeutic target in neurofibromatosis type 1. Am J Med Genet. 1999;89(1):14–22.
70. Dasgupta B, et al. Proteomic analysis reveals hyperactivation of the mammalian target of rapamycin pathway in neurofibromatosis 1-associated human and mouse brain tumors. Cancer Res. 2005;65(7):2755–60.
71. Johannessen CM, et al. The NF1 tumor suppressor critically regulates TSC2 and mTOR. Proc Natl Acad Sci U S A. 2005;102(24):8573–8.
72. Johansson G, et al. Effective in vivo targeting of the mammalian target of rapamycin pathway in malignant peripheral nerve sheath tumors. Mol Cancer Ther. 2008;7(5):1237–45.
73. Khalaf WF, et al. K-ras is critical for modulating multiple c-kit-mediated cellular functions in wild-type and Nf1+/– mast cells. J Immunol. 2007;178(4):2527–34.
74. Yang FC, et al. Nf1-dependent tumors require a microenvironment containing Nf1+/–– and c-kit-dependent bone marrow. Cell. 2008;135(3):437–48.
75. Yang FC, Staser K, Clapp DW. The plexiform neurofibroma microenvironment. Cancer Microenviron. 2012;5(3):307–10.
76. Plotkin SR, et al. Achieving consensus for clinical trials: The REiNS International Collaboration. Neurology. 2013;81(Supp):S1–5.
77. Gutmann DH, et al. Optimizing biologically targeted clinical trials for neurofibromatosis. Expert Opin Investig Drugs. 2013;22(4):443–62.
78. Widemann BC, et al. Phase 2 randomized, flexible crossover, double-blinded, placebo-controlled trial of the farnesyltransferase inhibitor tipifarnib in children and young adults with neurofibromatosis type 1 and progressive plexiform neurofibromas. Neuro-Oncology. 2014;16(5):707–18.
79. Babovic-Vuksanovic D, et al. Phase II trial of pirfenidone in adults with neurofibromatosis type 1. Neurology. 2006;67(10):1860–2.
80. Babovic-Vuksanovic D, et al. Phase I trial of pirfenidone in children with neurofibromatosis 1 and plexiform neurofibromas. Pediatr Neurol. 2007;36(5):293–300.
81. Widemann BC, et al. Phase II trial of pirfenidone in children and young adults with neurofibromatosis type 1 and progressive plexiform neurofibromas. Pediatr Blood Cancer. 2014;61(9):1598–602.
82. Weiss B, et al. Sirolimus for progressive neurofibromatosis type 1-associated plexiform neurofibromas: a Neurofibromatosis Clinical Trials Consortium phase II study. Neuro-Oncology. 2014;17(4):596–603.
83. Weiss B, et al. Sirolimus for non-progressive NF1-associated plexiform neurofibromas: an NF clinical trials consortium phase II study. Pediatr Blood Cancer. 2014;61(6):982–6.

84. Jakacki RI, et al. Phase I trial of pegylated interferon-alpha-2b in young patients with plexiform neurofibromas. Neurology. 2011;76(3):265–72.
85. Jakacki RI, et al. Phase II trial of pegylated interferon alfa-2b in young patients with neurofibromatosis type 1 and unresectable plexiform neurofibromas. Neuro-Oncology. 2017;19(2):289–97.
86. Widemann BC, et al. Phase II trial of pirfenidone in children and young adults with neurofibromatosis type 1 and progressive plexiform neurofibroma. Pediatr Blood Cancer. 2014;61:1598–602.
87. Weiss B, et al. Sirolimus for progressive neurofibromatosis type 1-associated plexiform neurofibromas: a neurofibromatosis Clinical Trials Consortium phase II study. Neuro-Oncology. 2015;17(4):596–603.
88. Jakacki R, et al. Preliminary results of a phase II trial of pegylated interferon-alfa-2B (PI) in pediatric patients with documented progression of neurofibromatosis type 1-related unresectable plexiform neurofibromas (PNF). Neuro-Oncology. 2012;14:16.
89. Mullin RL, et al. Reliability of functional outcome measures in adults with neurofibromatosis 1. SAGE Open Med. 2018;6:2050312118786860.
90. Martin S, et al. Development and validation of the English pain interference index and pain interference index-parent report. Pain Med. 2015;16(2):367–73.
91. Friday BB, Adjei AA. Advances in targeting the Ras/Raf/MEK/Erk mitogen-activated protein kinase cascade with MEK inhibitors for cancer therapy. Clin Cancer Res. 2008;14(2):342–6.
92. Lauchle JO, et al. Response and resistance to MEK inhibition in leukaemias initiated by hyperactive Ras. Nature. 2009;461(7262):411–4.
93. Gross A. M, et al. Selumetinib in Children with Inoperable Plexiform Neurofibromas. N Engl J Med. 2020. https://doi.org/10.1056/NEJMoa1912735.
94. Gross A, et al. SPRINT: phase II study of the MEK 1/2 inhibitor selumetinib (AZD6244, ARRY-142886) in children with neurofibromatosis type 1 (NF1) and inoperable plexiform neurofibromas (PN). J Clin Oncol. 2018;36(15):10503. Abstract presented at ASCO June 2, 2018, Chicago IL.
95. McCowage GB, et al. Trametinib in pediatric patients with neurofibromatosis type 1 (NF-1)-associated plexiform neurofibroma: a phase I/IIa study. J Clin Oncol. 2018;36(15):10504.
96. Weiss B, et al. NF106: Phase 2 Trial Of The Mek Inhibitor PD-0325901 in Adolescents and Adults with NF1-Related Plexiform Neurofibromas: an NF Clinical Trials Consortium Study; Abstracts from the 18th International Symposium on Pediatric Neuro-Oncology (ISPNO 2018) June 30 – July 3, 2018 Hyatt Regency Hotel Denver, Colorado, USA. Neuro-Oncology. 2018;20(suppl_2):i27–i213.
97. Banerjee A, et al. A phase I trial of the MEK inhibitor selumetinib (AZD6244) in pediatric patients with recurrent or refractory low-grade glioma: a Pediatric Brain Tumor Consortium (PBTC) study. Neuro-Oncology. 2017;19(8):1135–44.
98. Fangusaro J, et al. Selumetinib in paediatric patients with BRAF-aberrant or neurofibromatosis type 1-associated recurrent, refractory, or progressive low-grade glioma: a multicentre, phase 2 trial. Lancet Oncol. 2019;20(7):1011–1022.
99. Shih C-S, et al. NF105: A Phase II Prospective Study Of cabozantinib (Xl184) for plexiform neurofibromas In Subjects with Neurofibromatosis Type 1: A Neurofibromatosis Clinical Trial Consortium (NFCTC) Study; abstracts from the 18th International Symposium on Pediatric Neuro-Oncology (ISPNO 2018) June 30 – July 3, 2018 Hyatt Regency Hotel Denver, Colorado, USA. Neuro-Oncology. 2018;20(suppl_2):i27–i213.
100. Gutmann DH, Hunter-Schaedle K, Shannon KM. Harnessing preclinical mouse models to inform human clinical cancer trials. J Clin Invest. 2006;116(4):847–52.
101. Wu J, et al. Preclinical testing of sorafenib and RAD001 in the Nf(flox/flox);DhhCre mouse model of plexiform neurofibroma using magnetic resonance imaging. Pediatr Blood Cancer. 2012;58(2):173–80.
102. Wu J, et al. Plexiform and dermal neurofibromas and pigmentation are caused by Nf1 loss in desert hedgehog-expressing cells. Cancer Cell. 2008;13(2):105–16.

Diagnosis and Management of Malignant Tumours in NF1: Evolution from Atypical Neurofibroma to Malignant Peripheral Nerve Sheath Tumour and Treatment Options

12

Rosalie E. Ferner

Contents

12.1 History

In 1840 the surgeon Frederick Hale Thomson esquire delivered a lecture to his medical colleagues, in which he described a 36-year-old coachman with longstanding multiple cutaneous tumours [5]. The patient sought help from Thomson for a rapidly increasing swelling of the right thigh that caused severe throbbing. Despite the best available treatment with iodide of mercury, opiates and lard followed by turpentine and sulphuric acid he succumbed to his illness in agony; in retrospect, his case is consistent with an early description of NF1 associated malignant peripheral nerve sheath tumour (MPNST).

R. E. Ferner (✉)
National Neurofibromatosis Service, Department of Neurology, Guy's and St. Thomas' NHS Foundation Trust, London, UK
e-mail: rosalie.ferner@kcl.ac.uk

G. Tadini et al. (eds.), *Multidisciplinary Approach to Neurofibromatosis Type 1*,
https://doi.org/10.1007/978-3-319-92450-2_12

12.2 Introduction

Neurofibromatosis 1 is an inherited tumour suppressor disease and affected individuals have an increased propensity to develop both benign and malignant tumours [1]. Neurofibromas are peripheral nerve sheath tumours that are emblematic of the disease and form as discrete cutaneous or subcutaneous lesions or plexiform growths that may involve multiple nerve fascicles. Benign neurofibromas are the source of significant morbidity as they may cause pain and itching, disfigurement, neurological deficit and haemorrhage [1]. Cutaneous neurofibromas are invariably benign, but subcutaneous and plexiform growths have malignant potential. There is a 15.8% lifetime risk of developing a malignant peripheral nerve sheath tumour (MPNST) and high grade tumours metastasize widely, frequently presaging a poor prognosis [2, 3]. NF1 associated MPNSTs usually arise in pre-existing plexiform neurofibromas, they can occur at any age but are commonest in people in their late 20s and early 30s and tend to develop earlier than in sporadic disease [3, 4].

12.3 Diagnosis of NF1 Associated MPNST

12.3.1 Risk Factors

A number of factors have been identified that potentially are associated with a higher risk of developing MPNST and indicate the need for meticulous surveillance (Table 12.1) [4].

In a self-reported questionnaire sent to 4801 NF1 individuals, there were 878 respondents [6]. Family history was a significant risk factor for developing MPNST in people with NF1 and 19.4% with a diagnosis of MPNST had an affected family member, compared with 7.5% with no family history of MPNST. The tumour was diagnosed at an earlier age than in NF1 patients without a family history.

MPNSTs have been identified in NF1 patients following radiotherapy; in one retrospective national study in England 18 people with NF1 were irradiated for optic pathway glioma and four MPNSTs were diagnosed in the radiation pathway with a mean duration of 21 years following treatment [7].

About 4.7–11% of individuals with NF1 have a severe clinical phenotype associated with large deletions that involve the whole of the *NF1* gene and flanking regions at 17q11.2 [8]. These patients have a high tumour burden and are reported to have an increased lifetime risk (16–26%) of developing MPNST that may occur earlier

Table 12.1 Risk factors for development of malignant peripheral nerve sheath tumours in NF1

Family history of MPNST
Previous treatment with radiotherapy
NF1 microdeletion
Large internal plexiform neurofibroma burden
NF1 neuropathy
Atypical neurofibroma

than in people without *NF1* microdeletions [9, 10]. Furthermore, the co-deletion of the *SUZ12* gene as part of polycomb repressive complex 2 (PRC2) further exacerbates the risk for MPNST in this group of patients [11, 12]. PRC2 has histone methyltransferase activity and is involved in chromatin silencing, thereby repressing transcription.

Previous studies have suggested that individuals with a large number of internal plexiform neurofibromas are at increased risk for developing MPNST. Mautner and colleagues performed whole body MRI on 13 patients with NF1 associated MPNST and on 26 matched controls without MPNST [13]. They reported that only three out of 11 patients under 30 years without MPNST had internal plexiform neurofibromas, whereas all six patients with MPNST of similar age had internal plexiform neurofibromas.

NF1 is associated with a length dependent sensory motor axonal neuropathy that is diagnosed in adults. Affected individuals have thickened peripheral nerves, early development of cutaneous neurofibromas and multiple spinal nerve root neurofibromas [14]. Although the clinical manifestations are mild and the neuropathy is indolent, it has been reported in patients who have developed malignant change in plexiform neurofibromas. The neuropathy may either pre-date or occur after the diagnosis of MPNST.

Atypical neurofibromas are considered to be neurofibromas with potential for malignant transformation, they may co-exist with MPNST in different sites of the body and may occur before or after the development of an MPNST [15]. Atypical neurofibroma is a histological diagnosis based on a combination of high cellularity, nuclear atypia and less than 3/10 mitoses per high powered field (HPF) [16]. Neurofibromas that exhibit nuclear atypia in isolation are defined as benign tumours; conversely, the presence of necrosis and high mitotic activity is indicative of malignancy [3, 4]. A recent working group proposed the term atypical neurofibroma tous neoplasm of uncertain biological potential (ANNUBP) to describe these lesions because of the overlap between the pathology of atypical neurofibromas and low grade MPNSTs; they proposed a retrospective study of atypical neurofibromas and low grade MPNST to help clarify the potential for malignancy [4]. Chromosomal copy number loss of the CDKN2A/B gene locus has been identified in atypical neurofibromas and malignant peripheral nerve sheath tumours, but is absent in benign neurofibroma, supporting the premise that atypical neurofibromas are pre-malignant lesions [17].

A multi-centre retrospective study of 63 NF1 individuals with 76 atypical neurofibromas reported that the median age of diagnosis of the atypical lesions was 27.1 years [15]. The atypical neurofibromas were detected throughout the body and were predominantly intramuscular and were multiple in 15 patients (24%). The majority of tumours caused symptoms and pain was the most frequent complaint and was mostly accompanied by tumour growth. Distinct nodular lesions predominated and most tumours were positive on ^{18}F fluorodeoxyglucose positron emission tomography computerised tomography (FDG PETCT). Four atypical neurofibromas transformed to high grade MPNST and 17 patients had an MPNST in another region of the body. Two incompletely excised lesions recurred, but resection of atypical neurofibromas without wide margins was curative in 57 tumours.

Table 12.2 Clinical Manifestations of MPNST
(N.B. the symptoms may overlap with symptoms from benign neurofibromas)

Persistent and/or nocturnal pain
Rapid growth
Change in texture from soft to hard
Weakness, tingling, numbness or incoordination
Difficulty swallowing or breathing
Bladder or bowel disturbance
Sexual dysfunction
Haemorrhage

12.4 Clinical Manifestations of MPNST

The majority of malignant tumours arise in pre-existing subcutaneous or plexiform neurofibromas, but occasionally develop de novo [1, 4]. Rarely, MPNSTs may be asymptomatic and diagnosed incidentally, but usually present with one or more symptoms or signs, which frequently overlap with symptoms experienced by people with benign neurofibromas (Table 12.2) [3, 4]. It may be difficult to identify which neurofibroma has undergone malignant change when there are multiple symptomatic neurofibromas in the same region of the body, and patients do not automatically regard the development of a new lump as unusual in the context of NF1. Furthermore, NF1 individuals may have multiple co-existing complications of the disease with symptoms that are difficult to disentangle and cause diagnostic confusion. For instance, back pain attributed to a symptomatic spinal neurofibroma may be difficult to distinguish from symptoms arising from scoliosis.

12.5 Diagnosis of NF1 Associated MPNST

A meticulous clinical history should be elicited from NF1 individuals presenting with symptoms suggestive of MPNST, and should include inquiry about risk factors (see section on risk factors) as well as general and neurological assessment. Visible neurofibromas should be measured and photographed and magnetic resonance imaging (MRI) should be undertaken to determine the site, extent and volume (or three linear measurements) of the tumour.

Whole body MRI (WBMRI) using a short Tau inversion recovery sequence (STIR) has been advocated as a useful monitoring tool for individuals with NF1, to detect internal disease burden and to image large plexiform neurofibromas that involve more than one anatomical site [18]. Lobulation within the tumour, irregular contrast enhancement on T1-weighted images and ill-defined margins have been identified as features on WBMRI that are associated with MPNSTs, but do not have as high a sensitivity as FDG PET CT. Both 1.5 Tesla and 3.0 Tesla magnet strengths have been used but there is currently no consensus as to whether axial or coronal approaches are the optimal imaging planes, or whether 2D is better than 3D acquisition. A small retrospective study was performed on 22 benign neurofibromas and 9 MPNSTs with functional MRI using diffusion weighted imaging or apparent diffusion coefficient (ADC) mapping, dynamic contrast enhanced MRI [19]. Minimal ADC and average tumour diameter were highlighted as potentially useful markers of malignancy, but further research is necessary.

The dynamic imaging technique FDG PET CT visualises and quantifies glucose metabolism in cells. FDG PET CT plays a role in distinguishing the increased glucose metabolism of malignant tumours compared with benign plexiform neurofibromas. Previously it has been shown that FDG PET CT with delayed imaging has a sensitivity of 0.95 (95% CI 0.76–0.96) and specificity of 0.89 (95% CI 0.88–0.98) [20]. The maximum standard uptake value (SUVmax) with early and delayed imaging is a semi-quantitative imaging technique that reflects the regional metabolic uptake of glucose. Warbey et al. used early imaging at 90 min and delayed imaging at 4 h to demonstrate a significant difference between benign and malignant tumours [21]. They showed a correlation between mean SUVmax and tumour grade, but there was significant overlap and the grade of tumour could not be predicted for an individual patient. There was a significant difference in the mean SUVmax between benign and atypical neurofibromas, reinforcing the premise that atypical neurofibromas are at the lower end of the malignant spectrum (see section on atypical neurofibroma). C-11 Methionine PET reflects cellular proliferation and Bredella et al. advocated using this tracer in combination with FDG PET in order to increase specificity in equivocal cases, but the tracer has not been adopted as a routine imaging modality in symptomatic plexiform neurofibromas [22].

Unfortunately, the use of PET as a diagnostic tool across different institutions has become increasingly difficult. The type of scanner, scanner performance, tracer, imaging protocols and time points vary between institutions, and interpretation of PET across different centres is problematic [4]. There does not appear to be any benefit in undertaking regular surveillance with FDG PET CT in asymptomatic people with NF1 because of the radiation dose, and tumours may undergo malignant transformation in the interval between scans.

Pre-surgical biopsy of potentially high grade MPNSTs in an expert centre is advocated to plan optimal surgical management [4]. Atypical and low grade MPNSTs may be resected without prior biopsy, based on clinical and imaging findings [16]. It is difficult to distinguish atypical neurofibromas from low grade MPNSTs on pathology (see section on atypical neurofibroma), but high grade MPNSTs exhibit a high mitotic rate >10/10 per HPF, increased cellularity, atypical nuclei, necrosis and rhabdomyoblastic change may be identified [16]. Biomarkers may be useful in indicating malignant change, including tumour suppressor genes, Tumour Protein (Tp) 53 and p16/ cyclin dependent kinase inhibitor (CDKN)2A, proliferation markers (ki67), loss of Schwann cell lineage markers (S100 /Sox10) and loss of cluster of differentiation fibroblastic framework (CD)34 [16].

12.6 Management

The aim is to excise atypical neurofibromas or low grade MPNST without causing significant pain or functional impairment, wide margins are not required as there is no evidence that these tumours recur once they have been excised [16]. The goal for high grade MPNST is complete removal with wide resection, amputation should be reserved for extensive lesions and nerve reconstruction is not recommended for brachial plexus or lumbosacral plexus MPNST, because of the potential for suboptimal tumour removal [3, 16]. Radiotherapy is recommended for large, high grade or inadequately excised lesions, preferably administered pre-operatively, so that a small radiation field can be used to minimise toxicity [3, 16].

Individuals with NF1 appear to have a worse response to chemotherapy than their sporadic counterparts and chemotherapy is usually employed for metastatic disease. Few drugs have proved to be effective and the mainstay of treatment is doxorubicin alone, or in combination with ifosfamide to improve symptom control or to reduce the size of the tumour to achieve surgical resection [3, 4].

A recent clinical trial included 34 patients with NF1 associated high grade MPNST and 14 individuals with sporadic disease who received 2 cycles of neoadjuvant ifosfamide and doxorubicin followed by 2 cycles of ifosfamide and etoposide [23]. Etoposide and doxorubicin are inhibitors of topoisomerase 2 alpha which has been expressed in high grade MPNSTs. Five of 28 evaluable NF1 patients had a partial response (17.9%) compared with four out of nine patients with sporadic disease (44.4%) and 22 NF1 patients had stable disease compared with 4 sporadic MPNSTs. The trial did not have sufficient power to differentiate the objective response of NF1 versus sporadic patients but most patients achieved stable disease.

12.7 Patient Education

The difficulty in diagnosing NF1 associated MPNST cannot be overstated, particularly as the symptoms overlap with problems arising from benign neurofibromas. and physicians in primary care encounter the tumour rarely, if at all. Neurofibromatosis clinics, clinical nurse specialists and NF lay organisations are the ideal forum to educate patients and families and to advise when to seek medical help for symptomatic plexiform neurofibromas. In our national neurofibromatosis service, we provide a card with the contact details for our unit on one side and important symptoms on the other side with the acronym HELP—*H*ard, *E*nlarging rapidly, *L*imb weakness, numbness or incoordination, *P*ain that is persistent or nocturnal. Attention should be focused on adequate psychological support for patients and families affected by, or at risk of this serious complication and patient focused quality of life measures may be helpful in evaluating individual need [24].

12.8 The Future

It is discouraging that the current therapeutic options remain limited for individuals with N1 and MPNST. There is a need for international collaboration to collect cohesive data from patients with these malignant tumours in order to improve our understanding of the natural history [4]. Diagnostic imaging including MRI, diffusion weighted imaging and PET require standardisation across different institutions and auditing for diagnostic efficacy. Terminology amongst pathologists should be uniform and informative for the treating physician. Central storage of blood and tumour samples should be set up to facilitate the search for biomarkers to predict patients at risk for MPNST, response to therapy and prognosis. Pre-clinical models including DNA-fingerprinted MPNST lines, animal models replicating disease onset and metastasis and to screen novel therapy, and patient derived-xenograft models will contribute to understand the disease. Clinical trials should evaluate novel therapy and explore combination therapy and the use of appropriate outcome measures, including disease specific patient focused quality of life questionnaires are essential.

Acknowledgements I am very grateful to the patients within our national neurofibromatosis service, my colleagues in the NF1 and sarcoma units and NHS England for funding the clinical service.

References

1. Ferner RE, Gutmann DH. Neurofibromatosis type 1 (NF1): diagnosis and management. Handb Clin Neurol. 2013;115:939–55.
2. Uusitalo E, Leppavirta J, Koffert A, Suominen S, Vahtera J, Vahlberg T, et al. Incidence and mortality of neurofibromatosis: a total population study in Finland. J Invest Dermatol. 2015;135(3):904–6.
3. Ferner RE, Gutmann DH. International consensus statement on malignant peripheral nerve sheath tumors in neurofibromatosis. Cancer Res. 2002;62(5):1573–7.
4. Reilly KM, Kim A, Blakely J, Ferner RE, Gutmann DH, Legius E, et al. Neurofibromatosis type 1-associated MPNST state of the science: outlining a research agenda for the future. J Natl Cancer Inst. 2017;109(8):djx124.
5. CLINICAL LECTURE ON MOLLUSCUM. Lancet. 1841;36(924):256–60.
6. Malbari F, Spira M, Knight PB, Zhu C, Roth M, Gill J, et al. Malignant peripheral nerve sheath tumors in neurofibromatosis: impact of family history. J Pediatr Hematol Oncol. 2018;40(6):e359–e63.
7. Evans DG, Birch JM, Ramsden RT, Sharif S, Baser ME. Malignant transformation and new primary tumours after therapeutic radiation for benign disease: substantial risks in certain tumour prone syndromes. J Med Genet. 2006;43(4):289–94.
8. Kehrer-Sawatzki H, Mautner VF, Cooper DN. Emerging genotype-phenotype relationships in patients with large NF1 deletions. Hum Genet. 2017;136(4):349–76.
9. De Raedt T, Brems H, Wolkenstein P, Vidaud D, Pilotti S, Perrone F, et al. Elevated risk for MPNST in NF1 microdeletion patients. Am J Hum Genet. 2003;72(5):1288–92.
10. Mautner VF, Kluwe L, Friedrich RE, Roehl AC, Bammert S, Hogel J, et al. Clinical characterisation of 29 neurofibromatosis type-1 patients with molecularly ascertained 1.4 Mb type-1 NF1 deletions. J Med Genet. 2010;47(9):623–30.
11. De Raedt T, Beert E, Pasmant E, Luscan A, Brems H, Ortonne N, et al. PRC2 loss amplifies Ras-driven transcription and confers sensitivity to BRD4-based therapies. Nature. 2014;514(7521):247–51.
12. Zhang M, Wang Y, Jones S, Sausen M, McMahon K, Sharma R, et al. Somatic mutations of SUZ12 in malignant peripheral nerve sheath tumors. Nat Genet. 2014;46(11):1170–2.
13. Mautner VF, Asuagbor FA, Dombi E, Funsterer C, Kluwe L, Wenzel R, et al. Assessment of benign tumor burden by whole-body MRI in patients with neurofibromatosis 1. Neuro-Oncology. 2008;10(4):593–8.
14. Ferner RE, Hughes RA, Hall SM, Upadhyaya M, Johnson MR. Neurofibromatous neuropathy in neurofibromatosis 1 (NF1). J Med Genet. 2004;41(11):837–41.

15. Higham CS, Dombi E, Rogiers A, Bhaumik S, Pans S, Connor SEJ, et al. The characteristics of 76 atypical neurofibromas as precursors to neurofibromatosis 1 associated malignant peripheral nerve sheath tumors. Neuro-Oncology. 2018;20(6):818–25.
16. Miettinen MM, Antonescu CR, Fletcher CDM, Kim A, Lazar AJ, Quezado MM, et al. Histopathologic evaluation of atypical neurofibromatous tumors and their transformation into malignant peripheral nerve sheath tumor in patients with neurofibromatosis 1-a consensus overview. Hum Pathol. 2017;67:1–10.
17. Beert E, Brems H, Daniels B, De Wever I, Van Calenbergh F, Schoenaers J, et al. Atypical neurofibromas in neurofibromatosis type 1 are premalignant tumors. Genes Chromosomes Cancer. 2011;50(12):1021–32.
18. Ahlawat S, Fayad LM, Khan MS, Bredella MA, Harris GJ, Evans DG, et al. Current whole-body MRI applications in the neurofibromatoses: NF1, NF2, and schwannomatosis. Neurology. 2016;87(7 Suppl 1):S31–9.
19. Demehri S, Belzberg A, Blakeley J, Fayad LM. Conventional and functional MR imaging of peripheral nerve sheath tumors: initial experience. AJNR Am J Neuroradiol. 2014;35(8):1615–20.
20. Ferner RE, Golding JF, Smith M, Calonje E, Jan W, Sanjayanathan V, et al. [18F]2-fluoro-2-deoxy-D-glucose positron emission tomography (FDG PET) as a diagnostic tool for neurofibromatosis 1 (NF1) associated malignant peripheral nerve sheath tumours (MPNSTs): a long-term clinical study. Ann Oncol. 2008;19(2):390–4.
21. Warbey VS, Ferner RE, Dunn JT, Calonje E, O'Doherty MJ. [18F]FDG PET/CT in the diagnosis of malignant peripheral nerve sheath tumours in neurofibromatosis type-1. Eur J Nucl Med Mol Imaging. 2009;36(5):751–7.
22. Bredella MA, Torriani M, Hornicek F, Ouellette HA, Plamer WE, Williams Z, et al. Value of PET in the assessment of patients with neurofibromatosis type 1. AJR Am J Roentgenol. 2007;189(4):928–35.
23. Higham CS, Steinberg SM, Dombi E, Perry A, Helman LJ, Schuetze SM, et al. SARC006: phase II trial of chemotherapy in sporadic and neurofibromatosis type 1 associated chemotherapy-naive malignant peripheral nerve sheath tumors. Sarcoma. 2017;2017:8685638.
24. Ferner RE, Thomas M, Mercer G, Williams V, Leschziner GD, Afridi SK, et al. Evaluation of quality of life in adults with neurofibromatosis 1 (NF1) using the impact of NF1 on Quality Of Life (INF1-QOL) questionnaire. Health Qual Life Outcomes. 2017;15(1):34.

Neurological Complications in NF1

13

Una-Marie Sheerin and Rosalie E. Ferner

Contents

13.1 Introduction

Neurological complications of neurofibromatosis type 1 (NF1) are an important source of morbidity and mortality. These complications derive from not only the neurofibromas themselves but also from central nervous system tumours and the secondary complications resulting from bony deformities of the skull and skeleton.

U.-M. Sheerin (✉) · R. E. Ferner
National Neurofibromatosis Service, Department of Neurology, Guy's and St Thomas' NHS Foundation Trust, Guy's Hospital, London, UK
e-mail: Una.Sheerin@gstt.nhs.uk; rosalie.ferner@kcl.ac.uk

G. Tadini et al. (eds.), *Multidisciplinary Approach to Neurofibromatosis Type 1*,
https://doi.org/10.1007/978-3-319-92450-2_13

Table 13.1 Frequency and age of onset of neurological complications of neurofibromatosis type 1

Neurological complication	Frequency (%)	Age of onset
Learning difficulties	30–60%	Birth
Severe cognitive impairment (IQ < 70)	4–8%	Birth
Optic pathway glioma	15% (only 5% symptomatic)	Typically birth to 7 years
Epilepsy	6–7%	Lifelong
Dysembryoplastic neuroepithelial tumour	<5%	Lifelong
Multiple sclerosis	<5%	Adulthood
Cerebral and spinal gliomas	2–3%	Lifelong
Sphenoid wing dysplasia	<1%	Congenital
Aqueduct stenosis	1.5%	Lifelong
Chiari 1 malformation	1.5%	Lifelong
Neurofibromatous neuropathy	1.3%	Adulthood
Malignant peripheral nerve sheath tumour	15.8% lifetime risk [2]	Lifelong
Cerebrovascular abnormality	2.5% [3]	Childhood

Neurological complications associated with NF1, frequency, and ages of onset are listed in Table 13.1. The commonest neurological complication of NF1 are learning disabilities and behavioural problems and are more extensively discussed in Chap. 14, optic pathway gliomas are also discussed in Chap. 6. Malignant peripheral nerve sheath tumours are highly aggressive sarcomas, frequently associated with a poor prognosis and are discussed in Chap. 12.

The purpose of regular clinical review of patients with NF1 is to recognise and manage complications. Neurological examination should be undertaken during annual assessment by a clinician familiar with NF1. Any unexplained neurological signs or symptoms merit referral to a neurologist. Urgent advice and review is necessary if individuals experience acute or progressive sensory disturbance, incoordination or motor deficit with or without sphincter disturbance, which could indicate an intracranial lesion or spinal cord compression. Headaches on waking, vomiting, and altered consciousness are suggestive of raised intracranial pressure and constitute a neurological emergency. Rare or potentially life threatening complications should be managed by expert multidisciplinary teams that can provide diagnosis and lifelong surveillance and care [1]. As complications are likely to become symptomatic between appointments, patient education is key, enabling patients to recognise symptoms that require prompt clinical review.

13.2 Cognitive Impairment (See Also Chap. 14)

Cognitive impairment is the commonest neurological symptom in childhood. Characteristically the intelligent quotient (IQ) is in the average range (~90.6) with the distribution of IQ scores shifted one standard deviation to the left of the normal distribution. Mental retardation (IQ < 70) is uncommon [4]. Nearly 20% of children with NF1 meet criteria for a specific learning disorder, which is more than double that observed in the typically developing paediatric population [4]. As many as 75% of children with NF1 will require some type of help at school or remedial teaching [5]. In addition to specific learning disorders, children with NF1 often have deficits in other specific cognitive domains, including verbal learning, visuospatial and visual perceptual processing, language deficits, and dysexecutive problems [6–10]. Children with NF1 have specific deficits in attention, [9] particularly in sustained attention [4] with as many as 60% of children meeting diagnostic criteria for attention deficit hyperactivity disorder (ADHD) [11]. In contrast with ADHD observed in the general population, children with NF1 rarely meet the criteria for hyperactive/impulsive-type ADHD, and are more likely to be diagnosed with inattentive-type or combined-type ADHD [11]. There is also strong evidence for decline in social functioning [12–14] as well as substantially higher incidence of clinical autistic spectrum disorder (ASD), with approximately 25–40% of individuals with NF1 meeting the diagnostic criteria compared with 1–2% of ASD observed in the general population [13, 14]. Early recognition of behavioural and learning difficulties helps implement appropriate early behavioural and academic interventions and/or timely medical treatment.

13.3 Epilepsy

There is a tenfold increase in the likelihood of seizures in NF1 compared with the general population. Seizure frequency varies from 4% to 13% depending on the study design and ascertainment of patients [15–17]. All seizure types are encountered; however, the commonest is complex partial seizures, suggesting underlying cortical dysgenesis [15]. This is supported by a pathological study in which abnormal cerebral architecture, subcortical heterotopia, and glial nodules were found in patients with NF1 and cognitive impairment [18]. Onset of epilepsy is reported from infancy to late middle age and is usually mild compared with other neurocutaneous disorders. As seizures may be secondary to other recognised complications of NF1 including parenchymal glioma and aqueduct stenosis, individuals presenting with a first seizure should have MRI brain imaging even if they have had previous normal neuroimaging. Children with NF1 and epilepsy are generally more difficult to treat with a single anti-epileptic drug than children with epilepsy in the general population. Conversely adults with NF1 usually have very mild seizures [17, 19]. Individuals with NF1 and seizures may be good candidates for epilepsy surgery [17]. In the largest series of 12 patients with NF1 undergoing epilepsy surgery, eight were seizure-free at 1-year follow-up, and another individual had decreased seizure burden [20].

Glioneuronal tumours, such as ganglioglioma and dysembryoplastic neuroepithelial tumours (DNETs), have been reported in patients with NF1 and are almost always associated with seizures [21–23]. In the largest epilepsy surgery series in NF1, 40% of the tumours resected were DNETs [20], whereas DNETs only account for 14–18% of histological diagnoses in other epilepsy series [24]. DNETs are glioneuronal tumours that are cortically based and found most frequently in the temporal lobes. They are frequently found to co-occur with adjacent focal cortical dysplasia, suggesting a common developmental aetiology for both structural abnormalities.

13.4 Brain Tumours

Gliomas can develop in any location in the central nervous system in patients with NF1 and are usually World Health Organization (WHO) grade 1 gliomas (pilocytic astrocytomas). The majority of pilocytic astrocytomas are indolent neoplasms; more aggressive behaviour has been associated with symptomatic tumours, presentation after 8 years of age and gliomas occurring outside of the optic pathway [25].

13.4.1 Optic Pathway Gliomas (OPG)

The commonest brain tumour in children with NF1 is the optic pathway glioma (OPG), accounting for two-thirds of all brain tumours in children with NF1. OPGs are typically WHO grade I pilocytic astrocytomas. OPGs are found in as many as 15–20% of children with NF1 but only 5–7% ever cause signs or symptoms [26]. OPGs are usually seen in children younger than 6 years of age [26–28], it is rare for a newly symptomatic OPG to arise after the age of 7 years [29, 30]. These tumours can occur anywhere along the optic pathway, including the optic nerves, chiasm and post-chiasmatic tracts and radiations; however, the majority of OPGs arise within the anterior optic pathway [31]. Bilateral OPGs are more frequent in NF1 patients than in the general population [32]. Sporadic OPGs occurring in individuals who do not have NF1 have a worse visual outcome, higher morbidity, and increased mortality. Poor visual outcome despite treatment is associated with location of the OPG in the optic tracts/radiations, female gender, optic pallor at the time of treatment and presentation before the age of 2 years or over 5 years [30, 33–37]. Studies have shown that radiographic tumour progression is neither necessary nor sufficient to cause vision loss [36, 38–41].

13.4.2 Screening for Symptomatic OPGs

Young children do not complain of visual impairment until it is advanced, therefore visual examination by an experienced ophthalmologist or neuro-ophthalmologist familiar with NF1 is essential. Signs of a symptomatic OPG include reduced visual acuity, impaired colour vision, strabismus, proptosis, relative afferent pupillary defect, optic disc swelling or atrophy, and visual field defects. Precocious puberty is suggestive of OPG impingement on the hypothalamus. Parents also need to be aware of symptoms of visual loss such as failure to pick up small toys and bumping into objects.

Visual screening is mandatory at least annually in all children under the age of 8 years and then preferably every 2 years until the age of 18 years of age; however, there are no specific recommendations for adults [26, 37]. Measurement of visual acuity is the most useful screening tool as impaired colour vision, strabismus, and nystagmus are usually associated with visual acuity loss when due to an NF1 related OPG (NF1-OPG) [26]. Baseline assessment of colour vision and visual fields should be undertaken when the child is mature enough to cope with the test. MRI screening for detecting OPGs is not indicated routinely as it does not affect outcome, but there may be a role for MRI in children in whom no useful visual assessment can be performed, for example, children too young or immature to cope with testing. Studies have shown that visual evoked potentials have been unable to identify OPGs that require treatment or monitor the visual response to treatment [42–44]. The usefulness of optical coherence tomography (OCT), which measures the peripapillary retinal nerve fibre layer (pRNFL) thickness, diffusion tensor imaging (DTI) which measures the diffusion of water molecules, and volumetric MRI is being investigated for NF1-OPG.

Once a clinician suspects the presence of an OPG an MRI brain and orbits should be performed. Typically, OPGs manifest on MRI as expansile masses with robust gadolinium contrast enhancement (see Fig. 13.1).

Frequency of imaging and radiological surveillance of children with an OPG depend on the site of the tumour, degree of visual impairment and associated symptoms, and evidence of progressive disease [26]. Following the identification of an OPG in a child with NF1 it is recommended that they be reassessed every 3 months by MRI and ophthalmological examinations for the first year [26, 37], as

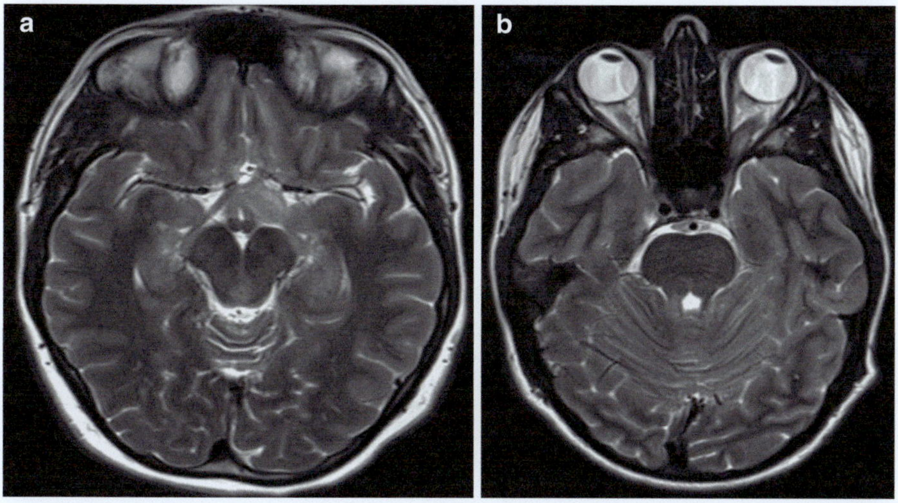

Fig. 13.1 (**a**) T2-weighted axial MRI demonstrates marked focal expansion of the left optic chiasm and proximal optic tract. (**b**) Tortuosity of the optic nerve sheath complexes, particularly on the left with expansion of the intraorbital, canalicular and pre-chiasmatic optic nerve in keeping with optic pathway glioma

treatment for NF1-OPG in the majority of children is initiated in the first year [36]. If the tumour is non-progressive after the first year, then the intervals between subsequent evaluations are lengthened to every 6 months. Tumours that remain stable for more than 3 years are less likely to become symptomatic [36] and can be monitored annually with MRI, but ophthalmology evaluations should continue every 6 months until at least 8 years of age before extending them to annually. OPGs that remain stable on ophthalmological assessment and MRI may undergo imaging less frequently. Ophthalmology evaluations should continue annually until 18 years of age and may be discontinued if clinically stable, as progression of OPG is rare in adulthood.

13.4.3 Treatment of OPGs

Amongst specialist NF centres there is no consensus regarding the indications for initiation of treatment of NF1-OPG. The most frequent primary indications for treatment included visual acuity loss and radiographic tumour progression [36]. Further studies are needed to delineate which indications for treatment are best able to prevent or mitigate visual loss in children with NF1-OPG. Guidelines for initiating treatment have recently been published [37]. The best indication for treatment is evidence of progressive, clinically significant vision loss. A difference of 0.2 logMAR or greater in visual acuity in a single eye from age-based normal values is considered abnormal, and a change in visual acuity of 0.2 logMAR or more is considered clinically significant [26, 45, 46]. As vision deficits due to NF1-OPG may go unnoticed and even precede a diagnosis of OPG, ophthalmological abnormalities found at tumour presentation which are thought to be chronic may not require therapy. Convincing evidence of new or progressive visual field loss (for instance, a new quadrantanopia) would also constitute clinically significant vision loss and indicate treatment. There are three other situations in which treatment is considered based on the potential impact of further visual loss. These include children who are blind or nearly blind (visual acuity worse than 1 logMAR in one eye) and visual acuity worse than 0.2 logMAR relative to age norms or tumour progression by MRI in the other eye. Secondly, children with visual acuity loss in a single eye near a functional threshold (0.6–1.0 logMAR relative to age norms) may benefit from chemotherapy to preserve or improve visual acuity because of the impact of any visual acuity change [36]. Lastly, treatment may be considered when there is suspected vision loss but unreliable visual acuity testing together with significant radiological tumour progression.

Changes in the eye examination such as new onset colour vision loss, disc pallor, optic nerve swelling, afferent pupillary defect, strabismus, or nystagmus in the absence of new visual acuity changes or new visual field defects should prompt more frequent surveillance but are not an indication for treatment. Numerous previous studies have shown that radiographic tumour progression is neither necessary nor sufficient to cause visual loss [36, 38–41]. Tumour progression with stable visual acuity and visual fields generally does not require treatment but is an indication for increased surveillance. Precocious puberty related to NF1-OPG is treated with gonadotrophin-releasing hormone antagonists but is not an indication for treatment with chemotherapy.

The aim of treatment for NF1-OPG is to reduce visual morbidity. First-line treatment is with chemotherapy (vincristine and carboplatin) and produces radiological tumour regression in many children. Radiotherapy is not recommended as patients with NF1 have a propensity to develop secondary tumours of the central nervous system as late sequelae of radiation exposure. In a longitudinal study of patients treated with radiotherapy for OPG, 50% developed secondary tumours including malignant peripheral nerve sheath tumours (MPNSTs) and other gliomas [47]. Use of radiotherapy is also associated with neurological problems including moya-moya syndrome, psychological, and endocrinological consequences [27, 48, 49]. Surgery is indicated only in unusual circumstances, such as disfiguring proptosis in a nearly blind eye or enlarging tumour mass with mass effect on critical structures [50]. Clinical trials are in progress assessing the use of mTOR and MEK inhibitors for the treatment of OPG.

13.4.4 Non-optic Pathway Gliomas in NF1

Brainstem tumours are the most frequently identified brain tumour outside of the optic pathway in NF1 patients and are mostly pilocytic astrocytomas, which are indolent with slow rates of growth [25]. NF1 brainstem gliomas typically arise in slightly older children (mean age 8–9.5 years), and are most commonly located in the medulla, in contrast to sporadically occurring brainstem gliomas, which typically arise in the pons. These tumours need to be distinguished from focal areas of signal intensity (FASI) on T2-weighted fluid-attenuated inversion recovery (FLAIR) MRI sequences commonly seen in most children with NF1 which sometimes persist into adulthood (Fig. 13.2) [51, 52]. These T2-hyperintensities typically arise in the basal ganglia, cerebellum, brainstem, and optic pathway. Similar to some low-grade gliomas, they do not enhance with contrast, making it challenging to differentiate them from a low-grade tumour. However, FASI are not space occupying lesions and do not exhibit mass effect. Due to these challenges it is recommended an experienced neuroradiologist with experience in NF1 review imaging to differentiate these two entities. Many gliomas do not require treatment and are followed by annual MRI surveillance.

Although most brainstem gliomas are indolent, they can result in neurologic dysfunction. Presenting symptoms can include cranial neuropathies, lethargy, diencephalic syndrome, gait instability, hydrocephalus, headache, and/or weight loss. Careful neurological examination is important to detect subtle abnormalities indicative of a brainstem glioma. Children with tumours that cause neurological signs or symptoms might require shunting, surgical resection, or chemotherapy.

The prevalence of newly diagnosed high-grade gliomas in adults with NF1 is 50–100 times higher than expected compared with the general population [53].

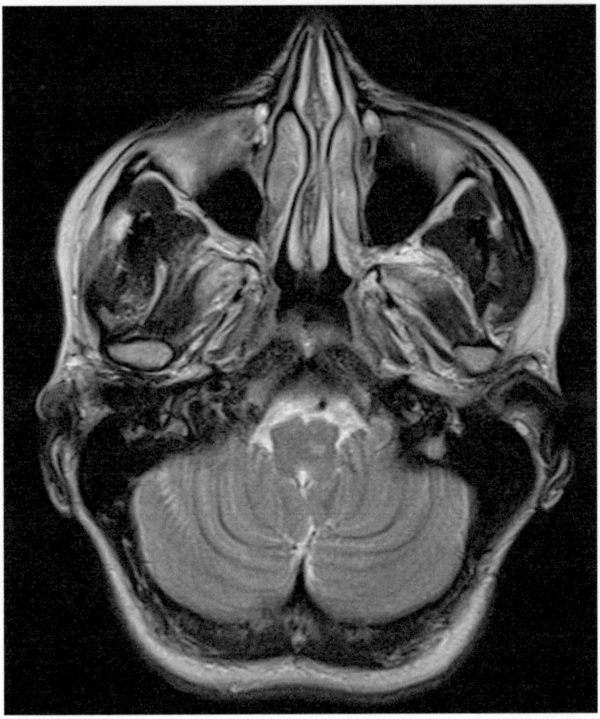

Fig. 13.2 T2-weighted axial MRI demonstrating a left medullary FASI

High-grade gliomas may either arise from a pre-existing low-grade glioma or less commonly occur without a low-grade glioma being identified. A number of risk factors for developing a high-grade glioma have been identified. Adults with prior radiotherapy as a child for OPG have an increased incidence of secondary glioma [47]. A large study of 100 adults and children with NF1 identified tumours in the thalamus are more likely to be associated with high-grade tumours and that surgical intervention is more likely with tumours in the thalamus, frontal lobes, and cerebellum, than in other anatomical locations [54] (Fig. 13.3).

The majority of tumours that progress are not pilocytic astrocytomas, but are other types of astrocytoma, that are associated with a more aggressive histological subtype [25, 54–56]. Overall, outcome is very favourable in NF1 patients with glioma, with 95% survival at 5 years, and 92% at 10 years with 65% patients being asymptomatic at follow-up. In cases where gliomas were detected incidentally on imaging for another indication, the risk of needing surgery was low (fewer than one fifth) [54]. The majority of tumours transforming to a high-grade glioma or requiring surgical intervention do so within 5 years of detection. No consensus guidelines exist, however, based on these findings; heightened surveillance with more frequent imaging should be considered in patients with thalamic tumours, and also in those with atypical histological findings for at least 5 years [54].

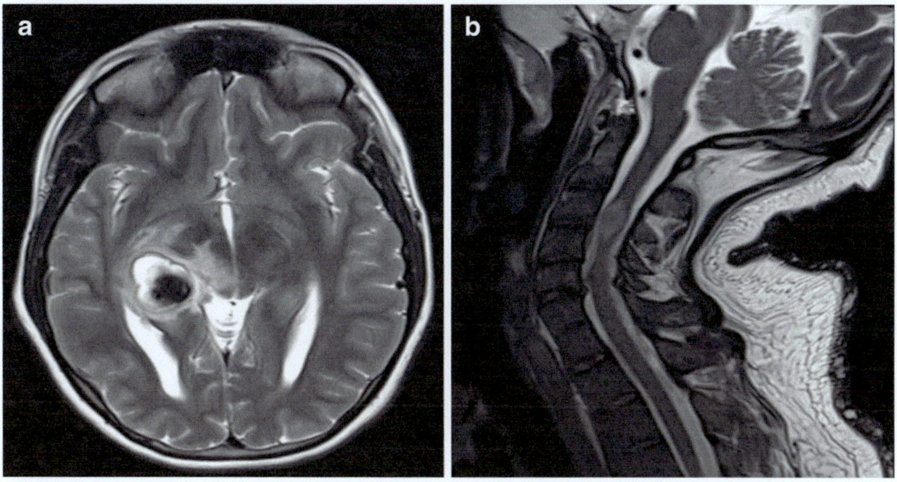

Fig. 13.3 (**a**) MRI axial T2 shows a right dorsolateral thalamic tumour with mass effect. (**b**) T2 weighted sagittal MRI shows a well-circumscribed expansile tumour centred on the right hemicord at C3

13.5 Spinal Cord Tumours

Spinal cord involvement in NF1 is typically from extramedullary growth of spinal root tumours. The association of intramedullary spinal cord tumours with NF1, although rare, has been reported [57, 58]. These tumours are typically astrocytomas and similar to brain gliomas in NF1 they appear to be generally indolent and only rarely cause symptoms. Careful neuroradiological review is needed to differentiate spinal cord tumours from spinal focal areas of T2 hyperintensity seen on MRI, which likely represent the spinal equivalent of the more commonly recognised brain FASI [59, 60].

13.6 Neurofibromatous Neuropathy

Neurofibromatous neuropathy is an indolent length-dependent sensorimotor axonal neuropathy with thickened peripheral nerves and early development of neurofibromas. Clinical manifestations are generally mild and not progressive but are accompanied by unusually early development of neurofibromas and increased risk of malignant peripheral nerve sheath tumours (MPNSTs) and therefore long-term follow-up is essential [61, 62]. Sural nerve biopsy in these patients has demonstrated diffuse neurofibromatous infiltration with disruption of the perineurium, which may be the consequence of aberrant signalling between Schwann cells, fibroblasts, and perineural cells [61].

13.7 Malformations of the Nervous System and Neurological Consequences of Bone Dysplasia

Hydrocephalus due to aqueduct stenosis is an uncommon complication of NF1 that results from periaqueductal proliferation of subependymal glial cells, or from a Chiari 1 malformation, or rarely with a tumour of the aqueduct [63, 64]. Sphenoid wing dysplasia may be detected incidentally on cranial imaging and is usually asymptomatic but can cause pulsating exophthalmos resulting from herniation of the temporal lobe into the orbit [63].

13.8 Vasculopathy

Vasculopathy associated with NF1 can affect any arterial vessel leading to systemic hypertension secondary to renal artery stenosis [65], cerebrovascular events [66], or peripheral vascular insufficiency [67]. Characteristic pathological changes have been described in all layers of the vascular wall that ultimately lead to narrowing of the arterial lumen. Cerebrovascular disease typically produces stenosis of the internal carotid artery, middle cerebral artery, or anterior cerebral artery and is often associated with a post-stenotic proliferation of small capillaries, which appears as a 'puff of smoke' ('moya-moya') on cerebral angiography. Moya-moya develops about three times more often than expected in children with NF1 after cranial irradiation for a primary brain tumour [68].

13.9 NF1 and Other Neurological Conditions

A number of other chronic neurological conditions are associated with NF1 including headache, multiple sclerosis, and sleep disorders [69, 70]. Increased frequency of migraine is reported in patients with NF1 (65% of NF1 patients in a systematic review) and had a significant impact on quality of life. Accurate phenotyping of the headache is important to offer appropriate treatment and advice [70]. There is an increased frequency of relapsing-remitting and primary progressive multiple sclerosis (MS) with a preponderance of primary progressive MS in NF1 [71–73]. The course of disease is usually indolent. The cause of the association between NF1 and MS is unknown, mutations in oligodendrocyte myelin glycoprotein (*OMGP*), a gene embedded within an intron of the *NF1* gene, have been excluded as the cause [74]. Other hypothesised mechanisms include proliferation of Schwann cells in the development of neurofibromas, results in abnormal exposure to peripheral myelin antigens, activating an autoimmune response to the same antigens in central nervous system (CNS) myelin. Alternatively, NF1 being a tumour suppression condition could result in a loss of control of immune system activity which might favour an autoimmune response to CNS myelin in susceptible patients [73]. Clinicians should be alert to possible overlap symptoms in NF1 and MS, for example, cord compression due to an intraspinal neurofibroma versus demyelination. Although NF1 is a tumour suppressor condition there is no contraindication to disease modifying immunosuppressive treatment in MS.

Children and adults with NF1 are also more likely to have experience sleep disturbances [69]. Higher rates of specific sleep disturbances, including sleep walking, sleep terrors, difficulty initiating and maintain sleep and abnormalities in arousal and sleep-wake transition [75, 76]. These problems lead to an overall increase in poor sleep quality and need careful assessment to determine underlying triggers and possible treatment strategies [77].

Superficial siderosis of the central nervous system is a rare disorder, which is the consequence of chronic subarachnoid haemorrhage. Clinical features include progressive sensorineural deafness and cerebellar ataxia, myelopathy, polyradiculopathy, anosmia, and dementia. There are several reports of superficial siderosis in patients with NF1, possibly as a result of distortion of the dura, leading to a weak point and a source of slow blood leakage through communication with the subarachnoid space [78–81].

Dural ectasia, which is widening of the vertebral sac, can be seen in individuals with NF1, may cause posterior vertebral scalloping typically extending over several vertebral levels. Typically, dural ectasia may be picked up incidentally on MRI imaging; however, rarely it can cause neurological complications.

13.10 Peripheral Nerve Sheath Tumours (See Also Chaps. 9 and 11)

Neurofibromas are benign peripheral nerve sheath tumours composed of neoplastic Schwann cells, fibroblasts, blood vessels, and mast cells. Neurofibromas present as dermal (cutaneous or subcutaneous), spinal nerve root, diffuse plexiform, nodular plexiform tumours or as neurofibromatous neuropathy. *Cutaneous neurofibromas* typically develop in adolescence, and typically increase in number with age (see chapter on neurofibromas). Discrete *subcutaneous neurofibromas* and spinal neurofibromas can cause pain or neurological deficits including sensory and motor loss and may rarely undergo malignant transformation [82]. *Plexiform neurofibromas* are benign tumours which develop as nodular lesions confined to the nerve or diffuse tumours that impinge on the surrounding soft tissue and may be associated with bone hypertrophy, vascular change, overlying pigmentation, or excess hair growth [1]. Plexiform neurofibromas cause significant morbidity due to the risk of malignant transformation to MPNST, disfigurement, pain and neurological deficit, and the potential for life threatening haemorrhage. Management of plexiform neurofibromas includes careful clinical monitoring, pain management, and excision for surgically amenable tumours. Surgery can be challenging due to the infiltration of surrounding tissue and nerves and the highly vascular nature of these tumours, which can lead to catastrophic haemorrhage.

Spinal nerve root neurofibromas can arise throughout the spine and at multiple levels, and likely represent plexiform tumours based on the involvement of multiple nerve fascicles. Spinal neurofibromas are common in patients with NF1, however, patients are mostly asymptomatic, [58] typically they are detected incidentally on neuroimaging performed for other indications. While neurofibromas can involve any of the cervical nerve roots, compression occurs most commonly in the upper spine at C2 and C3 (Fig. 13.4).

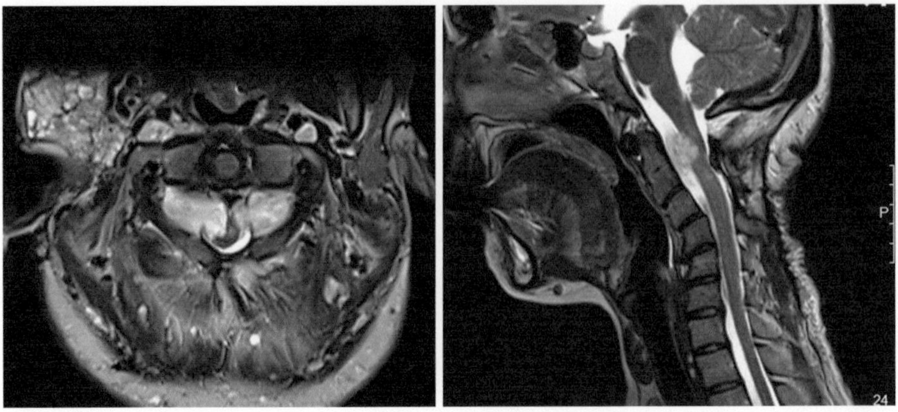

Fig. 13.4 Significant compression of the cord at the C2 level from bilateral neurofibromas with T2 hyperintense signal within the cervical cord at C2/C3 in keeping with chronic myelopathic signal change

The reason for high cervical cord compression is not known; it is possible that it reflects vulnerability of the C2 root to repeated low-grade trauma as it exits from the neural foramen and runs over the superior aspect of the C2 lamina [83]. When arising from the nerve root, the tumour grows in a dumbbell-shaped pattern as it passes through the foramen. Patients at any age are prone to developing signs or symptoms of cervical cord compression [83]. The most common presenting symptom of cord compression from cervical neurofibromas is progressive quadriparesis. Other symptoms include paraparesis, numbness, sphincter dysfunction, and neck pain. Symptomatic patients require prompt neurological assessment within a NF1 multidisciplinary team including both neurologists and neurosurgeons. Careful review of neuroradiology is needed to determine the level of the symptomatic neurofibroma as frequently these patients have spinal neurofibromas at multiple levels. The decision to undertake surgical decompression should be based on the progressive nature of neurological symptoms and deficits. Patients found to have radiological spinal cord compression from a neurofibroma but who are clinically asymptomatic should not have surgery based solely on the radiological findings but should be clinically monitored closely for progressive symptoms and signs.

13.11 Atypical Neurofibromas and Malignant Peripheral Nerve Sheath Tumour (MPNST) (See Also Chap. 12)

Atypical neurofibromas are symptomatic, hypercellular peripheral nerve sheath tumours, composed of cells with hyperchromatic nuclei in the absence of mitoses. Atypical neurofibromas have been shown to be premalignant tumours and

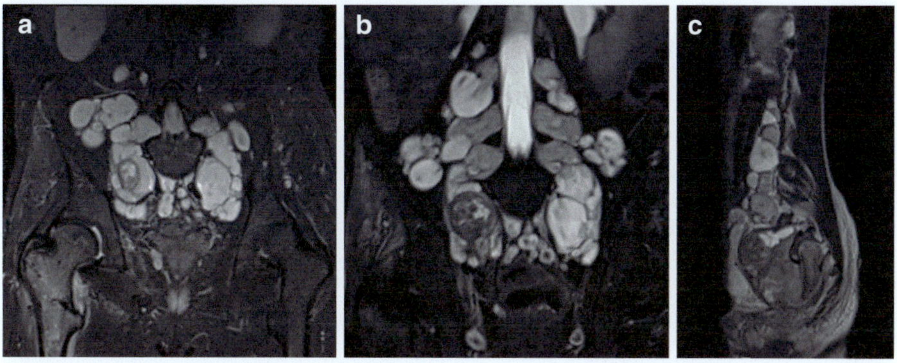

Fig. 13.5 (**a**) Nerve sheath tumour related to sciatic nerve with intra-lesion haemorrhage. Rapid growth over 2 months (**b**) and 4 months (**c**). Biopsy confirmed a grade 2 malignant peripheral nerve sheath tumour

exhibit molecular changes that are also found in malignant peripheral nerve sheath tumours (MPNST) [84]. Management is complete resection, which may reduce the risk of malignant transformation [85]. (see Chap. 12 on atypical neurofibromas).

MPNSTs are highly aggressive lesions associated with a poor prognosis [86]. (see Chap. 12) MPNSTs usually arise within pre-existing plexiform neurofibromas [87]. These tumours can develop at any age, but highest risk is in the third decade [86]. Symptoms which are concerning for risk of malignant transformation of a neurofibroma include a rapidly growing neurofibroma causing persistent or nocturnal pain, or a neurological deficit, or change in texture of a neurofibroma from soft to hard. As symptoms of MPNST are likely to occur between appointments, patients should be educated as to the symptoms suggestive of an MPNST, which should prompt them to make urgent contact with their specialist NF1 service. MPNSTs are difficult to diagnose as individuals with NF1 may have multiple tumours and symptoms of MPNSTs overlap with benign symptomatic plexiform neurofibromas. MRI can be used to characterise the site and size of symptomatic lesions but does not always detect malignancy (Fig. 13.5). The aim of treatment is complete excision with tumour-free margins. Low-grade MPNSTs treated appropriately are compatible with long-term survival. High-grade MPNSTs metastasize widely and have a poor prognosis [86].

References

1. Ferner RE, Huson SM, Thomas N, Moss C, Willshaw H, Evans DG, et al. Guidelines for the diagnosis and management of individuals with neurofibromatosis 1. J Med Genet. 2007;44(2):81–8.
2. Uusitalo E, Rantanen M, Kallionpaa RA, Poyhonen M, Leppavirta J, Yla-Outinen H, et al. Distinctive cancer associations in patients with neurofibromatosis type 1. J Clin Oncol. 2016;34(17):1978–86.

3. Rosser TL, Vezina G, Packer RJ. Cerebrovascular abnormalities in a population of children with neurofibromatosis type 1. Neurology. 2005;64(3):553–5.
4. Hyman SL, Shores A, North KN. The nature and frequency of cognitive deficits in children with neurofibromatosis type 1. Neurology. 2005;65(7):1037–44.
5. Krab LC, Oostenbrink R, de Goede-Bolder A, Aarsen FK, Elgersma Y, Moll HA. Health-related quality of life in children with neurofibromatosis type 1: contribution of demographic factors, disease-related factors, and behavior. J Pediatr. 2009;154(3):420–5, 5 e1.
6. Dilts CV, Carey JC, Kircher JC, Hoffman RO, Creel D, Ward K, et al. Children and adolescents with neurofibromatosis 1: a behavioral phenotype. J Dev Behav Pediatr. 1996;17(4):229–39.
7. Hyman SL, Arthur Shores E, North KN. Learning disabilities in children with neurofibromatosis type 1: subtypes, cognitive profile, and attention-deficit-hyperactivity disorder. Dev Med Child Neurol. 2006;48(12):973–7.
8. North KN, Riccardi V, Samango-Sprouse C, Ferner R, Moore B, Legius E, et al. Cognitive function and academic performance in neurofibromatosis. 1: consensus statement from the NF1 cognitive disorders task force. Neurology. 1997;48(4):1121–7.
9. North K, Hyman S, Barton B. Cognitive deficits in neurofibromatosis 1. J Child Neurol. 2002;17(8):605–12; discussion 27-9, 46-51.
10. Pride N, Payne JM, Webster R, Shores EA, Rae C, North KN. Corpus callosum morphology and its relationship to cognitive function in neurofibromatosis type 1. J Child Neurol. 2010;25(7):834–41.
11. Lidzba K, Granstrom S, Lindenau J, Mautner VF. The adverse influence of attention-deficit disorder with or without hyperactivity on cognition in neurofibromatosis type 1. Dev Med Child Neurol. 2012;54(10):892–7.
12. Walsh KS, Velez JI, Kardel PG, Imas DM, Muenke M, Packer RJ, et al. Symptomatology of autism spectrum disorder in a population with neurofibromatosis type 1. Dev Med Child Neurol. 2013;55(2):131–8.
13. Garg S, Green J, Leadbitter K, Emsley R, Lehtonen A, Evans DG, et al. Neurofibromatosis type 1 and autism spectrum disorder. Pediatrics. 2013;132(6):e1642–8.
14. Morris SM, Acosta MT, Garg S, Green J, Huson S, Legius E, et al. Disease burden and symptom structure of autism in neurofibromatosis type 1: a study of the international NF1-ASD consortium team (INFACT). JAMA Psychiat. 2016;73(12):1276–84.
15. Korf BR, Carrazana E, Holmes GL. Patterns of seizures observed in association with neurofibromatosis 1. Epilepsia. 1993;34(4):616–20.
16. Ferner RE, Jackson MJ. The neurofibromatoses. In: Shorvon SD, Anderman R, Rea G, editors. The causes of epilepsy. Cambridge: Cambridge University Press; 2011. p. 183–8.
17. Ostendorf AP, Gutmann DH, Weisenberg JL. Epilepsy in individuals with neurofibromatosis type 1. Epilepsia. 2013;54(10):1810–4.
18. Rosman NP, Pearce J. The brain in multiple neurofibromatosis (von Recklinghausen's disease): a suggested neuropathological basis for the associated mental defect. Brain. 1967;90(4):829–38.
19. Jackson REFaMJ. Neurocutaneous syndromes: neurofibromatoses. In: Simon D. Shorvon FA, Renzo Guerrini, editor. The causes of epilepsy: Cambridge University PressCambridge; 2011. p. 183–188.
20. Barba C, Jacques T, Kahane P, Polster T, Isnard J, Leijten FS, et al. Epilepsy surgery in neurofibromatosis type 1. Epilepsy Res. 2013;105(3):384–95.
21. Lellouch-Tubiana A, Bourgeois M, Vekemans M, Robain O. Dysembryoplastic neuroepithelial tumors in two children with neurofibromatosis type 1. Acta Neuropathol. 1995;90(3):319–22.
22. Fedi M, Anne Mitchell L, Kalnins RM, Gutmann DH, Perry A, Newton M, et al. Glioneuronal tumours in neurofibromatosis type 1: MRI-pathological study. J Clin Neurosci. 2004;11(7):745–7.
23. Parizel PM, Martin JJ, Van Vyve M, van den Hauwe L, De Schepper AM. Cerebral ganglioglioma and neurofibromatosis type I. case report and review of the literature. Neuroradiology. 1991;33(4):357–9.

24. Pasquier B, Peoc HM, Fabre-Bocquentin B, Bensaadi L, Pasquier D, Hoffmann D, et al. Surgical pathology of drug-resistant partial epilepsy. A 10-year-experience with a series of 327 consecutive resections. Epileptic Disord. 2002;4(2):99–119.
25. Guillamo JS, Creange A, Kalifa C, Grill J, Rodriguez D, Doz F, et al. Prognostic factors of CNS tumours in neurofibromatosis 1 (NF1): a retrospective study of 104 patients. Brain. 2003;126(Pt 1):152–60.
26. Listernick R, Ferner RE, Liu GT, Gutmann DH. Optic pathway gliomas in neurofibromatosis-1: controversies and recommendations. Ann Neurol. 2007;61(3):189–98.
27. Listernick R, Louis DN, Packer RJ, Gutmann DH. Optic pathway gliomas in children with neurofibromatosis 1: consensus statement from the NF1 optic pathway glioma task force. Ann Neurol. 1997;41(2):143–9.
28. King A, Listernick R, Charrow J, Piersall L, Gutmann DH. Optic pathway gliomas in neurofibromatosis type 1: the effect of presenting symptoms on outcome. Am J Med Genet A. 2003;122A(2):95–9.
29. Leonard JR, Perry A, Rubin JB, King AA, Chicoine MR, Gutmann DH. The role of surgical biopsy in the diagnosis of glioma in individuals with neurofibromatosis-1. Neurology. 2006;67(8):1509–12.
30. Listernick R, Ferner RE, Piersall L, Sharif S, Gutmann DH, Charrow J. Late-onset optic pathway tumors in children with neurofibromatosis 1. Neurology. 2004;63(10):1944–6.
31. Listernick R, Charrow J, Greenwald M, Mets M. Natural history of optic pathway tumors in children with neurofibromatosis type 1: a longitudinal study. J Pediatr. 1994;125(1):63–6.
32. Chateil JF, Soussotte C, Pedespan JM, Brun M, Le Manh C, Diard F. MRI and clinical differences between optic pathway tumours in children with and without neurofibromatosis. Br J Radiol. 2001;74(877):24–31.
33. Balcer LJ, Liu GT, Heller G, Bilaniuk L, Volpe NJ, Galetta SL, et al. Visual loss in children with neurofibromatosis type 1 and optic pathway gliomas: relation to tumor location by magnetic resonance imaging. Am J Ophthalmol. 2001;131(4):442–5.
34. Zeid JL, Charrow J, Sandu M, Goldman S, Listernick R. Orbital optic nerve gliomas in children with neurofibromatosis type 1. J AAPOS. 2006;10(6):534–9.
35. Diggs-Andrews KA, Brown JA, Gianino SM, Rubin JB, Wozniak DF, Gutmann DH. Sex is a major determinant of neuronal dysfunction in neurofibromatosis type 1. Ann Neurol. 2014;75(2):309–16.
36. Fisher MJ, Loguidice M, Gutmann DH, Listernick R, Ferner RE, Ullrich NJ, et al. Visual outcomes in children with neurofibromatosis type 1-associated optic pathway glioma following chemotherapy: a multicenter retrospective analysis. Neuro-Oncology. 2012;14(6):790–7.
37. de Blank PMK, Fisher MJ, Liu GT, Gutmann DH, Listernick R, Ferner RE, et al. Optic pathway gliomas in neurofibromatosis type 1: an update: surveillance, treatment indications, and biomarkers of vision. J Neuroophthalmol. 2017;37(Suppl 1):S23–32.
38. Shofty B, Ben-Sira L, Freedman S, Yalon M, Dvir R, Weintraub M, et al. Visual outcome following chemotherapy for progressive optic pathway gliomas. Pediatr Blood Cancer. 2011;57(3):481–5.
39. Grill J, Laithier V, Rodriguez D, Raquin MA, Pierre-Kahn A, Kalifa C. When do children with optic pathway tumours need treatment? An oncological perspective in 106 patients treated in a single Centre. Eur J Pediatr. 2000;159(9):692–6.
40. Campagna M, Opocher E, Viscardi E, Calderone M, Severino SM, Cermakova I, et al. Optic pathway glioma: long-term visual outcome in children without neurofibromatosis type-1. Pediatr Blood Cancer. 2010;55(6):1083–8.
41. Kelly JP, Weiss AH. Detection of tumor progression in optic pathway glioma with and without neurofibromatosis type 1. Neuro-Oncology. 2013;15(11):1560–7.
42. Ng YT, North KN. Visual-evoked potentials in the assessment of optic gliomas. Pediatr Neurol. 2001;24(1):44–8.
43. Falsini B, Ziccardi L, Lazzareschi I, Ruggiero A, Placentino L, Dickmann A, et al. Longitudinal assessment of childhood optic gliomas: relationship between flicker visual evoked potentials and magnetic resonance imaging findings. J Neuro-Oncol. 2008;88(1):87–96.

44. Kelly JP, Leary S, Khanna P, Weiss AH. Longitudinal measures of visual function, tumor volume, and prediction of visual outcomes after treatment of optic pathway gliomas. Ophthalmology. 2012;119(6):1231–7.
45. Avery RA, Ferner RE, Listernick R, Fisher MJ, Gutmann DH, Liu GT. Visual acuity in children with low grade gliomas of the visual pathway: implications for patient care and clinical research. J Neuro-Oncol. 2012;110(1):1–7.
46. Fisher MJ, Avery RA, Allen JC, Ardern-Holmes SL, Bilaniuk LT, Ferner RE, et al. Functional outcome measures for NF1-associated optic pathway glioma clinical trials. Neurology. 2013;81(21 Suppl 1):S15–24.
47. Sharif S, Ferner R, Birch JM, Gillespie JE, Gattamaneni HR, Baser ME, et al. Second primary tumors in neurofibromatosis 1 patients treated for optic glioma: substantial risks after radiotherapy. J Clin Oncol. 2006;24(16):2570–5.
48. Packer RJ, Ater J, Allen J, Phillips P, Geyer R, Nicholson HS, et al. Carboplatin and vincristine chemotherapy for children with newly diagnosed progressive low-grade gliomas. J Neurosurg. 1997;86(5):747–54.
49. Desai SS, Paulino AC, Mai WY, Teh BS. Radiation-induced moyamoya syndrome. Int J Radiat Oncol Biol Phys. 2006;65(4):1222–7.
50. Avery RA, Fisher MJ, Liu GT. Optic pathway gliomas. J Neuroophthalmol. 2011; 31(3):269–78.
51. Ferner RE, Chaudhuri R, Bingham J, Cox T, Hughes RA. MRI in neurofibromatosis 1. The nature and evolution of increased intensity T2 weighted lesions and their relationship to intellectual impairment. J Neurol Neurosurg Psychiatry. 1993;56(5):492–5.
52. DeBella K, Poskitt K, Szudek J, Friedman JM. Use of "unidentified bright objects" on MRI for diagnosis of neurofibromatosis 1 in children. Neurology. 2000;54(8):1646–51.
53. Gutmann DH, Rasmussen SA, Wolkenstein P, MacCollin MM, Guha A, Inskip PD, et al. Gliomas presenting after age 10 in individuals with neurofibromatosis type 1 (NF1). Neurology. 2002;59(5):759–61.
54. Byrne S, Connor S, Lascelles K, Siddiqui A, Hargrave D, Ferner RE. Clinical presentation and prognostic indicators in 100 adults and children with neurofibromatosis 1 associated non-optic pathway brain gliomas. J Neuro-Oncol. 2017;133(3):609–14.
55. Pollack IF, Shultz B, Mulvihill JJ. The management of brainstem gliomas in patients with neurofibromatosis 1. Neurology. 1996;46(6):1652–60.
56. Molloy PT, Bilaniuk LT, Vaughan SN, Needle MN, Liu GT, Zackai EH, et al. Brainstem tumors in patients with neurofibromatosis type 1: a distinct clinical entity. Neurology. 1995;45(10):1897–902.
57. Lee M, Rezai AR, Freed D, Epstein FJ. Intramedullary spinal cord tumors in neurofibromatosis. Neurosurgery. 1996;38(1):32–7.
58. Thakkar SD, Feigen U, Mautner VF. Spinal tumours in neurofibromatosis type 1: an MRI study of frequency, multiplicity and variety. Neuroradiology. 1999;41(9):625–9.
59. D'Amico A, Mazio F, Ugga L, Cuocolo R, Cirillo M, Santoro C, et al. Medullary unidentified bright objects in neurofibromatosis type 1: a case series. BMC Pediatr. 2018;18(1):91.
60. Ruegger AD, Coleman L, Hansford JR, McLean N, Dabscheck G. Spinal cord hyperintensities in neurofibromatosis type 1: are they the cord equivalent of unidentified bright objects in the brain? Pediatr Neurol. 2018;86:63–5.
61. Ferner RE, Hughes RA, Hall SM, Upadhyaya M, Johnson MR. Neurofibromatous neuropathy in neurofibromatosis 1 (NF1). J Med Genet. 2004;41(11):837–41.
62. Drouet A, Wolkenstein P, Lefaucheur JP, Pinson S, Combemale P, Gherardi RK, et al. Neurofibromatosis 1-associated neuropathies: a reappraisal. Brain. 2004;127(Pt 9): 1993–2009.
63. Huson SM, Harper PS, Compston DA. Von Recklinghausen neurofibromatosis. A clinical and population study in South-East Wales. Brain. 1988;111(Pt 6):1355–81.
64. Afifi AK, Dolan KD, Van Gilder JC, Fincham RW. Ventriculomegaly in neurofibromatosis-1. Association with Chiari type I malformation. Neurofibromatosis. 1988;1(5–6):299–305.

65. Han M, Criado E. Renal artery stenosis and aneurysms associated with neurofibromatosis. J Vasc Surg. 2005;41(3):539–43.
66. Terry AR, Jordan JT, Schwamm L, Plotkin SR. Increased risk of cerebrovascular disease among patients with neurofibromatosis type 1: population-based approach. Stroke. 2016;47(1): 60–5.
67. Farmakis SG, Han M, White F, Khanna G. Neurofibromatosis 1 vasculopathy manifesting as a peripheral aneurysm in an adolescent. Pediatr Radiol. 2014;44(10):1328–31.
68. Ullrich NJ, Robertson R, Kinnamon DD, Scott RM, Kieran MW, Turner CD, et al. Moyamoya following cranial irradiation for primary brain tumors in children. Neurology. 2007;68(12):932–8.
69. Madubata CC, Olsen MA, Stwalley DL, Gutmann DH, Johnson KJ. Neurofibromatosis type 1 and chronic neurological conditions in the United States: an administrative claims analysis. Genet Med. 2015;17(1):36–42.
70. Afridi SK, Leschziner GD, Ferner RE. Prevalence and clinical presentation of headache in a National neurofibromatosis 1 service and impact on quality of life. Am J Med Genet A. 2015;167A(10):2282–5.
71. Ferner RE, Hughes RA, Johnson MR. Neurofibromatosis 1 and multiple sclerosis. J Neurol Neurosurg Psychiatry. 1995;58(5):582–5.
72. Etemadifar M, Fatehi F, Sahraian MA, Borhanihaghighi A, Ardestani PM, Kaji-Esfahani M, et al. Multiple sclerosis and neurofibromatosis type 1: report of seven patients from Iran. Mult Scler. 2009;15(9):1126–30.
73. Perini P, Gallo P. The range of multiple sclerosis associated with neurofibromatosis type 1. J Neurol Neurosurg Psychiatry. 2001;71(5):679–81.
74. Johnson MR, Ferner RE, Bobrow M, Hughes RA. Detailed analysis of the oligodendrocyte myelin glycoprotein gene in four patients with neurofibromatosis 1 and primary progressive multiple sclerosis. J Neurol Neurosurg Psychiatry. 2000;68(5):643–6.
75. Johnson H, Wiggs L, Stores G, Huson SM. Psychological disturbance and sleep disorders in children with neurofibromatosis type 1. Dev Med Child Neurol. 2005;47(4): 237–42.
76. Licis AK, Vallorani A, Gao F, Chen C, Lenox J, Yamada KA, et al. Prevalence of sleep disturbances in children with neurofibromatosis type 1. J Child Neurol. 2013;28(11): 1400–5.
77. Leschziner GD, Golding JF, Ferner RE. Sleep disturbance as part of the neurofibromatosis type 1 phenotype in adults. Am J Med Genet A. 2013;161A(6):1319–22.
78. Manfredi M, De Togni L, Beltramello A. Superficial siderosis of the central nervous system in a patient with neurofibromatosis type I. Eur Neurol. 2000;43(2):121–2.
79. Matsumoto A, Suzuki H, Tobita M, Hisanaga K. An autopsy case of superficial siderosis of the central nervous system accompanied by anterior sacral polycystic meningocele in neurofibromatosis type 1. Rinsho Shinkeigaku. 2016;56(7):486–94.
80. O'Hare M, Fearon C, Kavanagh EC, Murray B, Lynch T. Superficial siderosis and dural ectasia: a case report. Neurology. 2016;87(16):1743–4.
81. Gonzalez-Pinto T, Perez Concha T, Moreno EA. Intracranial arterial dolichoectasia and superficial siderosis associated to neurofibromatosis type 1: report of one case. Neurol Sci. 2018;39(12):2209–11.
82. Tucker T, Wolkenstein P, Revuz J, Zeller J, Friedman JM. Association between benign and malignant peripheral nerve sheath tumors in NF1. Neurology. 2005;65(2): 205–11.
83. Leonard JR, Ferner RE, Thomas N, Gutmann DH. Cervical cord compression from plexiform neurofibromas in neurofibromatosis 1. J Neurol Neurosurg Psychiatry. 2007;78(12): 1404–6.
84. Beert E, Brems H, Daniels B, De Wever I, Van Calenbergh F, Schoenaers J, et al. Atypical neurofibromas in neurofibromatosis type 1 are premalignant tumors. Genes Chromosomes Cancer. 2011;50(12):1021–32.

85. Higham CS, Dombi E, Rogiers A, Bhaumik S, Pans S, Connor SEJ, et al. The characteristics of 76 atypical neurofibromas as precursors to neurofibromatosis 1 associated malignant peripheral nerve sheath tumors. Neuro-Oncology. 2018;20(6):818–25.
86. Ferner RE, Gutmann DH. International consensus statement on malignant peripheral nerve sheath tumors in neurofibromatosis. Cancer Res. 2002;62(5):1573–7.
87. McCarron KF, Goldblum JR. Plexiform neurofibroma with and without associated malignant peripheral nerve sheath tumor: a clinicopathologic and immunohistochemical analysis of 54 cases. Mod Pathol. 1998;11(7):612–7.

Learning Disabilities and Behaviour in Neurofibromatosis Type 1 Patients

14

Shruti Garg and Jonathan Green

Contents

14.1 Cognitive and Language Impairments

14.1.1 Intellectual Ability

Early studies overestimated the prevalence of intellectual impairment suggesting rates of about 30% in the NF1 population. Prevalence estimates from these studies were skewed due to ascertainment and assessment biases; the study population was recruited from mental institutions and hospitals, and crude measures of intelligence such as the number of years in education were used [1]. More recent studies have demonstrated the mean full scale IQ in NF1 to be between 80 and 90;

S. Garg (✉) · J. Green
Child and Adolescent Psychiatry, University of Manchester, Manchester, UK
e-mail: shruti.garg@manchester.ac.uk; Jonathan.Green@manchester.ac.uk

G. Tadini et al. (eds.), *Multidisciplinary Approach to Neurofibromatosis Type 1*,
https://doi.org/10.1007/978-3-319-92450-2_14

prevalence estimates of intellectual impairment (defined as IQ < 70 and associated impairments in adaptive functioning) are generally accepted as being between 4% and 8% [2, 3] compared to 3% in the general population. Significant learning disability is often associated with microdeletions on the *NF1* gene [4]. There is a verbal/performance IQ discrepancy [5], with NF1 children displaying significantly better verbal IQ but this has not been universally replicated [6]. Specific learning impairments (defined as a discrepancy of two standard deviations between IQ and achievement on co-normed standardised tests) are much more prevalent with estimates of at least 20% [7]. About 75% of all children with NF1 perform one standard deviation below age-matched peers in one or more academic domains of spelling, mathematics or reading and are four times more likely to be attending a special educational provision [2]. Longitudinal cohort studies suggest that the *NF1* mutation confers a general vulnerability for cognitive difficulties, which is observable in the pre-school years [8].

14.1.2 Visual-Spatial and Perceptual Skills

Impairments in visual-spatial functioning had long been considered as a hallmark characteristic of NF1 but recent studies suggest that these impairments are a part of a wider spectrum of cognitive impairments [9]. These impairments, which are characterised by difficulty organising and accurately interpreting visual information, have traditionally been measured across different NF1 studies by the Judgement of Line orientation (JLO) test and Rey-Osterrieth Complex Figure tasks [10], with poor performance a consistent feature across a number of different studies [6, 11]. Hyman et al. found that 56% of children with NF1 scored at least 1 standard deviation (SD) lower than the general population mean on the JLO. However, a recent study that undertook a detailed investigation into specific sub-processes underlying visuospatial functioning concluded that visuospatial impairments are in fact due to underlying deficits in executive function. In a case–control study of 39 NF1 children with age /gender matched controls, Van Eylen et al. found intact visual form discrimination and visual integration and typical visual processing style when executive function impairments are taken into consideration [9].

14.1.3 Executive Function

Executive function has been defined by Lezak as ‘capacities that enable a person to engage in independent, purposive, self-serving behaviour’ [12]. It refers to skills such as planning, attention, inhibition, cognitive flexibility, organisation and self-monitoring. Planning, inhibitory control, working memory and attention are some of the executive function domains that have been studied in detail and found to be impaired in the NF1 group [6, 13]. Roy et al. carried out a case-control study of 36 NF1 children matched to healthy controls using three action-planning tasks. They found that as compared to healthy controls, the NF1 group performed poorly on the action-planning tasks. Deficits are also seen in 'cognitive control', which is equivalent to executive function but incorporating levels of complexity in tasks [14, 15]. Huijbregts et al. found that cognitive control deficits remained evident even after excluding children with NF1 and Attention-Deficit Hyperactivity Disorder (ADHD), suggesting that hyperactivity/inattention do not fully explain the cognitive control deficits in NF1. A detailed investigation into five domains of executive function (inhibition, cognitive flexibility, generativity, working memory and planning) using an extended test battery in 42 NF1 children compared to normative and autistic controls found that executive deficits are a core feature of NF1 rather than a secondary effect of lower IQ or ASD symptoms [16].

14.1.4 Speech and Language Impairments

A wide range of language deficits are associated with NF1, such that a global language deficit is seen as a key feature of the NF1 cognitive phenotype [10]. These impairments may include deficits in language structure, semantic language, receptive and expressive language, verbal working memory and comprehension, noted in at least one-third of children with NF1 impacting on functional social communication [17–19]. These impairments are noted very early on in development. For example, a cross sectional case–control study of 39 NF1 toddlers aged 21–30 months suggested delayed language development, reduced productive vocabulary and sentence complexity in almost three- quarters of the sample according to parental reports. Further, a recent pilot study of ten infants with NF1 suggested expressive and receptive language delay at 10 months both on parent report and Mullen's Scale of Early Learning [20].

Speech alteration affecting speech sounds including abnormal speaking rate, volume, pitch and hoarseness and hypernasality have also been noted [21]. A case-control study of 62 NF1 participants suggested problems with pitch regulation resulting in monotone speech, deviance in phonation, misarticulation and disfluency; these difficulties being worse in children and men as compared to adults and women, respectively [22]. These results are suggestive of a motoric dyspraxia of the different anatomical parts of the vocal tract. Speech and language impairments in NF1 are often comorbid with ADHD and social communication impairments.

14.2 Behavioural Impairments

14.2.1 ADHD

ADHD is the most commonly reported psychiatric disorder in NF1, with prevalence estimates of 30–67% [23–25] compared with 3–7% for ADHD in the general population [26]. Further, the frequency of ADHD in NF1 is equally distributed across the genders, as opposed to the general population where it presents with a male bias in a ratio of about 3:1 [27]. In-depth investigation of attentional impairments in NF1 suggests deficits in all of the attentional domains including sustained visual and auditory attention, divided attention, selective attention and response inhibition [28]. Substantial majority of studies suggest a predominantly combined or inattentive sub-type of ADHD. Children with NF1 frequently present with poor psychosocial functioning, poor social competence and social skills [29, 30]. NF1 with ADHD is associated with more emotional difficulties and aggression than NF1 without ADHD [31]. The ADHD symptoms can persist through to adulthood and can significantly impact quality of life and occupational functioning. In a study of 26 adults with NF1 + ADHD compared with NF1 without ADHD and a sample of adults with ADHD only, Mautner et al. found that the NF1 + ADHD group presented with an emotionally unstable psychological phenotype similar to the group with ADHD only [32]. Payne et al. have demonstrated poor correlation between functional measures (such as the Conners scale) and conventional neuropsychological tests of executive function. In a study of 199 NF1 children and 55 matched sibling controls, the authors demonstrated that cognitive tests for executive function were a poor predictor of functional impairments in attention/concentration at home or school [25]. These results suggest that both neuropsychological tests and functional measures should be incorporated into clinical assessment for ADHD.

Findings from Nf1 animal model studies suggest attention system abnormality is due to reduced dopamine in the striatum, which is normalised following methylphenidate or L-dopa administration [33].

14.2.2 Autism Spectrum Disorder and Social Communication Impairments

There is substantial comorbidity of Autism Spectrum Disorder with NF1 as compared to the ASD prevalence of 1% seen in the general population [34]. Social communication impairments have been commonly reported in NF1 including impaired social skills, social isolation, peer rejection and poorer performance on tasks measuring social information processing as compared to normative controls [29, 30, 35]. The link between NF1 and ASD, however, has only been systematically investigated over the last decade with prevalence of between 10 and 30% ASD. Using an epidemiological design, detailed parental interviews and child assessment measures, Garg et al. demonstrated a population prevalence of 25% ASD in children with NF1. A number of publications have since replicated this result [36, 37]. A recent retrospective study of 128 clinic referred children found a lower prevalence rates of about 11% ASD in NF1 and additional 16.5% with sub-clinical ASD symptoms [38]. Similarly a recent large international consortium sample of 531 NF1 individuals found ASD prevalence of 13% and additional 26% sub-clinical symptoms using parent rated screening instruments [39]. Similar to the general population, there is a 3:1 male sex bias in prevalence rates for ASD in NF1 [38, 40]. The prevalence of ASD in NF1 does not correlate with physical phenotypic severity or intellectual impairment [38, 41]. There is also substantial comorbidity of ASD and ADHD with 25% children meeting clinical criteria for both disorders [42].

The ASD symptomatology has been replicated in NF1 animal models. Molosh et al. studied the social learning deficits in $Nf1^{+/-}$ mice using the well-validated three-chamber social memory test. The $Nf1^{+/-}$ mice showed abnormal amygdala glutamate, GABA and specific disruptions in the expression of two proteins associated with glutamate and GABA. Deletion of the p21 protein activated kinase gene, which is a positive regulator of Ras MAPK activity, normalised the disruptions in the amygdala and rescued the social learning deficits. Further pharmacological blockade of Pak1 activity produced a similar effect [43].

14.2.3 Internalising and Externalising Disorders

Research investigating emotional behavioural difficulties in children with NF1 has shown significantly higher scores on CBCL (Child Behaviour Check List) than the normative population particularly for anxiety, depression and aggression [30, 44]. Using parent, teacher and self-report measures, a large study of 183 NF1 children aged 6–17 years reported 32% clinical range emotional/behavioural problems. Parental perception of these difficulties was much higher than that reported by teachers or on self-report [45]. A cross sectional study of 53 children with NF1 and plexiform neurofibromas found 32% were at risk of internalising problems and 11% at risk of externalising problems on parent-reported measures. Moreover, lower IQ, greater physical disease severity, higher stressful life events were related to more behavioural impairment [46]. Adults with NF1 are at increased risk of psychiatric morbidity with significant mental illness reported in at least 33% [47]. Using internet based questionnaires, a cross sectional study of 498 adults with NF1 suggested 55% participants rated themselves as having a high likelihood of clinical depression [48]. Individuals with NF1 also self-report poorer quality of life, anxiety, distorted self-image as compared to normative controls [49].

14.2.4 Sleep

Sleep disturbance is a commonly reported clinical problem in NF1 but has not yet been investigated in detail by research studies. Higher rates of parasomnias including sleepwalking and night terrors have been reported in NF1, which correlate with conduct problems, hyperactivity and emotional problems [50]. A large cross sectional study of 129 NF1 children and their unaffected siblings found significantly more disturbances in initiating and maintaining sleep, arousal, sleep-wake transitions and hyperhidrosis in the NF1 group. In this study, the sleep problems did not correlate with IQ or ADHD [51]. Studies in NF1 drosophila/animal models suggest aberrant calcium cycling in the neurons of circadian circuits required for rest: activity rhythms [52]. A similar mechanism may be relevant in explaining the sleep phenotype in NF1 patients.

14.3 Imaging Correlates of Cognitive and Behavioural Deficits

Both structural and functional brain imaging are suggestive of brain abnormalities that correlate with neuropsychological phenotype. There is increase in brain volume and macrocephaly both on imaging and head circumference measurements, most likely driven by increase in white matter in the frontal region and corpus callosum and increase in grey matter volume in posterior brain regions [53]. The corpus collosum is enlarged relative to total brain volume; larger corpus callosum volume is related to academic underachievement, lower IQ, executive function and visuospatial impairments [13]. High intensity focal areas are observed on T2-weighted brain MRI in up to 90% of all children. These T2 hyperintensities (T2H) appear most commonly in the basal ganglia, cerebellum, thalamus, brain stem and sub-cortical white matter. The relationship between the T2H and cognitive function is unclear but recent studies demonstrate that T2H in the thalamus or thalamo-striatal region is associated with more severe cognitive impairment [54], suggesting that T2H in this region may contribute to cognitive impairment through thalamo-cortical dysfunction [55]. A small longitudinal follow-up study from childhood to adulthood over an 18-year period suggested that discrete T2H located in the basal ganglia, thalamus and brainstem tend to resolve in adulthood. Further, the resolution of T2H is associated with improvement in cognitive function possibly as a result of increased efficiency within the white matter tracts [56].

Functional MRI studies are still in its infancy in NF1 but have been used to investigate the neural basis of visuospatial processing and working memory deficits in NF1. Using the JLO task, Clements-Stephens et al. demonstrated greater right than left hemisphere activation in comparison with healthy controls possibly suggestive of inefficient right hemisphere network in NF1 [57]. Violante et al. found a link between aberrant default mode network activation and visual processing in NF1 [58]. In a more recent study, Ibrahim et al. investigated the neural basis of spatial working memory deficits in NF1 and found significant hypoactivation of working memory circuitry, particularly the left dorsolateral prefrontal cortex and right intraparietal sulcus and aberrant functional connectivity in the NF1 group [59].

14.4 Mechanism Based Treatment Approaches for Cognitive Impairments in NF1

NF1 animal models have proved invaluable in modelling the cognitive and behavioural deficits seen in NF1, elucidating the underlying neurobiology and aiding the development of targeted interventions. Findings from *Nf1*$^{+/-}$ heterozygous mouse models suggest learning impairments in NF1 are caused by excessive Ras /MAPK pathway activity, which in turn results in increased MAPK dependent phosphorylation of synapsin I, increase in GABA release in the interneurons with consequent deficits in synaptic plasticity and cognitive/behavioural phenotype in mice [43, 60]. Further, the cognitive phenotype in mice can be rescued by downregulating Ras activity using farnesyl transferase inhibitors or statins [61]. Translational clinical trials of statins in human participants with Nf1, however, have been disappointing [62]. A large RCT of simvastatin of 84 children, aged 8–16 years found no improvements in cognitive deficits or parent-reported behavioural problems [63]. Similarly, a 16-week RCT of lovastatin in 146 8–15-year-olds with NF1 and visuospatial learning/attention deficits found no improvements on a paired associate learning task [64]. More recently, a small RCT of Simvastatin in 30 young children aged 4–10 years with NF1 and ASD using multi-parametric imaging was suggestive of Simvastatin effects in brain areas associated with NF1 pathophysiology and social brain network [65].

The role of defective dopaminergic function has also been implicated as a contributing factor for underling attentional problems in NF1 although the precise mechanisms are unclear. Animal model studies suggest reduced dopaminergic signalling in the hippocampal region, which can be normalised by using dopamine-elevating drugs such as methylphenidate [66, 67]. Small scale RCTs of methylphenidate in children with NF1 suggest good clinical benefit [31, 68].

14.4.1 Summary and Implications for Clinical Practice

The last few years have seen a considerable acceleration in research into the cognitive and behavioural manifestations of NF1. This is a welcome development, since it turns out that cognitive, social and behavioural morbidity is the most prevalent morbidity in NF1 in early childhood, one that greatly concerns families and impacts on children's developmental adaptation. In concert with all neurodevelopmental disorders, the cognitive and behavioural manifestations of the primary genetic disorder are various, often comorbid, and unlikely that they represent a specific phenotype. The recognition of a high prevalence of autistic spectrum disorder has been an important advance in recent years with rates comparable but separate to those for ADHD. In the past, cognitive and behavioural capabilities were often under recognised due to 'diagnostic overshadowing' [42] and this meant that specific relevant interventions were not accessible to families affected children. Recent research should make this a thing of the past: the cognitive and behavioural comorbidities of ADHD, ASD, anxiety all have specific evidenced remediation strategies which can be applied by psychiatrists and other mental health professionals expert in this area. This plus general awareness and specific educational management should improve early adaptation for families of children with the disorder.

An important methodological advance has been the establishment of two prospective longitudinal infancy cohort studies beginning in early infancy and following the cognitive [69] and neurodevelopmental/behavioural [20] trajectories, respectively, of these infants. The combination of these prospective studies, along with descriptive studies at different stages of development in affected children has important clinical implications for services. Early cognitive and behavioural symptoms identified by these studies could act as 'red flags' for later problems and should be subject to active surveillance or offered primary prevention intervention.

In addition to these clinical implications, the fact that NF1 is a single gene disorder with mechanistic understanding from animal models has great relevance for our understanding of the development of the cognitive and behavioural phenotypes in this disorder and more widely. Animal models of NF1 show cognitive and behavioural atypicalities that can be understood as analogous to the human phenotypes and have been responsive to various intervention strategies, which reverse the core pathophysiology of the disorder [43, 61]. While there has been no simple translational benefit as yet into human therapeutics, recent trials have shown relevant effects on neural functioning [70], and other specific brain-based therapeutics are currently being tested [71]. From both animal and human models we have the opportunity to learn a great deal about neural system functioning from the perturbation consequent on *NF1* gene disruption. We know already from animal work the effect of NF1 on GABA, excitation/inhibition imbalance, synaptic protein expression and long-term potentiation. How these system effects are expressed both regionally in brain and temporally over development will be key to understanding the emergence of specific phenotypes as well as their co-occurrence. As similar work is done across other single gene and other neurodevelopmental disorders, it becomes less likely that we will find cognitive and behavioural phenotypes that are specific to discrete disorders such as NF1. Instead the rule is for common final pathways to phenotypes across different neural system disruptions. This has been understood theoretically as in the nature of common developmental adaptations to different primary neural system disruptions [72]. Since primary disruptions are understood in single gene disorders, they provide causal anchors to understand the neurobiological basis of complex neurodevelopmental disorders.

In this way, the neuropsychiatric and neurodevelopmental approach to NF1 has begun an exciting new phase, which will have both theoretical and practical clinical implications going forward.

References

1. Cole WG, Myers NA. Neurofibromatosis in childhood. Aust N Z J Surg. 1978;48(4):360–5.
2. Krab LC, Aarsen FK, de Goede-Bolder A, Catsman-Berrevoets CE, Arts WF, Moll HA, et al. Impact of neurofibromatosis type 1 on school performance. J Child Neurol. 2008;23(9): 1002–10.
3. North K, Joy P, Yuille D, Cocks N, Hutchins P. Cognitive function and academic performance in children with neurofibromatosis type 1. Dev Med Child Neurol. 1995;37(5):427–36.
4. Pasmant E, Vidaud M, Vidaud D, Wolkenstein P. Neurofibromatosis type 1: from genotype to phenotype. J Med Genet. 2012;49(8):483–9.
5. Legius E, Descheemaeker MJ, Spaepen A, Casaer P, Fryns JP. Neurofibromatosis type 1 in childhood: a study of the neuropsychological profile in 45 children. Genet Couns. 1994;5(1):51–60.
6. Hyman S, Shores A, North K. The nature and frequency of cognitive deficits in children with neurofibromatosis type 1. Neurology. 2005;65(7):1037–44. Developmental medicine and child neurology 4812 (2007): 973-7.
7. Hyman SL, Arthur Shores E, North KN. Learning disabilities in children with neurofibromatosis type 1: subtypes, cognitive profile, and attention-deficit-hyperactivity disorder. Dev Med Child Neurol. 2006;48(12):973–7.

8. Klein-Tasman BP, Colon AM, Brei N, van der Fluit F, Casnar CL, Janke KM, et al. Adaptive behavior in young children with neurofibromatosis type 1. Int J Pediatr. 2013;2013:690432.
9. Van Eylen L, Plasschaert E, Wagemans J, Boets B, Legius E, Steyaert J, et al. Visuoperceptual processing in children with neurofibromatosis type 1: true deficit or artefact? Am J Med Genet B Neuropsychiatr Genet. 2017;174(4):342–58.
10. Payne J, North K. Neurofibromatosis type 1. In: Goldstein S, Reynolds CR, editors. Handbook of neurodevelopmental and genetic disorders in children. New York: Guilford Press; 2010. p. 588.
11. Lehtonen A, Garg S, Roberts SA, Trump D, Evans DG, Green J, et al. Cognition in children with neurofibromatosis type 1: data from a population-based study. Dev Med Child Neurol. 2015;57(7):645–51.
12. Lezak M, Howieson D, Loring D, Hannay J, Fischer J. Neuropsychological assessment. Oxford: Oxford University Press; 2004.
13. Pride N, Payne JM, Webster R, Shores EA, Rae C, North KN. Corpus callosum morphology and its relationship to cognitive function in neurofibromatosis type 1. J Child Neurol. 2010;25(7):834–41.
14. Rowbotham I, Pit-ten Cate IM, Sonuga-Barke EJ, Huijbregts SC. Cognitive control in adolescents with neurofibromatosis type 1. Neuropsychology. 2009;23(1):50–60.
15. Huijbregts S, Swaab H, de Sonneville L. Cognitive and motor control in neurofibromatosis type I: influence of maturation and hyperactivity-inattention. Dev Neuropsychol. 2010;35(6):737–51.
16. Plasschaert E, Van Eylen L, Descheemaeker MJ, Noens I, Legius E, Steyaert J. Executive functioning deficits in children with neurofibromatosis type 1: the influence of intellectual and social functioning. Am J Med Genet B Neuropsychiatr Genet. 2016;171B(3):348–62.
17. Brei NG, Klein-Tasman BP, Schwarz GN, Casnar CL. Language in young children with neurofibromatosis-1: relations to functional communication, attention, and social functioning. Res Dev Disabil. 2014;35(10):2495–504.
18. Thompson HL, Viskochil DH, Stevenson DA, Chapman KL. Speech-language characteristics of children with neurofibromatosis type 1. Am J Med Genet A. 2010;152A(2):284–90.
19. Dilts C, Carey J, Kircher J, Hoffman R, Creel D, Ward K, et al. Children and adolescents with neurofibromatosis1: a behavioral phenotype. J Dev Behav Pediatr. 1996;17:229–39.
20. Kolesnik AM, Jones EJH, Garg S, Green J, Charman T, Johnson MH, et al. Early development of infants with neurofibromatosis type 1: a case series. Mol Autism. 2017;8:62.
21. Lorch M, Ferner R, Golding J, Whurr R. The nature of speech and language impairment in adults with neurofibromatosis 1. J Neurolinguistics. 1999;12(3–4):157–65.
22. Alivuotila L, Hakokari J, Visnapuu V, Korpijaakko-Huuhka AM, Aaltonen O, Happonen RP, et al. Speech characteristics in neurofibromatosis type 1. Am J Med Genet A. 2010;152A(1):42–51.
23. Hofman K, Harris E, Bryan R, Denckla M. Neurofibromatosis type 1: the cognitive phenotype. J Pediatr. 1994;124:S1–8.
24. Coude F, Mignot C, Lyonnet S, Munnich A. Early grade repetition and inattention associated with Neurofibromatosis type 1. J Atten Disord. 2007;11:101–5.
25. Payne JM, Hyman SL, Shores EA, North KN. Assessment of executive function and attention in children with neurofibromatosis type 1: relationships between cognitive measures and real-world behavior. Child Neuropsychol. 2011;17(4):313–29.
26. Polanczyk G, de Lima MS, Horta BL, Biederman J, Rohde LA. The worldwide prevalence of ADHD: a systematic review and metaregression analysis. Am J Psychiatry. 2007;164(6):942–8.
27. Gaub M, Carlson CL. Gender differences in ADHD: a meta-analysis and critical review. J Am Acad Child Adolesc Psychiatry. 1997;36(8):1036–45.
28. Isenberg JC, Templer A, Gao F, Titus JB, Gutmann DH. Attention skills in children with neurofibromatosis type 1. J Child Neurol. 2013;28(1):45–9.
29. Noll R, Reiter-Purtill J, Moore B, Schorry E, Lovell A, Vannatta K, et al. Social, emotional, and behavioral functioning of children with NF1. Am J Med Genet A. 2007;143A:2261–73.
30. Barton B, North K. Social skills of children with neurofibromatosis type 1. Dev Med Child Neurol. 2004;46:553–63.

31. Mautner V, Kluwe L, Thakker S, Leark R. Treatment of ADHD in neurofibromatosis type 1. Dev Med Child Neurol. 2002;44(3):164–70.
32. Mautner VF, Granstrom S, Leark RA. Impact of ADHD in adults with neurofibromatosis type 1: associated psychological and social problems. J Atten Disord. 2015;19(1):35–43.
33. Brown JA, Emnett RJ, White CR, Yuede CM, Conyers SB, O'Malley KL, et al. Reduced striatal dopamine underlies the attention system dysfunction in neurofibromatosis-1 mutant mice. Hum Mol Genet. 2010;19(22):4515–28.
34. Baird G, Simonoff E, Pickles A, Chandler S, Loucas T, Meldrum D, et al. Prevalence of disorders of the autism spectrum in a population cohort of children in South Thames: the special needs and autism project (SNAP). Lancet. 2006;15(9531):210–5.
35. Huijbregts S, Jahja R, De Sonneville L, De Breij S, Swaab-Barneveld H. Social information processing in children and adolescents with neurofibromatosis type 1. Dev Med Child Neurol. 2010;52(7):620–5.
36. Plasschaert E, Descheemaeker MJ, Van Eylen L, Noens I, Steyaert J, Legius E. Prevalence of autism spectrum disorder symptoms in children with neurofibromatosis type 1. Am J Med Genet B Neuropsychiatr Genet. 2014;168(1):72–80.
37. Walsh KS, Velez JI, Kardel PG, Imas DM, Muenke M, Packer RJ, et al. Symptomatology of autism spectrum disorder in a population with neurofibromatosis type 1. Dev Med Child Neurol. 2013;55(2):131–8.
38. Eijk S, Mous SE, Dieleman GC, Dierckx B, Rietman AB, de Nijs PFA, et al. Autism spectrum disorder in an unselected cohort of children with Neurofibromatosis type 1 (NF1). J Autism Dev Disord. 2018;48(7):2278–85.
39. Morris SM, Acosta MT, Garg S, Green J, Huson S, Legius E, et al. Disease burden and symptom structure of autism in neurofibromatosis type 1: a study of the international NF1-ASD consortium team (INFACT). JAMA Psychiat. 2016;73(12):1276–84.
40. Garg S, Heuvelman H, Huson S, Tobin H, Green J, Northern UKNFRN. Sex bias in autism spectrum disorder in neurofibromatosis type 1. J Neurodev Disord. 2016;8:26.
41. Garg S, Green J, Leadbitter K, Emsley R, Lehtonen A, Evans DG, et al. Neurofibromatosis type 1 and autism spectrum disorder. Pediatrics. 2013;132(6):e1642–8.
42. Garg S, Lehtonen A, Huson SM, Emsley R, Trump D, Evans DG, et al. Autism and other psychiatric comorbidity in neurofibromatosis type 1: evidence from a population-based study. Dev Med Child Neurol. 2013;55(2):139–45.
43. Molosh AI, Johnson PL, Spence JP, Arendt D, Federici LM, Bernabe C, et al. Social learning and amygdala disruptions in Nf1 mice are rescued by blocking p21-activated kinase. Nat Neurosci. 2014;17(11):1583–90.
44. Descheemaeker MJ, Ghesquiere P, Symons H, Fryns JP, Legius E. Behavioural, academic and neuropsychological profile of normally gifted Neurofibromatosis type 1 children. J Intellect Disabil Res. 2005;49(Pt 1):33–46.
45. Rietman AB, van der Vaart T, Plasschaert E, Nicholson BA, Oostenbrink R, Krab LC, et al. Emotional and behavioral problems in children and adolescents with neurofibromatosis type 1. Am J Med Genet B Neuropsychiatr Genet. 2018;177(3):319–28.
46. Martin S, Wolters P, Baldwin A, Gillespie A, Dombi E, Walker K, et al. Social-emotional functioning of children and adolescents with neurofibromatosis type 1 and plexiform neurofibromas: relationships with cognitive, disease, and environmental variables. J Pediatr Psychol. 2012;37(7):713–24.
47. Samuelsson B, Riccardi V. Neurofibromatosis in Gothenburg, Sweden. III. Psychiatric and social aspects. Neurofibromatosis. 1989;2:84–106.
48. Cohen JS, Levy HP, Sloan J, Dariotis J, Biesecker BB. Depression among adults with neurofibromatosis type 1: prevalence and impact on quality of life. Clin Genet. 2015;88(5):425–30.
49. Cipolletta S, Spina G, Spoto A. Psychosocial functioning, self-image, and quality of life in children and adolescents with neurofibromatosis type 1. Child Care Health Dev. 2018;44(2):260–8.
50. Johnson H, Wiggs L, Stores G, Huson S. Psychological disturbance and sleep disorders in children with neurofibromatosis type 1. Dev Med Child Neurol. 2005;47:237–42.

51. Licis AK, Vallorani A, Gao F, Chen C, Lenox J, Yamada KA, et al. Prevalence of sleep disturbances in children with neurofibromatosis type 1. J Child Neurol. 2013;28(11):1400–5.
52. Bai L, Lee Y, Hsu CT, Williams JA, Cavanaugh D, Zheng X, et al. A conserved circadian function for the neurofibromatosis 1 gene. Cell Rep. 2018;22(13):3416–26.
53. Greenwood RS, Tupler LA, Whitt JK, Buu A, Dombeck CB, Harp AG, et al. Brain morphometry, T2-weighted hyperintensities, and IQ in children with neurofibromatosis type 1. Arch Neurol. 2005;62(12):1904–8.
54. Hyman SL, Gill DS, Shores EA, Steinberg A, North KN. T2 hyperintensities in children with neurofibromatosis type 1 and their relationship to cognitive functioning. J Neurol Neurosurg Psychiatry. 2007;78(10):1088–91.
55. Chabernaud C, Sirinelli D, Barbier C, Cottier JP, Sembely C, Giraudeau B, et al. Thalamo-striatal T2-weighted hyperintensities (unidentified bright objects) correlate with cognitive impairments in neurofibromatosis type 1 during childhood. Dev Neuropsychol. 2009;34(6):736–48.
56. Payne JM, Pickering T, Porter M, Oates EC, Walia N, Prelog K, et al. Longitudinal assessment of cognition and T2-hyperintensities in NF1: an 18-year study. Am J Med Genet A. 2014;164A(3):661–5.
57. Clements-Stephens AM, Rimrodt SL, Gaur P, Cutting LE. Visuospatial processing in children with neurofibromatosis type 1. Neuropsychologia. 2008;46(2):690–7.
58. Violante IR, Ribeiro MJ, Edden RA, Guimaraes P, Bernardino I, Rebola J, et al. GABA deficit in the visual cortex of patients with neurofibromatosis type 1: genotype-phenotype correlations and functional impact. Brain J Neurol. 2013;136(Pt 3):918–25.
59. Ibrahim AFA, Montojo CA, Haut KM, Karlsgodt KH, Hansen L, Congdon E, et al. Spatial working memory in neurofibromatosis 1: altered neural activity and functional connectivity. NeuroImage Clin. 2017;15:801–11.
60. Costa R, Federov N, Kogan J, Murphy G, Stern J, Ohno M, et al. Mechanism for the learning deficits in a mouse model of neurofibromatosis type 1. Nature. 2002;415:526–30.
61. Li W, Cui Y, Kushner S, Brown R, Jentsch J, Frankland P, et al. The HMG-CoA reductase inhibitor lovastatin reverses the learning and attention deficits in a mouse model of neurofibromatosis type 1. Curr Biol. 2005;15(21):1961–7.
62. Krab L, de Goede-Bolde RA, Aarsen F, Pluijm S, Bouman M, van der Geest J, et al. Effect of simvastatin on cognitive functioning in children with neurofibromatosis type 1: a randomized controlled trial. JAMA. 2008;300(3):287–94.
63. van der Vaart T, Plasschaert E, Rietman AB, Renard M, Oostenbrink R, Vogels A, et al. Simvastatin for cognitive deficits and behavioural problems in patients with neurofibromatosis type 1 (NF1-SIMCODA): a randomised, placebo-controlled trial. Lancet Neurol. 2013;12(11):1076–83.
64. Payne JM, Barton B, Ullrich NJ, Cantor A, Hearps SJ, Cutter G, et al. Randomized placebo-controlled study of lovastatin in children with neurofibromatosis type 1. Neurology. 2016;87(24):2575–84.
65. Stivaros S, Garg S, Tziraki M, Cai Y, Thomas O, Mellor J, et al. Randomised controlled trial of simvastatin treatment for autism in young children with neurofibromatosis type 1 (SANTA). Mol Autism. 2018;9:12.
66. Diggs-Andrews KA, Gutmann DH. Modeling cognitive dysfunction in neurofibromatosis-1. Trends Neurosci. 2013;36(4):237–47.
67. Diggs-Andrews KA, Tokuda K, Izumi Y, Zorumski CF, Wozniak DF, Gutmann DH. Dopamine deficiency underlies learning deficits in neurofibromatosis-1 mice. Ann Neurol. 2013;73(2):309–15.
68. Lion-Francois L, Gueyffier F, Mercier C, Gerard D, Herbillon V, Kemlin I, et al. The effect of methylphenidate on neurofibromatosis type 1: a randomised, double-blind, placebo-controlled, crossover trial. Orphanet J Rare Dis. 2014;9:142.
69. Lorenzo J, Barton B, Acosta MT, North K. Mental, motor, and language development of toddlers with neurofibromatosis type 1. J Pediatr. 2011;158(4):660–5.

70. Mainberger F, Jung NH, Zenker M, Wahllander U, Freudenberg L, Langer S, et al. Lovastatin improves impaired synaptic plasticity and phasic alertness in patients with neurofibromatosis type 1. BMC Neurol. 2013;13:131.
71. Omrani A, van der Vaart T, Mientjes E, van Woerden GM, Hojjati MR, Li KW, et al. HCN channels are a novel therapeutic target for cognitive dysfunction in Neurofibromatosis type 1. Mol Psychiatry. 2015;20(11):1311–21.
72. Johnson MH, Gliga T, Jones E, Charman T. Annual research review: infant development, autism, and ADHD--early pathways to emerging disorders. J Child Psychol Psychiatry. 2015;56(3):228–47.

Mosaic NF1

15

Gianluca Tadini, Teresa Schgor, and Michela Brena

Contents

G. Tadini (✉) · M. Brena
Pediatric Dermatology Unit, Fondazione IRCCS Ca' Granda, Ospedale Maggiore Policlinico, Department of Physiopathology and Transplantation, Milan, Italy

Paediatric Highly Intensive Care Unit, Fondazione IRCCS Ca' Granda Ospedale Maggiore Policlinico, Milan, Italy

Center for Inherited Cutaneous Diseases, University of Milan, Milan, Italy
e-mail: gtadinicmce@unimi.it

T. Schgor
Pediatric Dermatology Unit, Fondazione IRCCS Ca' Granda, Ospedale Maggiore Policlinico, Department of Physiopathology and Transplantation, University of Milan, Milan, Italy

G. Tadini et al. (eds.), *Multidisciplinary Approach to Neurofibromatosis Type 1*,
https://doi.org/10.1007/978-3-319-92450-2_15

15.1 Definition

Mosaic NF1 (MNF1) is a clinical variant of NF1, so far called “segmental” or “localized” or NF type V, due to post-zygotic mutations in the NF1 gene [1].

This condition has an estimated prevalence of 0.0014–0.002 (1/36.000–1/40.000) [2], roughly 10–20 times less frequent than NF1 due to germline mutations, but may be largely underrepresented.

15.2 Clinical Manifestations

The clinical presentation is traditionally divided into four types:

1. Pigmentary lesions only
2. Neurofibromas only
3. Mixed forms
4. Plexiform tumors

In our cohort of about 250 cases of MNF1 group 1 accounts for 65%, group 2 for 25%, group 3 for less than 5%, and group 4 for 10–15%, confirming the previous data of the literature [3].

In particular, it must be underlined that the number and the dimension of pigmentary lesions are not so relevant for the diagnosis of MNF1.

Group 1 MNF1 follows a checkerboard distribution (“quadrants”) that is normally the most frequent pattern for mosaic pigmentary lesions. Superior (scapular) girdle, both anterior and posterior, seems to be the preferred site of occurrence of MNF1, followed by inferior (pelvic) girdle and other body sites.

Group 1 MNF1 may be visible at birth and is diagnosed usually within the first years of life. MNF1 showing only CALMs of small dimensions (“freckling”) may have a late onset during infancy. Mixed pattern presenting together freckling with intermingled CALMs of major dimension is also visible. (Fig. 15.1).

Fig. 15.1

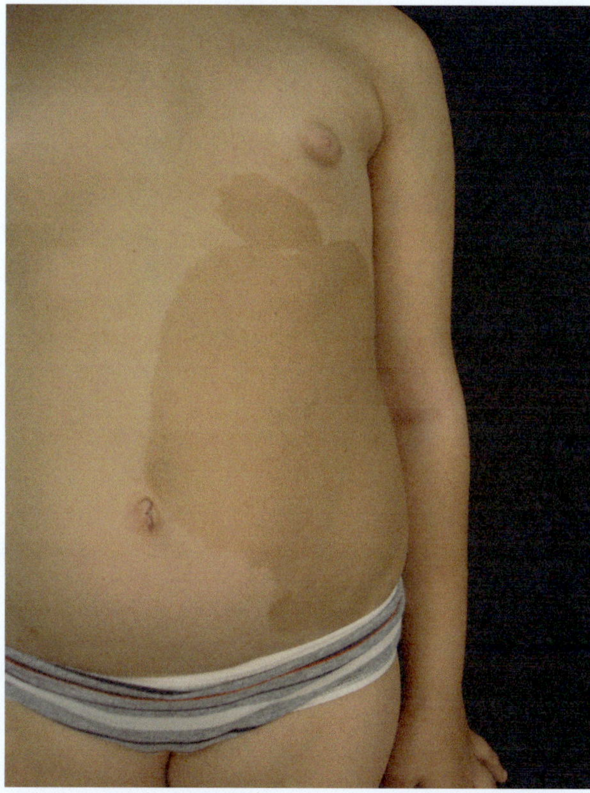

An underreported finding in pigmentary MNF1 is that an easily recognizable background pigmentation that sharply demarcate the affected area is common. Usually, a sharp midline border is visible but is frequently seen that affected areas override the midline border as it often occurs in non-NF1 pigmentary mosaicism and is not so rare to spot some pigmentary lesions in the neighboring skin, perhaps reflecting a more complex mosaic condition (Fig. 15.2) [4, 5].

Fig. 15.2

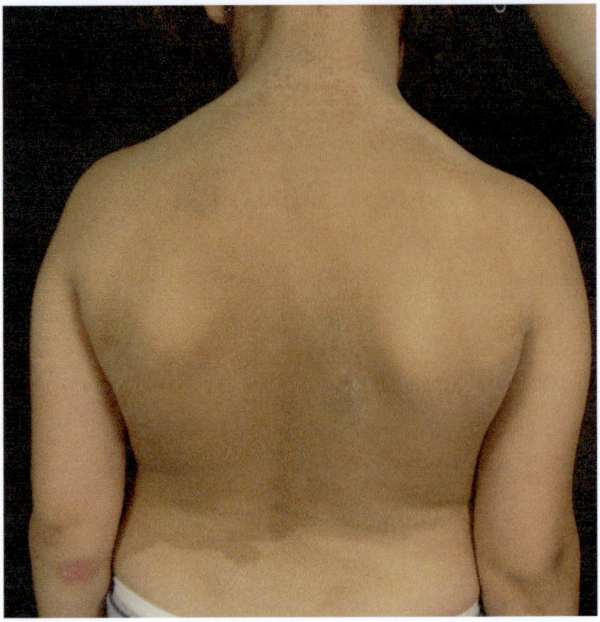

Group 2 (neurofibromas only) shows a distribution of lesions following the lines of Blaschko (Fig. 15.3) [6]. This pattern may be not so obvious to recognize, due to the fact that neurofibromas are often in a very small number. Neurofibromas in MNF1 are usually late-onset lesions, developing after third–fourth decade (Figs. 15.4 and 15.5).

Fig. 15.3

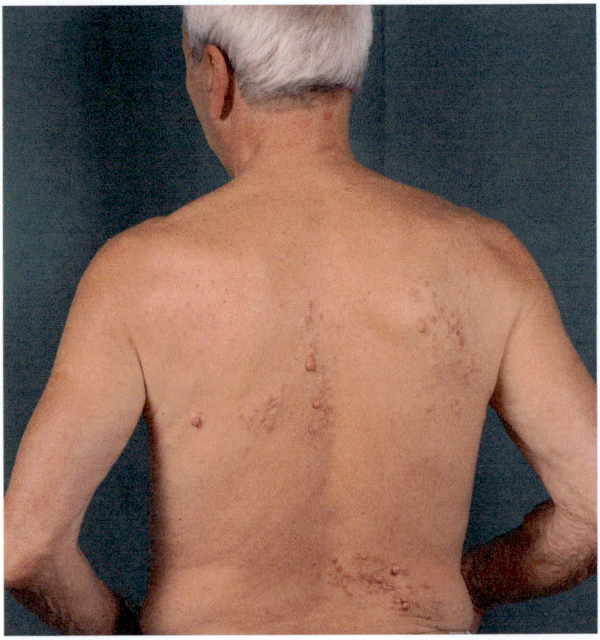

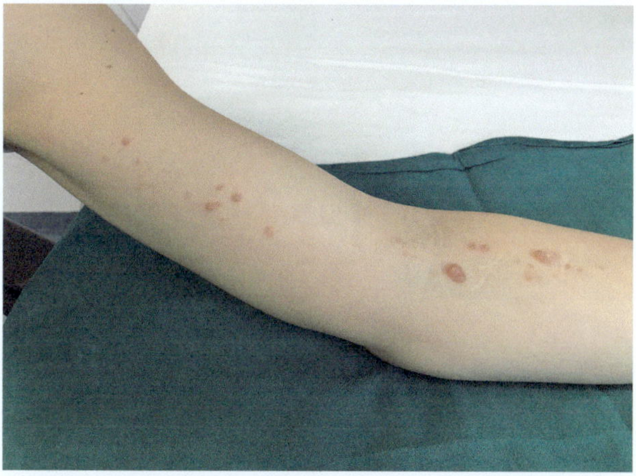

Fig. 15.4

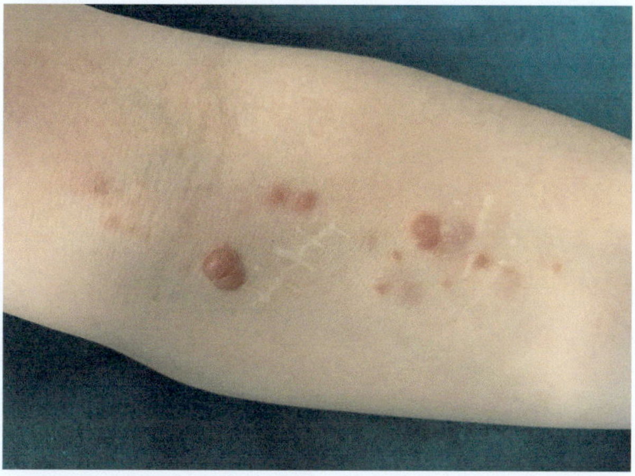

Fig. 15.5

Group 3 is very rare and may represent allelic twin-spot due to somatic recombination. In few patients, you may find pigmentary lesions in a checkerboard pattern and neurofibromas distributed along Blaschko lines with unilateral or bilateral, symmetric or asymmetric distribution (Fig. 15.6).

Fig. 15.6

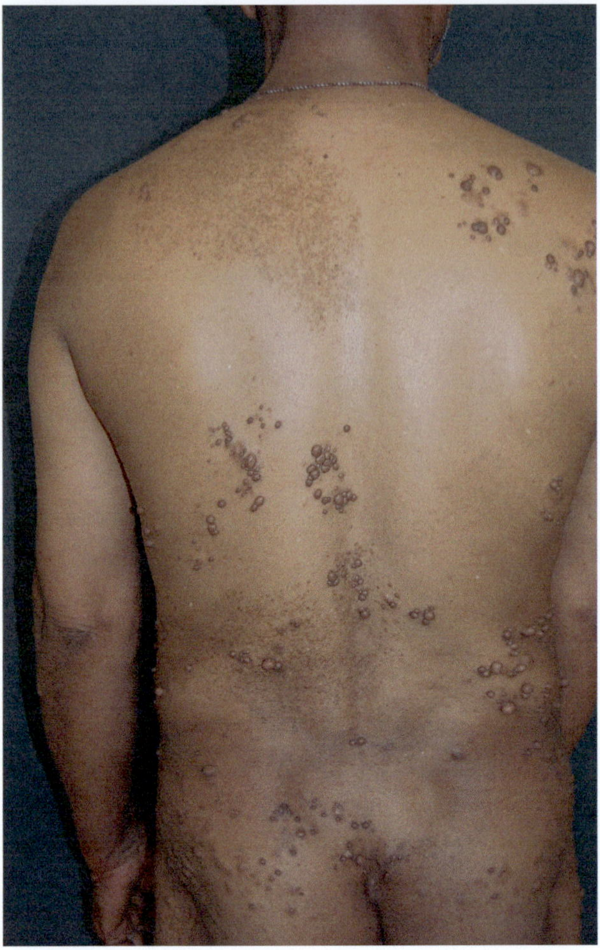

Group 4 lesions are called "plexiform neurofibromas" due to their histopathological pattern. They are visible at birth as "herald patches" and are distributed along a checkerboard pattern (see Fig. 15.7 and Chap. 5). Checkerboard pattern of distribution is clearly visible on the trunk, neck, and head but on the contrary is not clearly appreciable on arms and legs, where it appears as a patchy or longitudinal lesion (Fig. 15.8).

Fig. 15.7

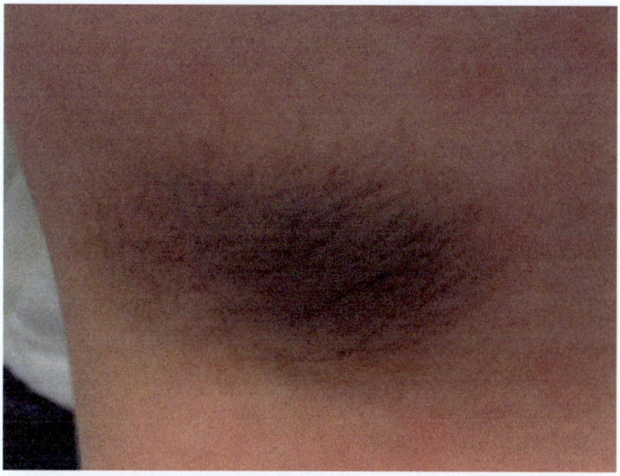

Fig. 15.8

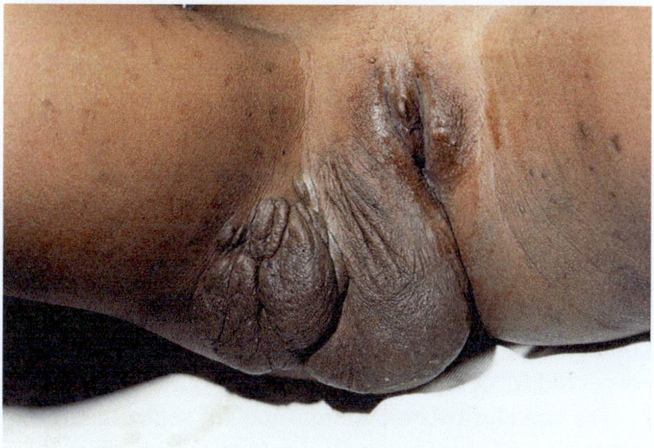

MNF1 follows the rules of cutaneous mosaicism delineate by Happle [6]. In particular, it is important to consider the timing of post-zygotic NF1 gene mutation and the cell type involved (final destination of the cell type). Depending on this, we may have a huge variability in the clinical presentation, ranging from the more frequent presentation of cutaneous lesions confined in a single area (80–90% of MNF1) to multiple areas involved, both unilateral or bilateral (2–6%) [4], in a symmetric or asymmetrical distribution (see Figs. 15.3 and 15.4) [7].

The time of occurrence of the post-zygotic mutations during embryonic development may lead to a very different phenotypes, ranging from late occurring mutations in patients with CALMs or neurofibromas in a localized body area to a very early somatic mutation that can give a phenotype called "generalized mosaic NF1": these patients exhibit typical symptoms of NF1 disease, usually in a rather mild form, without any recognizable mosaic pattern making them indistinguishable from NF1 patients due to germinal mutations.

The real prevalence of this particular subset of MNF1 is not predictable but they may account for up to 5% of NF1 patients overall. In a large NF1 cohort (3500 patients) studied molecularly by the group of Ludwine Messiaen [8] they found 146 "gross" NF1 deletions (referred often as NF1 microdeletions); 14 of these 146 were due to somatic mosaicism, supporting the concept that there is a direct relationship between the high new mutation rate in NF1 gene and the frequency of mosaicism.

These patients with "generalized" "non-pattern" MNF1 may account also for a percentage of patients fulfilling the diagnostic criteria for NF1 without NF1 gene mutations detected with standard molecular techniques, given the putative low rate of the mutation presence in blood cells used for the screening [9].

It must also be noted that there is a frequent occurrence of acquired, somatic "second hit" mutations resulting in loss of heterozygosity at the NF1 locus, demonstrated in melanocytes derived from café-au-lait macules, neurofibromas, and plexiform neurofibromas [10–13]. Identical mechanism is found in osseous tissue from tibial abnormalities [14] and is also responsible for malignant peripheral nerve sheath tumors (MPNST) and many of the NF1-associated malignancies.

Anemic nevus (AN) and juvenile xanthogranulomas, that are frequent and precocious cutaneous signs that may help for early diagnosis in NF1, are absent in our cohort and in other large series examined. Only one case of AN is reported in a suspected MNF1 patient [15].

The last clinical consideration is for segmental lentiginoses (SL): are they a form of MNF1 or not? Known also as Partial Unilateral Lentiginoses, it is a rare pigmentation disorder characterized by numerous freckle-like lesions in a mosaic checkerboard distribution, often with a background of hyperpigmented skin. They have usually sharp borders on the midline but many exceptions are visible. They may be unique or multiple and may be unilateral or bilateral, more often localized in the upper part of the body (Fig. 15.9). They may have intermingled café-au-lait macules within the area occupied by freckle-like lesions (Fig. 15.10). Recently Yasar [16] described associated Lisch nodules and a single patient with associated neurofibromas.

Fig. 15.9

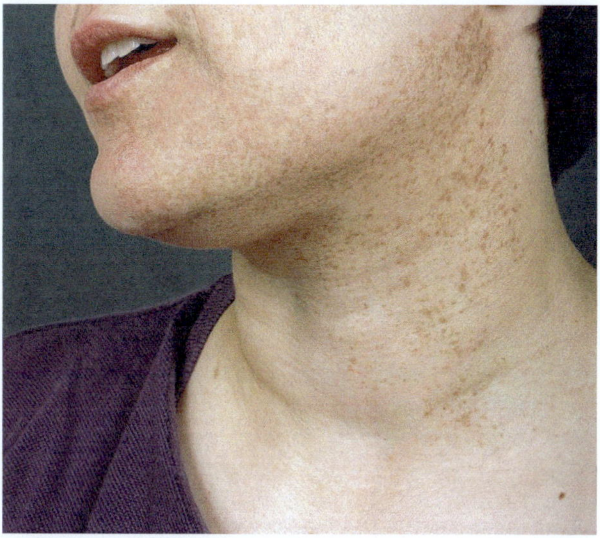

Fig. 15.10

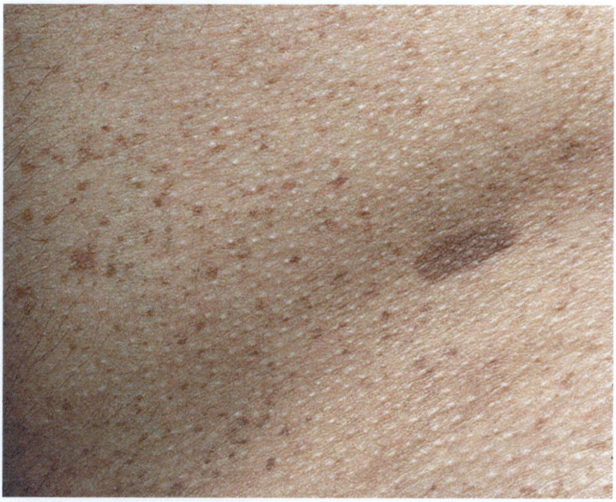

Unfortunately, there are no report of NF1 mutations in these cases but we believe that with NGS techniques SL should be easily confirmed as a variant of MNF1.

15.3 Associated Signs

Usually MNF1 is regarded as a benign clinical situation and in the vast majority of patients, this concept holds true. Analyzing large series of MNF1 [reviewed by Romero in 2016, 17] it must be noted that some associated sign may be present [4, 18].

Rarely Lisch nodules are detected (2–5% of MNF1 patients) and there is a single report of optic way glioma. In the same percentage bony abnormalities are detected, namely scoliosis and fibrous osseous dysplasia (sphenoid and tibia). Seizures are reported in 2–3% of MNF1 patients as well as learning disabilities. Associated malignancies in two patients are reported [4].

In the reviewed single case reports, the 28% of patients with "pigmentary" MNF1 had associated signs: this large number may be explained by the fact that published cases are more likely to be complex enough to be accepted. On the contrary, pediatric series may underestimate associated signs due to the peculiar development during time of NF1 signs and symptoms.

Some associated malignancies are reported in MNF1, namely MPNST (second hit Knudson hypothesis-loss of heterozygosity) [19] and gastric cancer [20]. Co-occurrence of malignancies in MNF1 is far lower than in patients harboring germinal mutations.

In our cohort (250 patients, age ranging from 1 to 76 years of age) the associated "extracutaneous" signs do not exceed the 10% of cases being ocular (Lisch nodules and choroidal hamartomas), neuropsychological findings (learning disabilities, dyslexia), and osseous lesions (sphenoid dysplasia - Fig. 15.11 - and scoliosis) the more frequent, confirming the data of the literature. No associated malignancies were detected.

Fig. 15.11

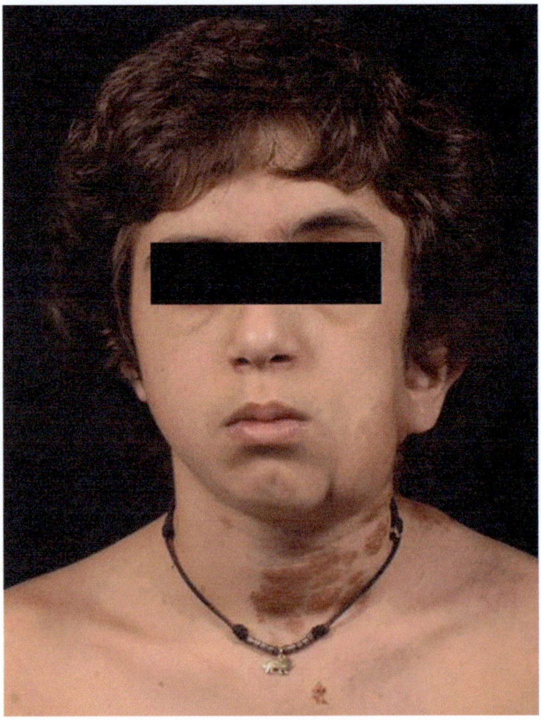

Considering all these data, patients affected by MNF1 should be attentively followed up for associated extracutaneous disorders. When available, blood and skin testing for NF1 mutations may confirm the MNF1 diagnosis.

Next generation sequences techniques may be the method of choice for mosaic detection, having high sensitivity and a quantitative aspect using adapted bioinformatics filtering parameters that are able to detect small percentage of cells carrying the NF1 somatic mutation. Finally, the frequency of mosaicism in sporadic NF1 affected patients is currently largely unknown [21].

There is a risk for MNF1 patients, even low, to transmit the mutation to the offspring in case of gonosomal of gonadic mosaicism. In literature, this risk is from 3 up to 6% [2]. All MNF1 patients must receive genetic counseling illustrating the risk to have children with NF1 [17].

In spite of the sporadic "per se" nature of MNF1, some familial proven case is reported [22, 23] and may be explained by a paradominant trait [24].

Sperm donors also must be analyzed clinically and donor bank must be aware of the risk for gonosomal mosaicism in sperm donors in order to avoid half siblings with NF1 [25].

15.4 Differential Diagnosis

Mosaic SPRED1 mutations leading to a mosaic form of Legius syndrome are reported in the literature and must be considered in differential diagnosis when suspecting MNF1 [26].

A recent study [27] confirmed that CALMs in Legius syndrome are caused by biallelic inactivating mutations in SPRED1 gene, as seen in CALMs in NF1 patients [13].

In our knowledge there is no report in literature of a mosaic distribution in Mismatch Repair syndrome associated pigmentary lesions.

Funding Sources None.

Conflict of Interest None declared.

References

1. Tinschert S, Naumann I, Stegmann E, Buske A, Kaufmann D, Thiel G, Jenne DE. Segmental neurofibromatosis is caused by somatic mutation of the neurofibromatosis type 1 (NF1) gene. Eur J Hum Genet. 2000;8(6):455–9.
2. Ruggieri M, Huson SM. The clinical and diagnostic implications of mosaicism in the neurofibromatoses. Neurology. 2001;56(11):1433–43.
3. Brena M, Unpublished data, personal observation.
4. Vázquez-Osorio I, Duat-Rodríguez A, García-Martínez FJ, Torrelo A, Noguera-Morel L, Hernández-Martín A. Cutaneous and systemic findings in mosaic neurofibromatosis type 1. Pediatr Dermatol. 2017;34(3):271–6.
5. Tadini G, Milani D, Menni F, Pezzani L, Sabatini C, Esposito S. Is it time to change the neurofibromatosis 1 diagnostic criteria? Eur J Intern Med. 2014;25(6):506–10.

6. Toberer F, Happle R, Schneiderbauer R, Hausser I, Kröhl V, Epple A, Moog U, Enk AH, Lonsdorf AS. At first sight or second glance: clinical presentation of mosaic manifestations of autosomal dominant skin disorders - a case series. J Eur Acad Dermatol Venereol. 2017;31(11):1912–5.
7. Tadini G, Brena M, Gelmetti C, Pezzani L. Atlas of genodermatoses. 2nd ed. London: CRC Press; 2015.
8. Messiaen L, Vogt J, Bengesser K, Fu C, Mikhail F, Serra E, Garcia-Linares C, Cooper DN, Lazaro C, Kehrer-Sawatzki H. Mosaic type-1 NF1 microdeletions as a cause of both generalized and segmental neurofibromatosis type-1 (NF1). Hum Mutat. 2011;32(2):213–9.
9. Vandenbroucke I, van Doorn R, Callens T, Cobben JM, Starink TM, Messiaen L. Genetic and clinical mosaicism in a patient with neurofibromatosis type 1. Hum Genet. 2004;114(3):284–90.
10. Upadhyaya M, Spurlock G, Thomas L, Thomas NS, Richards M, Mautner VF, Cooper DN, Guha A, Yan J. Microarray-based copy number analysis of neurofibromatosis type-1 (NF1)-associated malignant peripheral nerve sheath tumors reveals a role for rho-GTPase pathway genes in NF1 tumorigenesis. Hum Mutat. 2012;33(4):763–76.
11. Emmerich D, Zemojtel T, Hecht J, Krawitz P, Spielmann M, Kühnisch J, Kobus K, Osswald M, Heinrich V, Berlien P, Müller U, Mautner VF, Wimmer K, Robinson PN, Vingron M, Tinschert S, Mundlos S, Kolanczyk M. Somatic neurofibromatosis type 1 (NF1) inactivation events in cutaneous neurofibromas of a single NF1 patient. Eur J Hum Genet. 2015;23(6):870–3.
12. Maertens O, De Schepper S, Vandesompele J, Brems H, Heyns I, Janssens S, Speleman F, Legius E, Messiaen L. Molecular dissection of isolated disease features in mosaic neurofibromatosis type 1. Am J Hum Genet. 2007;81(2):243–51.
13. De Schepper S, Maertens O, Callens T, Naeyaert JM, Lambert J, Messiaen L. Somatic mutation analysis in NF1 café au lait spots reveals two NF1 hits in the melanocytes. J Invest Dermatol. 2008;128(4):1050–3.
14. Kobus K, Hartl D, Ott CE, Osswald M, Huebner A, von der Hagen M, Emmerich D, Kühnisch J, Morreau H, Hes FJ, Mautner VF, Harder A, Tinschert S, Mundlos S, Kolanczyk M. Double NF1 inactivation affects adrenocortical function in NF1Prx1 mice and a human patient. PLoS One. 2015;10(3):e0119030.
15. Marque M, Roubertie A, Jaussent A, Carneiro M, Meunier L, Guillot B, Pinson L, Pinson S, Bessis D. Nevus anemicus in neurofibromatosis type 1: a potential new diagnostic criterion. J Am Acad Dermatol. 2013;69(5):768–75.
16. Yaşar Ş, Ersanli A, Göktay F, Aytekin S, Cebeci D, Güneş P. Partial unilateral lentiginosis is mosaic neurofibromatosis type 1 or not? J Dermatol. 2017;44(1):29–35.
17. García-Romero MT, Parkin P, Lara-Corrales I. Mosaic Neurofibromatosis type 1: a systematic review. Pediatr Dermatol. 2016;33(1):9–17.
18. Tanito K, Ota A, Kamide R, Nakagawa H, Niimura M. Clinical features of 58 Japanese patients with mosaic neurofibromatosis 1. J Dermatol. 2014;41(8):724–8.
19. Li K, Won CH, Moon SE. A superficial form of malignant peripheral nerve sheath tumour associated with segmental neurofibromatosis. Acta Derm Venereol. 2005;85(6):540–1.
20. Kajimoto A, Oiso N, Fukai K, Ishii M. Bilateral segmental neurofibromatosis with gastric carcinoma. Clin Exp Dermatol. 2007;32(1):43–4.
21. Pasmant E, Parfait B, Luscan A, Goussard P, Briand-Suleau A, Laurendeau I, Fouveaut C, Leroy C, Montadert A, Wolkenstein P, Vidaud M, Vidaud D. Neurofibromatosis type 1 molecular diagnosis: what can NGS do for you when you have a large gene with loss of function mutations? Eur J Hum Genet. 2015 May;23(5):596–601.
22. Jankovic I, Kovacevic P, Visnjic M, Jankovic D, Velickovic M. A unique case of hereditary bilateral segmental neurofibromatosis on the face. An Bras Dermatol. 2012;87(6):895–8.
23. Oguzkan S, Cinbis M, Ayter S, Anlar B, Aysun S. Familial segmental neurofibromatosis. J Child Neurol. 2004;19(5):392–4.
24. Happle R. What is paradominant inheritance? J Med Genet. 2009;46(9):648.

25. Ejerskov C, Farholt S, Skovby F, Vestergaard EM, Haagerup A. Clinical presentations of 23 half-siblings from a mosaic neurofibromatosis type 1 sperm donor. Clin Genet. 2016;89(3):346–50.
26. Brems H, Pasmant E, Van Minkelen R, Wimmer K, Upadhyaya M, Legius E, Messiaen L. Review and update of SPRED1 mutations causing Legius syndrome. Hum Mutat. 2012;33(11):1538–46.
27. Jobling RK, Lara-Corrales I, Hsiao MC, Shugar A, Hedges S, Messiaen L, Kannu P. Mosaicism for a SPRED1 deletion revealed in a patient with clinically suspected mosaic neurofibromatosis. Br J Dermatol. 2017;176(4):1077–8.

Legius Syndrome, Other Café-au-lait Diseases and Differential Diagnosis of NF1

16

Ellen Denayer, Eric Legius, and Hilde Brems

Contents

E. Denayer
Clinical Department of Human Genetics, KU Leuven-University of Leuven, University Hospitals Leuven, Leuven, Belgium
e-mail: ellen.denayer@uzleuven.be

E. Legius · H. Brems (✉)
Clinical Department of Human Genetics, KU Leuven-University of Leuven, University Hospitals Leuven, Leuven, Belgium

Department of Human Genetics, KU Leuven-University of Leuven, Leuven, Belgium
e-mail: eric.legius@uzleuven.be; hilde.brems@kuleuven.be

G. Tadini et al. (eds.), *Multidisciplinary Approach to Neurofibromatosis Type 1*,
https://doi.org/10.1007/978-3-319-92450-2_16

Neurofibromatosis type 1 (NF1) is characterized by typical clinical manifestations including multiple café-au-lait spots (CALs), skin fold freckling, Lisch nodules in the iris, optic pathway gliomas, and neurofibromas. The condition is inherited in an autosomal dominant manner and is caused by inactivating mutations in the *NF1* gene located on chromosome band 17q11.2. It is estimated that about half of patients have NF1 as a result of a de novo *NF1* pathogenic mutation. Clinical diagnostic criteria for NF1 were established at the National Institutes of Health Consensus Development Conference (1988). In young children without family history, however, it is often difficult to make a definitive diagnosis based on clinical grounds, because these children often only manifest multiple CALMs, whereas other manifestations of the disease frequently only present later on in childhood or in adulthood. Moreover differential diagnosis with other CALM-manifesting disorders is often difficult on clinical grounds.

In 2007 Brems et al. reported a NF1-like syndrome which showed clinical overlap with the NF1 phenotype and was caused by heterozygous germline loss-of-function mutations in the *SPRED1* gene. In the first report affected patients were described presenting multiple CALMs, axillary freckling, macrocephaly and in some individuals Noonan-like facial features, lipomas, learning problems, and/or attention deficit [1]. The typical neurofibromas and other tumoral manifestations of NF1 seemed to be absent in these patients and overall a milder phenotype was present in individuals with NF1-like syndrome. To clearly differentiate between both disorders and to avoid confusion in diagnosis and counselling between NF1 and NF1-like syndrome, The NF1-like syndrome was renamed after expert consensus at the 13th European Neurofibromatosis Meeting (2008) to be "Legius syndrome," referring to Eric Legius, the senior author of the initial publication describing this condition. It is estimated that about 1–4% of individuals with multiple CALMs and fulfilling NIH clinical diagnostic criteria for NF1 in fact have Legius syndrome [2].

The other most important differential diagnosis for patients presenting with multiple CALs is Constitutive Mismatch Repair Deficiency (CMMRD). This is an autosomal recessive condition caused by homozygous or compound heterozygous mutations in one of the mismatch repair genes (*MLH1, MSH2, MSH6, PMS2*). Heterozygous mutations in one of these mismatch repair genes are the cause of the autosomal dominant Lynch cancer syndrome. Pigmentary findings present in at least half of the CMMRD cases are difficult to distinguish from those in NF1 or Legius syndrome. However, individuals with CMMRD usually develop tumors in childhood. This condition should be considered in children from consanguineous parents, where parents do not show clinical findings of NF1, but can have symptoms or family history compatible with Lynch syndrome.

CALMs can also be found in other genetic conditions, including piebaldism, neurofibromatosis type 2 (NF2), schwannomatosis, Noonan syndrome with multiple lentigines, and McCune-Albright syndrome. The cutaneous phenotype in these latter conditions is, however, often distinguishable from NF1 for trained clinicians. In this chapter a short introduction to Legius syndrome, CMMRD, and other CALM-manifesting disorders will be given. In addition differential diagnoses of NF1 will be described.

16.1 Legius Syndrome

16.1.1 Clinical Features

In the original report describing NF1-like syndrome five families with an autosomal dominant inherited condition presenting with multiple CALMs, axillary freckling, macrocephaly, and at times a Noonan-like facial appearance were described. Learning difficulties and/or attention deficit were observed in several children and multiple lipomas were present in several adults. Some typical NF1 features such as Lisch nodules of the iris, neurofibromas, and central nervous system tumors were systematically absent [1].

Following this first report several other patients' cohorts with this syndrome were published. Pasmant et al. identified five probands with a *SPRED1* mutation in 61 index cases. They confirmed a high prevalence of CALMs, freckling and learning disability as well as absence of neurofibromas and Lisch nodules [3]. Noonan-like dysmorphism was not observed and macrocephaly was reported in only one individual. Lipomas were seen in one family. Spurlock et al. identified six probands with *SPRED1* mutations in 85 unrelated patients referred for *NF1* gene testing who were *NF1* mutation negative and had no cutaneous neurofibromas [4]. All affected probands but one satisfied NF1 diagnostic criteria. They all had CALMs. None had Noonan-like features, macrocephaly, Lisch nodules, or cutaneous neurofibromas. No significant developmental or learning problems were observed.

Messiaen et al. performed a genotype-phenotype study in 22 unrelated probands carrying a *SPRED1* mutation identified through clinical testing [5]. Fifty percent of *SPRED1* positive individuals fulfilled NF1 NIH diagnostic criteria based on the presence of more than five CALMs with or without freckling or a NF1 family history. Symptomatic optic pathway gliomas, neurofibromas, or typical NF1 osseous lesions were absent in the affected individuals and there was no increased prevalence of lipomas. Relative macrocephaly was documented in 27% of individuals and language/speech difficulties in 25% of children. In a second cross-sectional study Messiaen et al. performed *SPRED1* mutation analysis in 1318 unrelated patients presenting with a broad range of signs typical for NF1 but no detectable *NF1* mutation [5]. They identified 26 pathogenic *SPRED1* mutations in 33 probands and 7 probable non-pathogenic missense mutations in 9 probands. A *SPRED1* mutation detection rate of 19% was found in families with an autosomal dominant phenotype of CALM with or without freckling and no other NF1 features.

Denayer et al. described 30 individuals from 14 families [6]. Their results confirmed that Legius syndrome is characterized by the presence of CALs with or without freckling and the absence of typical NF1 complications such as Lisch nodules and neurofibromas. In a subset of patients learning difficulties, ADHD and Noonan-like facial features and/or sternal abnormalities were found. One vestibular schwannoma and one benign tumor of the abdominal wall (desmoid tumor) were observed. Both tumor types had not been reported before in association with Legius syndrome and it is unclear whether there is a causal relationship between these tumors and the germline *SPRED1* mutation. Learning difficulties were mentioned in 14/25 patients (56%), three patients were diagnosed with ADHD and one with ADD. Aspecific hyperintense T2 lesions on brain MRI were reported in two individuals. Unilateral postaxial polydactyly was found in two patients in this study and in one patient reported by Messiaen et al.

Since then several case reports have been published describing patients with *SPRED1* pathogenic mutations.

Learning difficulties [1, 3, 7], hyperactivity [1, 5], and language or speech delay [3, 5] have been reported in several children with Legius syndrome. Whether Legius syndrome is associated with a specific neurocognitive profile, this was investigated in a small study by Denayer et al. [6]. In 15 patients with Legius syndrome a mean FSIQ of 101.57 (SD = 17.57; median = 107; IQR = 23) was reported, which did not differ significantly from the control group (unaffected siblings), and is higher than the mean FSIQ in 103 patients with NF1. These preliminary data suggest that in addition to the somatic phenotype [5], the cognitive phenotype is milder in Legius syndrome than in NF1 and other RASopathies. In Legius syndrome, the standard deviation was larger than expected, indicating a large variability in mean FSIQ in patients with Legius syndrome. A significantly lower performance IQ in children with Legius syndrome was found than in unaffected family members. In comparison with NF1, there were few behavioral problems as assessed by the CBCL.

Whether Legius syndrome is associated with an increased risk for malignancies is still not resolved yet. Only one patient was reported with one of the following tumors:giant cell tumor, dermoid tumor of the ovary, breast cancer [5], vestibular schwannoma, desmoid tumor [6]. Pasmant et al. reported a child that presented acute myeloblastic leukemia [3, 8]. In the blast cells of this child no somatic *SPRED1* mutation or loss of heterozygosity was found. This research group subsequently screened 230 pediatric lymphoblastic and acute myeloblastic leukemias and found a loss-of-function frameshift *SPRED1* variant in a patient with Legius syndrome. In this patient the karyotype of white blood cell blasts showed a *SPRED1* loss of heterozygosity [9]. However, no other *SPRED1* pathogenic variants were found in the cohort although SPRED1 protein and *SPRED1* mRNA levels were decreased in the majority of acute myeloblastic leukemias at diagnosis [9]. Further studies are needed to assess the potential risk for malignancies in Legius syndrome, particularly given that *SPRED1* is part of the RAS-MAPK signalling transduction pathway, a pathway involved in several neoplasms.

Combined data in the literature suggest that the highest chances of finding a *SPRED1* mutation are in familial cases of CALMs with or without freckling.

Sporadic cases of CALMs are more likely due to mosaicism for NF1 [10]. Nevus anemicus has been suggested to be a clinical sign possibly differentiating NF1 from other CALM disorders [11]. They found a prevalence of 51% of nevus anemicus in patients with NF1, compared to a prevalence of 2% in control subjects and suggested to add this feature tot the list of clinical diagnostic criteria for NF1. However, we identified a nevus anemicus in a patient with Legius syndrome due to pathogenic *SPRED1* mutation as well as in a patient with Noonan syndrome with multiple lentigines due to *PTPN11* mutation, suggesting nevus anemicus is characteristic of a broader group of RASopathies and cannot be used to differentiate clinically between NF1 and Legius syndrome [12].

In 2000, choroidal abnormalities were described in NF1 individuals by Yasunari et al. [13] as multiple bright patchy nodules of choroidal origin at and around the posterior pole detectable with a scanning laser ophthalmoscope. Histologically they represent ovoid bodies clustered around axons and consisting of hyperplastic Schwann cells and melanocytes. Although single choroidal nodules are frequently noticed in healthy individuals, multiple choroidal nodules seem to be specific for NF1, emerging the debate to include choroidal nodules as a new diagnostic criterion in the NIH diagnostic criteria for NF1. Cassiman et al. investigated whether these nodules could be used to differentiate NF1 from other CALM syndromes, especially Legius syndrome. They concluded that although the presence of a single choroidal nodule is more frequent in patients with Legius syndrome than in the general population, the presence of more than one choroidal nodule is typical and pathognomonic for NF1 [14].

16.1.2 Molecular Features

After linkage analysis in two families with multiple CALs and freckling and without *NF1* mutation this NF1-like phenotype was mapped to a region on chromosome 15 where *SPRED1* was localized. The *SPRED1* gene was considered a good candidate gene since it had been shown that the encoded SPRED1 protein negatively regulates the RAS-MAPK signalling pathway, as neurofibromin does. Indeed inactivating germline mutations in the *SPRED1* gene were detected in the affected individuals of these two families as well as in three other families and an additional six unrelated patients with a similar phenotype [1]. The *SPRED1* gene (Sprouty-related, EVH1 domain containing 1) was discovered in 2001 by Yoshimura et al. in a mouse cDNA osteoclast library [15]. The human *SPRED1* gene is located on chromosome band 15q13.2 and spans 104.4 kb of genomic sequence. It consists of seven exons coding for 444 amino acids. In the SPRED1 protein three functional domains have been identified: an N-terminal EVH1-domain, a central c-KIT-binding domain, and a C-terminal SPRY-related domain. Human SPRED1 is highly expressed in lung, brain, spinal cord, and spleen and lower expression is present in liver, pancreas, prostate, kidney, heart, thymus, muscle, and bone marrow. SPRED1 is an inhibitor of the RAS-MAPK signalling pathway by interacting with neurofibromin and suppressing RAF activation by active RAS (RAS-GTP). The molecular details of this interaction and the effects of the mutations identified in Legius syndrome and NF1 on this interaction was first identified by Stowe et al. [16] and afterwards further investigated by Hirata et al. [17]. In this study, using a yeast two-hybrid system and an immunoprecipitation assay in HEK293 cells, it was demonstrated that the SPRED1 EVH1 domain interacts with the N-terminal 16 amino acids and the C-terminal 20 amino acids of the GTPase-activating protein (GAP)-related domain (GRD) of neurofibromin, which form two crossing α-helix coils outside the GAP domain. These regions have been shown to be dispensable for GAP activity and are not present in p120(GAP). Several mutations in these N- and C-terminal regions of the GRD in NF1 patients and pathogenic missense mutations in the EVH1 domain of SPRED1 in Legius syndrome reduced the binding affinity between the EVH1 domain and the GRD. EVH1 domain mutations with reduced binding to the GRD also disrupted the MAPK suppression activity of SPRED1. These data demonstrate that SPRED1 inhibits the RAS-MAPK pathway by recruiting neurofibromin to RAS through the EVH1-GRD interaction.

All identified mutations and polymorphisms in the *SPRED1* gene are summarized in the Leiden Open Variation Database, which is accessible online at http://www.lovd.nl/SPRED1. No clear mutational hotspots in the gene have been identified. Most of the pathogenic mutations are predicted to be truncating (nonsense or frameshift mutations). A minority are missense mutations. Most of the missense mutations are classified as polymorphisms. For some missense mutations functional characterization was able to classify them as pathogenic [1, 17]. Spencer et al. [18] reported that deletions comprise approximately 10% of *SPRED1* pathogenic variants and include multi-exon deletions and whole *SPRED1* gene deletions. In the original study by Brems et al. a somatic frameshift *SPRED1* mutation was identified in cultured melanocytes from a CAL from an individual with Legius syndrome in addition to the known germline *SPRED1* mutation in this patient. This showed that CALMs in patients with Legius syndrome are caused by biallelic inactivation of the *SPRED1* gene, a mechanism similar to the biallelic inactivation of the *NF1* gene in cultured melanocytes from patients with NF1 [1].

16.1.3 Animal Models

The SPRED1 protein is conserved during evolution and a Spred1 homolog with >90% protein identity exists in mouse, where the *Spred1* gene is located on the second chromosome. Expression during fetal development in mouse was shown in brain, heart, lung, liver, and bone, whereas in adult mice Spred1 is predominantly expressed in brain [19, 20]. A Spred1 knockout mouse model was generated by homologous recombination resulting in the KBD and SPR being homozygously deleted [21]. In contrast to Nf1−/− mice that are embryonically lethal, Spred1−/− mice are viable and they are clinically recognizable from their wild-type littermates by their lower body weight and shortened face. These mice are fertile although there is higher mortality in Spred1−/− pups than in the wild-type and heterozygous littermates. The Spred1 knockout mouse model was first studied in an allergic asthma model, where Spred1−/− mice developed a more severe allergic reaction due to increased numbers of eosinophils in the lungs [21]. After discovery of *SPRED1* mutations as a cause of Legius syndrome and reports suggesting increased risk for learning difficulties and developmental delay in individuals with this condition, the cognitive phenotype, more specifically hippocampus-dependent learning and memory and synaptic plasticity in the Spred1 knockout mouse model was studied [22]. Spred1−/− mice showed decreased learning and memory performance in the Morris water maze and visual discrimination defects in the T-mice, with normal basic neuromotor and sensory abilities. No difference in performance between Spred1+/− mice and wild-types was observed in the Morris water maze. However, during the final mixed-trial visual discrimination tasks of the T-maze the Spred1+/− mice performed at an intermediate level between Spred1−/− mice and wild-types. Electrophysiological recordings on brain slices from Spred1−/− mice identified defects in short- and long-term synaptic hippocampal plasticity. Biochemical analysis, 4 h after LTP induction, demonstrated increased Mapk-phosphorylation in these Spred1−/− slices compared to wild-type brain slices.

These findings are very similar to the learning and synaptic plasticity defects observed in the Nf1+/− mice and stress the importance of the RAS-MAPK pathway in learning and memory.

16.2 Constitutive Mismatch Repair Deficiency (CMMRD)

Lynch syndrome is an autosomal dominant cancer predisposition syndrome characterized by increased risk for adult malignancy, including colorectal cancer, gynecological tumors (ovarian cancer and endometrial cancer), and urinary tumors. The syndrome is caused by heterozygous mutations in one of the mismatch repair genes *MLH1, MSH2, MSH6, PMS2* or deletion of the 3′ end of *EPCAM*. These genes are responsible for correcting base substitution mismatches or insertion-deletion mismatches generated during DNA replication. Tumors in individuals with Lynch syndrome frequently demonstrate microsatellite instability (MSI) and lack of expression of the mutated MMR gene by immunohistochemistry.

In 1999 Wang et al. reported two siblings with homozygous mutations in the mismatch repair gene *MLH1*. They presented with respectively non-Hodgkin lymphoma and acute myeloid leukemia followed by medulloblastoma. They also had clinical features resembling NF1 such as CALMs in both siblings and respectively pseudoarthrosis of the tibia in one and multiple cutaneous neurofibromas in the other sibling [23]. These children originated from consanguineous mating in a family with a highly penetrant Lynch syndrome phenotype, presenting multiple colorectal tumors in adult family members. During the same year three children from consanguineous parents were described that presented with early diagnosis of hematological malignancy by the age of 3 years. In addition two of the three children had clinical features of NF1. Both their parents had been diagnosed with colon cancer and several other family members had colon cancer. The family history was consistent with Lynch syndrome and heterozygous *MLH1* mutation was found in adult family members. In DNA from the deceased children there was strong evidence for homozygosity for this *MLH1* mutation [24].

Subsequently several reports described homozygous or compound heterozygous mutations in MMR genes in a distinct childhood cancer predisposition syndrome termed constitutional mismatch repair deficiency CMMRD. Most frequently described malignancies in these children are non-Hodgkin's lymphomas, high-grade gliomas, and colorectal carcinomas, but also low-grade gliomas and premalignant gastro-intestinal lesions have been identified. The most prevalent non-neoplastic features in CMMRD are CALMs and other pigmentary alterations. Wimmer et al. showed that 60% of CMMRD patients have at least 1 CALM or hyperpigmented skin area and 18% presented (often in addition to CALMs) with other NF1 diagnostic features (freckling, neurofibromas, Lisch nodules, bone lesion, optic pathway glioma) [25]. Interestingly in up to 75% of families with CMMRD no Lynch-associated malignancies were identified in adult family members carrying the heterozygous MMR gene mutation [26, 27]. This is probably related to the fact that mostly mutations in *PMS2* and *MSH6* are found in CMMRD pedigrees. These genes are known to be associated with a less penetrant Lynch syndrome phenotype. It is possible that the highly penetrant *MSH2* or *MLH1* mutations are embryonically lethal in the homozygous state.

16.3 Other Conditions That Can Present with Café-au-lait Spots

16.3.1 Piebaldism

Piebaldism is a rare autosomal dominant condition that is characterized by the congenital absence of melanocytes in affected areas of the skin and hair. Patients often have a white forelock of hair and the underlying forehead may be involved. Irregularly shaped white areas without pigmentation can be present on the face, trunk, and extremities, usually in a symmetrical distribution. Islands of hyperpigmentation can be present within or at the border of these depigmented areas, which can mimic CALMs. The condition is caused by heterozygous mutation in the *KIT* proto-oncogene or sometimes in the zinc finger transcription factor *SNAI2*. Several case reports describe patients said to have both piebaldism and NF1. Stevens et al. reported on a large family with piebaldism in which two members met diagnostic criteria for NF1 based on the presence of >5 CALMs and intertriginous freckling. Interestingly, only these two family members were of mixed race. A *KIT* mutation responsible for the piebaldism phenotype was present in several family members. Comprehensive *NF1* and *SPRED1* mutation analysis in the proband meeting diagnostic criteria for NF1, however, revealed no mutation, indicating that the clinical phenotype of piebaldism may occasionally include CALMs and intertriginous freckling, possibly creating diagnostic confusion especially in the absence of a family history of piebaldism. However, careful clinical evaluation and molecular testing if necessary should distinguish between piebaldism and NF1 [28].

16.3.2 Neurofibromatosis Type 2 (NF2)

NF2 is an autosomal dominant condition characterized by bilateral vestibular schwannomas, schwannomas of other cranial and peripheral nerves, cutaneous schwannomas, meningiomas and ependymomas. Posterior subcapsular lens opacities that rarely progress to visually significant cataract can be the first manifesting symptom of the condition. Almost all affected individuals develop bilateral vestibular schwannomas by the age of 30. Mononeuropathy occurring in childhood is increasingly been recognized and may present as facial nerve palsy, third nerve palsy, or hand/foot drop. NF2 is caused by mutations of the *NF2* gene located on the long arm of chromosome 22 (chromosome band 22q12.2). Multiple CALMs can be present in children with NF2, although usually there are less than five CALM and they are smaller than those seen in NF1. Moreover in NF2 they tend to be paler and have more irregular borders. Hypopigmented areas can also occur [29].

16.3.3 Familial Schwannomatosis

Familial schwannomatosis is a rare autosomal dominant condition characterized by multiple schwannomas, predominantly occurring in the spine, but also in the peripheral nerves and cranial nerves. Unilateral vestibular schwannomas, meningiomas, and lipomas can occur, but the most differentiating feature from NF2 is the absence of bilateral vestibular schwannomas and germline *NF2* mutations. The condition can be caused by heterozygous germline mutations in *SMARCB1* or *LZTR1*, both located on chromosome band 22q11 [30, 31]. The tumors do not follow the Knudson's two hit hypothesis but follow a 3 step 4 hit hypothesis, with involvement of the *NF2* locus. Merker et al. reported that 23% of patients had at least one CAL >1.5 cm; None had more than four. No intertriginous freckling was reported in this cohort of patients [32]. Some patients with schwannomatosis do not have germline mutations in *SMARCB1* or *LZTR1*.

16.3.4 Noonan Syndrome with Multiple Lentigines

Noonan syndrome with multiple lentigines is an autosomal dominant condition previously referred to as LEOPARD syndrome and characterized by multiple lentigines, dysmorphic facial features including ocular hypertelorism and ptosis, short stature, pectus deformity, and congenital heart disease, mostly hypertrophic cardiomyopathy or pulmonic stenosis. Sensorineural hearing loss is present in about 20% of patients and intellectual disability, usually mild in 30%. The condition can be caused by heterozygous mutations in *PTPN11 or RAF1*. Lentigines are small (usually <5 mm) brown flat spots mostly located on the face, neck, and upper part of the trunk, not affecting the mucosa. In general, lentigines do not appear until age 4–5 years but then increase to the thousands by puberty. CALMs are also observed in the majority of patients, usually preceding the appearance of lentigines [33].

16.3.5 McCune-Albright Syndrome

Fibrous Dysplasia/McCune-Albright syndrome (FD/MAS) is characterized by large CALMs with irregular margins, polyostotic fibrous dysplasia, and endocrine problems. FD/MAS is the result of an early embryonic postzygotic somatic activating mutation of *GNAS (*encoding the cAMP pathway-associated G-protein, $G_s\alpha$) [34]. There are no verified instances of vertical transmission of FD/MAS. CALMs are common and are usually the first manifestation of the disease, apparent at or shortly after birth. Broad bands of hypermelanosis are present, the CALMs follow Blaschko's lines. The CALMs are often unilateral localized ending at the midline, these CALMs have rough borders, this in contrast to the smooth borders of the NF1 associated CALMs. Fibrous dysplasia (FD) may occur in many bones but often limited to one side of the body. These lesions may lead to uneven growth, deformities and even fractures causing scoliosis, craniofacial deformities, limited mobility, vision, and/or hearing loss. Endocrinological complications can include gonadotropin-independent precocious puberty, thyroid abnormalities, and growth hormone excess.

16.3.6 Isolated CALMs

Children with fair hair and pale skin and freckles (phototype 1) often can manifest multiple CALMs, which are usually paler and with more irregular borders than those seen in NF1.

16.4 Differential Diagnosis of NF1

16.4.1 Infantile Myofibromatosis

Infantile myofibromatosis is a rare autosomal dominant disorder, mostly congenital. The majority of cases are sporadic; however, familial cases are described. The disorder is characterized by the growth of one or multiple hard tumors of the skin, bone, soft tissue, skeletal muscle, and more rare of the viscera.

Solitary myofibromas are the commonest form and most often occur in the skin and subcutaneous tissue of the head and neck, these myofibromas can regress. Generalized myofibromatosis is associated with visceral involvement and this condition has serious prognostic implications. Two genes have been identified in infantile myofibromatosis *PDGFRB* and *NOTCH3* [35, 36].

16.4.2 Proteus Syndrome

The majority of patients have no or minimal clinical features at birth, normally the disease manifests between 6 and 18 months with asymmetric overgrowth as main clinical feature. Most frequently hands and feet are involved and the overgrowth severely can progress. Bones of limbs, skull, and spine are often affected as well as the central nervous system, vascular and adipose tissue. Cerebriform connective tissue nevi are present in most individuals with Proteus syndrome. Proteus syndrome is caused by a somatic mosaic *AKT1* mutation [37] and it is hypothesized that a germline *AKT1* mutation is lethal.

16.4.3 Orbital Neurofibromas

In 2012 four patients were described with multiple orbital neurofibromas, painful peripheral nerve tumors, a distinctive face, and marfanoid habitus [38]. These patients showed enlarged corneal nerves as well as neuronal migration defects on brain MRI. No pathogenic mutation was identified in *NF1*, *NF2,* or *SMARCB1,* therefore a new syndrome was hypothesized.

16.4.4 Hyaline Fibromatosis Syndrome

Hyaline fibromatosis syndrome is a rare autosomal recessive disorder with homozygous or compound heterozygous mutations in *ANTRX2* [39, 40]. Several body regions may be involved: skin, joints, bone, and internal organs. It is a painful and disfiguring syndrome with hyaline accumulation in the body with small pearly papules predominantly in face, neck, and skull. The main clinical feature is joint stiffness, the syndrome is also characterized by gingival hypertrophy. Severe cases may present at birth or the first months of life, while milder cases present at childhood.

16.4.5 Hybrid Nerve Sheath Tumors

Hybrid nerve sheath tumors are benign peripheral nerve sheath tumors with combined features of more than one conventional type (neurofibroma, schwannoma, perineurioma). Neurofibromas are the hallmark of NF1 and schwannomas the hallmark of NF2 or schwannomatosis. Hybrid neurofibromas/schwannomas were described in tumor syndromes such as NF1, NF2, and especially in schwannomatosis [41], it is a challenge to molecularly characterize the different parts of these tumors. In 2016, a cohort of hybrid neurofibromas/schwannomas was molecularly investigated [42]. A major alteration detected in 44% of the tumors was loss or partial loss of chromosome 22 (including *LZTR1*, *SMARCB1,* and *NF2*) and secondly a focal deletion of *CTNNA3* was detected in one tumor. More research should be done to better understand the underlying mechanism in the initiation and growth of these hybrid tumors. Recently targetable activating mutations were reported in ERBB2 in four hybrid nerve sheath tumors [43].

16.5 Conclusions

CALs are the most frequent and an early manifestation of NF1. In young children without other manifestations of NF1 establishing a correct diagnosis can be difficult. Differential diagnoses to consider are Legius syndrome, especially in familial cases of CALM with or without freckling and without other typical NF1 features and CMMRD [25]. Other CALM-manifesting disorders and other syndromes can usually be distinguished by their disease-specific manifestations and different aspect of the CALMs.

References

1. Brems H, Chmara M, Sahbatou M, Denayer E, Taniguchi K, Kato R, Somers R, Messiaen L, De Schepper S, Fryns JP, Cools J, Marynen P, Thomas G, Yoshimura A, Legius E. Germline loss-of-function mutations in SPRED1 cause a neurofibromatosis 1-like phenotype. Nat Genet. 2007;39(9):1120–6.
2. Brems H, Pasmant E, Van Minkelen R, Wimmer K, Upadhyaya M, Legius E, Messiaen L. Review and update of SPRED1 mutations causing Legius syndrome. Hum Mutat. 2012;33(11):1538–46.
3. Pasmant E, Sabbagh A, Hanna N, Masliah-Planchon J, Jolly E, Goussard P, Ballerini P, Cartault F, Barbarot S, Landman-Parker J, Soufir N, Parfait B, Vidaud M, Wolkenstein P, Vidaud D, France RN. SPRED1 germline mutations caused a neurofibromatosis type 1 overlapping phenotype. J Med Genet. 2009a;46(7):425–30.
4. Spurlock G, Bennett E, Chuzhanova N, Thomas N, Jim HP, Side L, Davies S, Haan E, Kerr B, Huson SM, Upadhyaya M. SPRED1 mutations (Legius syndrome): another clinically useful genotype for dissecting the neurofibromatosis type 1 phenotype. J Med Genet. 2009;46(7):431–7.
5. Messiaen L, Yao S, Brems H, Callens T, Sathienkijkanchai A, Denayer E, Spencer E, Arn P, Babovic-Vuksanovic D, Bay C, Bobele G, Cohen BH, Escobar L, Eunpu D, Grebe T, Greenstein R, Hachen R, Irons M, Kronn D, Lemire E, Leppig K, Lim C, McDonald M, Narayanan V, Pearn A, Pedersen R, Powell B, Shapiro LR, Skidmore D, Tegay D, Thiese H, Zackai EH, Vijzelaar R, Taniguchi K, Ayada T, Okamoto F, Yoshimura A, Parret A, Korf B, Legius E. Clinical and mutational spectrum of neurofibromatosis type 1-like syndrome. JAMA. 2009;302(19):2111–8.
6. Denayer E, Chmara M, Brems H, Kievit AM, van Bever Y, Van den Ouweland AM, Van Minkelen R, de Goede-Bolder A, Oostenbrink R, Lakeman P, Beert E, Ishizaki T, Mori T, Keymolen K, Van den Ende J, Mangold E, Peltonen S, Brice G, Rankin J, Van Spaendonck-Zwarts KY, Yoshimura A, Legius E. Legius syndrome in fourteen families. Hum Mutat. 2011;32(1):E1985–98.
7. Muram-Zborovski TM, Stevenson DA, Viskochil DH, Dries DC, Wilson AR, Mao R. SPRED 1 mutations in a neurofibromatosis clinic. J Child Neurol. 2010;25(10):1203–9.
8. Pasmant E, Ballerini P, Lapillonne H, Perot C, Vidaud D, Leverger G, Landman-Parker J. SPRED1 disorder and predisposition to leukemia in children. Blood. 2009b;114(5):1131.
9. Pasmant E, Gilbert-Dussardier B, Petit A, de Laval B, Luscan A, Gruber A, Lapillonne H, Deswarte C, Goussard P, Laurendeau I, Uzan B, Pflumio F, Brizard F, Vabres P, Naguibvena I, Fasola S, Millot F, Porteu F, Vidaud D, Landman-Parker J, Ballerini P. SPRED1, a RAS MAPK pathway inhibitor that causes Legius syndrome, is a tumour suppressor downregulated in paediatric acute myeloblastic leukaemia. Oncogene. 2015;34(5):631–8.
10. Kehrer-Sawatzki H, Cooper DN. Mosaicism in sporadic neurofibromatosis type 1: variations on a theme common to other hereditary cancer syndromes? J Med Genet. 2008;45(10):622–31.

11. Tadini G, Brena M, Pezzani L, Gelmetti C, Santagada F, Boldrini MP. Anemic nevus in neurofibromatosis type 1. Dermatology. 2013;226(2):115–8.
12. Bulteel C, Morren MA, De Haes P, Denayer E, Legius E, Brems H. Nevus anemicus and RASopathies. JAAD Case Rep. 2018;4(4):390–1.
13. Yasunari T, Shiraki K, Hattori H, Miki T. Frequency of choroidal abnormalities in neurofibromatosis type 1. Lancet. 2000;356(9234):988–92.
14. Cassiman C, Casteels I, Jacob J, Plasschaert E, Brems H, Dubron K, Keer KV, Legius E. Choroidal abnormalities in café-au-lait syndromes: a new differential diagnostic tool? Clin Genet. 2017;91(4):529–35.
15. Wakioka T, Sasaki A, Kato R, Shouda T, Matsumoto A, Miyoshi K, Tsuneoka M, Komiya S, Baron R, Yoshimura A. Spred is a sprouty-related suppressor of Ras signalling. Nature. 2001;412(6847):647–51.
16. Stowe IB, Mercado EL, Stowe TR, Bell EL, Oses-Prieto JA, Hernández H, Burlingame AL, McCormick F. A shared molecular mechanism underlies the human rasopathies Legius syndrome and Neurofibromatosis-1. Genes Dev. 2012;26(13):1421–6.
17. Hirata Y, Brems H, Suzuki M, Kanamori M, Okada M, Morita R, Llano-Rivas I, Ose T, Messiaen L, Legius E, Yoshimura A. Interaction between a domain of the negative regulator of the Ras-ERK pathway, SPRED1 protein, and the GTPase-activating protein-related domain of neurofibromin is implicated in Legius syndrome and neurofibromatosis type 1. J Biol Chem. 2016;291(7):3124–34.
18. Spencer E, Davis J, Mikhail F, Fu C, Vijzelaar R, Zackai EH, Feret H, Meyn MS, Shugar A, Bellus G, Kocsis K, Kivirikko S, Pöyhönen M, Messiaen L. Identification of SPRED1 deletions using RT-PCR, multiplex ligation-dependent probe amplification and quantitative PCR. Am J Med Genet A. 2011;155A(6):1352–9.
19. Engelhardt CM, Bundschu K, Messerschmitt M, Renné T, Walter U, Reinhard M, Schuh K. Expression and subcellular localization of Spred proteins in mouse and human tissues. Histochem Cell Biol. 2004;122(6):527–38.
20. Kato R, Nonami A, Taketomi T, Wakioka T, Kuroiwa A, Matsuda Y, Yoshimura A. Molecular cloning of mammalian Spred-3 which suppresses tyrosine kinase-mediated Erk activation. Biochem Biophys Res Commun. 2003;302(4):767–72.
21. Inoue H, Kato R, Fukuyama S, Nonami A, Taniguchi K, Matsumoto K, Nakano T, Tsuda M, Matsumura M, Kubo M, Ishikawa F, Moon BG, Takatsu K, Nakanishi Y, Yoshimura A. Spred-1 negatively regulates allergen-induced airway eosinophilia and hyperresponsiveness. J Exp Med. 2005;201(1):73–82.
22. Denayer E, Ahmed T, Brems H, Van Woerden G, Borgesius NZ, Callaerts-Vegh Z, Yoshimura A, Hartmann D, Elgersma Y, D'Hooge R, Legius E, Balschun D. Spred1 is required for synaptic plasticity and hippocampus-dependent learning. J Neurosci. 2008;28(53):14443–9.
23. Wang Q, Lasset C, Desseigne F, Frappaz D, Bergeron C, Navarro C, Ruano E, Puisieux A. Neurofibromatosis and early onset of cancers in hMLH1-deficient children. Cancer Res. 1999;59(2):294–7.
24. Ricciardone MD, Ozçelik T, Cevher B, Ozdağ H, Tuncer M, Gürgey A, Uzunalimoğlu O, Cetinkaya H, Tanyeli A, Erken E, Oztürk M. Human MLH1 deficiency predisposes to hematological malignancy and neurofibromatosis type 1. Cancer Res. 1999;59(2):290–3.
25. Wimmer K, Kratz CP, Vasen HF, Caron O, Colas C, Entz-Werle N, Gerdes AM, Goldberg Y, Ilencikova D, Muleris M, Duval A, Lavoine N, Ruiz-Ponte C, Slavc I, Burkhardt B. Brugieres L; EU-consortium care for CMMRD (C4CMMRD). Diagnostic criteria for constitutional mismatch repair deficiency syndrome: suggestions of the European consortium 'care for CMMRD' (C4CMMRD). J Med Genet. 2014;51(6):355–65.
26. Bakry D, Aronson M, Durno C, Rimawi H, Farah R, Alharbi QK, Alharbi M, Shamvil A, Ben-Shachar S, Mistry M, Constantini S, Dvir R, Qaddoumi I, Gallinger S, Lerner-Ellis J, Pollett A, Stephens D, Kelies S, Chao E, Malkin D, Bouffet E, Hawkins C, Tabori U. Genetic and clinical determinants of constitutional mismatch repair deficiency syndrome: report from the constitutional mismatch repair deficiency consortium. Eur J Cancer. 2014;50(5):987–96.

27. Ripperger T, Beger C, Rahner N, Sykora KW, Bockmeyer CL, Lehmann U, Kreipe HH, Schlegelberger B. Constitutional mismatch repair deficiency and childhood leukemia/lymphoma--report on a novel biallelic MSH6 mutation. Haematologica. 2010;95(5):841–4.
28. Stevens CA, Chiang PW, Messiaen LM. Café-au-lait macules and intertriginous freckling in piebaldism: clinical overlap with neurofibromatosis type 1 and Legius syndrome. Am J Med Genet A. 2012;158A(5):1195–9.
29. Ruggieri M, Iannetti P, Polizzi A, La Mantia I, Spalice A, Giliberto O, Platania N, Gabriele AL, Albanese V, Pavone L. Earliest clinical manifestations and natural history of neurofibromatosis type 2 (NF2) in childhood: a study of 24 patients. Neuropediatrics. 2005;36(1):21–34.
30. Hulsebos TJ, Plomp AS, Wolterman RA, Robanus-Maandag EC, Baas F, Wesseling P. Germline mutation of INI1/SMARCB1 in familial schwannomatosis. Am J Hum Genet. 2007;80(4):805–10.
31. Piotrowski A, Xie J, Liu YF, Poplawski AB, Gomes AR, Madanecki P, Fu C, Crowley MR, Crossman DK, Armstrong L, Babovic-Vuksanovic D, Bergner A, Blakeley JO, Blumenthal AL, Daniels MS, Feit H, Gardner K, Hurst S, Kobclka C, Lee C, Nagy R, Rauen KA, Slopis JM, Suwannarat P, Westman JA, Zanko A, Korf BR, Messiaen LM. Germline loss-of-function mutations in LZTR1 predispose to an inherited disorder of multiple schwannomas. Nat Genet. 2014;46(2):182–7.
32. Merker VL, Esparza S, Smith MJ, Stemmer-Rachamimov A, Plotkin SR. Clinical features of schwannomatosis: a retrospective analysis of 87 patients. Oncologist. 2012;17(10):1317–22.
33. Digilio MC, Sarkozy A, de Zorzi A, Pacileo G, Limongelli G, Mingarelli R, Calabrò R, Marino B, Dallapiccola B. LEOPARD syndrome: clinical diagnosis in the first year of life. Am J Med Genet A. 2006;140(7):740–6.
34. Weinstein LS, Shenker A, Gejman PV, Merino MJ, Friedman E, Spiegel AM. Activating mutations of the stimulatory G protein in the McCune-Albright syndrome. N Engl J Med. 1991;325(24):1688–95.
35. Cheung YH, Gayden T, Campeau PM, LeDuc CA, Russo D, Nguyen VH, Guo J, Qi M, Guan Y, Albrecht S, Moroz B, Eldin KW, Lu JT, Schwartzentruber J, Malkin D, Berghuis AM, Emil S, Gibbs RA, Burk DL, Vanstone M, Lee BH, Orchard D, Boycott KM, Chung WK, Jabado N. A recurrent PDGFRB mutation causes familial infantile myofibromatosis. Am J Hum Genet. 2013;92(6):996–1000.
36. Martignetti JA, Tian L, Li D, Ramirez MC, Camacho-Vanegas O, Camacho SC, Guo Y, Zand DJ, Bernstein AM, Masur SK, Kim CE, Otieno FG, Hou C, Abdel-Magid N, Tweddale B, Metry D, Fournet JC, Papp E, McPherson EW, Zabel C, Vaksmann G, Morisot C, Keating B, Sleiman PM, Cleveland JA, Everman DB, Zackai E, Hakonarson H. Mutations in PDGRFB cause autosomal dominant infantile myofibromatosis. Am J Hum Genet. 2013;92:1001–7.
37. Lindhurst MJ, Sapp JC, Teer JK, Johnston JJ, Finn EM, Peters K, Turner J, Cannons JL, Bick D, Blakemore L, Blumhorst C, Brockmann K, Calder P, Cherman N, Deardorff MA, Everman DB, Golas G, Greenstein RM, Kato BM, Keppler-Noreuil KM, Kuznetsov SA, Miyamoto RT, Newman K, Ng D, O'Brien K, Rothenberg S, Schwartzentruber DJ, Singhal V, Tirabosco R, Upton J, Wientroub S, Zackai EH, Hoag K, Whitewood-Neal T, Robey PG, Schwartzberg PL, Darling TN, Tosi LL, Mullikin JC, Biesecker LG. A mosaic activating mutation in AKT1 associated with the Proteus syndrome. N Engl J Med. 2011;365(7):611–9.
38. Babovic-Vuksanovic D, Messiaen L, Nagel C, Brems H, Scheithauer B, Denayer E, Mao R, Sciot R, Janowski KM, Schuhmann MU, Claes K, Beert E, Garrity JA, Spinner RJ, Stemmer-Rachamimov A, Gavrilova R, Van Calenbergh F, Mautner V, Legius E. Multiple orbital neurofibromas, painful peripheral nerve tumors, distinctive face and marfanoid habitus: a new syndrome. Eur J Hum Genet. 2012;20(6):618–25.
39. Dowling O, Difeo A, Ramirez MC, Tukel T, Narla G, Bonafe L, Kayserili H, Yuksel-Apak M, Paller AS, Norton K, Teebi AS, Grum-Tokars V, Martin GS, Davis GE, Glucksman MJ, Martignetti JA. Mutations in capillary morphogenesis gene-2 result in the allelic disorders juvenile hyaline fibromatosis and infantile systemic hyalinosis. Am J Hum Genet. 2003;73(4):957–66.

40. Hanks S, Adams S, Douglas J, Arbour L, Atherton DJ, Balci S, Bode H, Campbell ME, Feingold M, Keser G, Kleijer W, Mancini G, McGrath JA, Muntoni F, Nanda A, Teare MD, Warman M, Pope FM, Superti-Furga A, Futreal PA, Rahman N. Mutations in the gene encoding capillary morphogenesis protein 2 cause juvenile hyaline fibromatosis and infantile systemic hyalinosis. Am J Hum Genet. 2003;73(4):791–800.
41. Harder A, Wesemann M, Hagel C, Schittenhelm J, Fischer S, Tatagiba M, Nagel C, Jeibmann A, Bohring A, Mautner VF, Paulus W. Hybrid neurofibroma/schwannoma is overrepresented among schwannomatosis and neurofibromatosis patients. Am J Surg Pathol. 2012;36(5):702–9.
42. Stahn V, Nagel I, Fischer-Huchzermeyer S, Oyen F, Schneppenheim R, Gesk S, Bohring A, Chikobava L, Young P, Gess B, Werner M, Senner V, Harder A. Molecular analysis of hybrid neurofibroma/schwannoma identifies common monosomy 22 and α-T-catenin/CTNNA3 as a novel candidate tumor suppressor. Am J Pathol. 2016;186(12):3285–96.
43. Michael W. Ronellenfitsch, Patrick N. Harter, Martina Kirchner, Christoph Heining, Barbara Hutter, Laura Gieldon, Jens Schittenhelm, Martin U. Schuhmann, Marcos Tatagiba, Gerhard Marquardt, Marlies Wagner, Volker Endris, Christian H. Brandts, Victor-Felix Mautner, Evelin Schröck, Wilko Weichert, Benedikt Brors, Andreas von Deimling, Michel Mittelbronn, Joachim P. Steinbach, David E. Reuss, Hanno Glimm, Albrecht Stenzinger, Stefan Fröhling. Targetable ERBB2 mutations identified in neurofibroma/schwannoma hybrid nerve sheath tumors. Journal of Clinical Investigation. 2020.

Cancer Risk and Spectrum in Individuals with RASopathies

17

Mwe Mwe Chao, Martin Zenker, and Christian Peter Kratz

Contents

17.1 Introduction

The identification of Ras emerged from the study of highly potent transforming retroviruses isolated from animals [1]. Specifically, in the 1960s, it was shown that the Harvey murine sarcoma virus and the Kirsten murine sarcoma virus induced sarcomas when injected into rats [2, 3]. It would later be established that two *ra*t *s*arcoma (ras; Harvey ras or Ha-ras or H-ras; Kirsten ras, or Ki-ras or K-ras) genes encoding for their respective 21 kD protein products were the transformative

M. M. Chao · C. P. Kratz (✉)
Center for Pediatrics and Adolescent Medicine, Pediatric Hematology Oncology, Hannover Medical School, Hannover, Germany
e-mail: kratz.christian@mh-hannover.de

M. Zenker
Institute of Human Genetics, University Hospital Magdeburg, Magdeburg, Germany
e-mail: martin.zenker@med.ovgu.de

G. Tadini et al. (eds.), *Multidisciplinary Approach to Neurofibromatosis Type 1*,
https://doi.org/10.1007/978-3-319-92450-2_17

elements of the viruses and that many cancers in man harbor mutations in the *HRAS* and *KRAS* human homologs [1]. Subsequently, additional studies elucidated over 150 related genes and their corresponding protein products that function as small guanosine nucleotide GTPases termed the Ras superfamily of proteins [4]. The Ras subfamily is a branch of the superfamily.

In humans, the RAS subfamily of proteins consists of 36 members [4]. HRAS, KRAS, and NRAS are the best studied because defects are associated with disease. These three RAS isoforms are key components of the RAS/mitogen-activated protein kinase (MAPK) signaling pathway which functions to relay extracellular signals into the cell. Notably, RAS and other components of RAS/MAPK pathway interact with other cellular proteins and pathways in an intricate and complex manner. Activation of the pathway is initiated when an extracellular ligand such as a growth factor binds to the transmembrane tyrosine kinase receptor (RTK), which leads to autophosphorylation and recruitment of adaptor proteins (GRB1, CBL, SHP2, and SOS1) to the intracellular domain. Thereafter, SOS1 performing as a guanosine nucleotide exchange factor (GEF) facilitates the exchange of GDP for GTP on RAS. The GTP-bound RAS then binds to and activates the first protein of the MAPK pathway, RAF (ARAF, BRAF, or CRAF). Next, MEK1/2 and then ERK1/2 are successively activated. The stimulated ERK1 and ERK2 interact with membrane, cytosolic, and nuclear substrates to regulate cell growth, differentiation, and proliferation. NF1 and SPRED1 serve as negative regulators of the RAS/MAPK pathway (Fig. 17.1). Dysregulation of the RAS/MAPK pathway has important

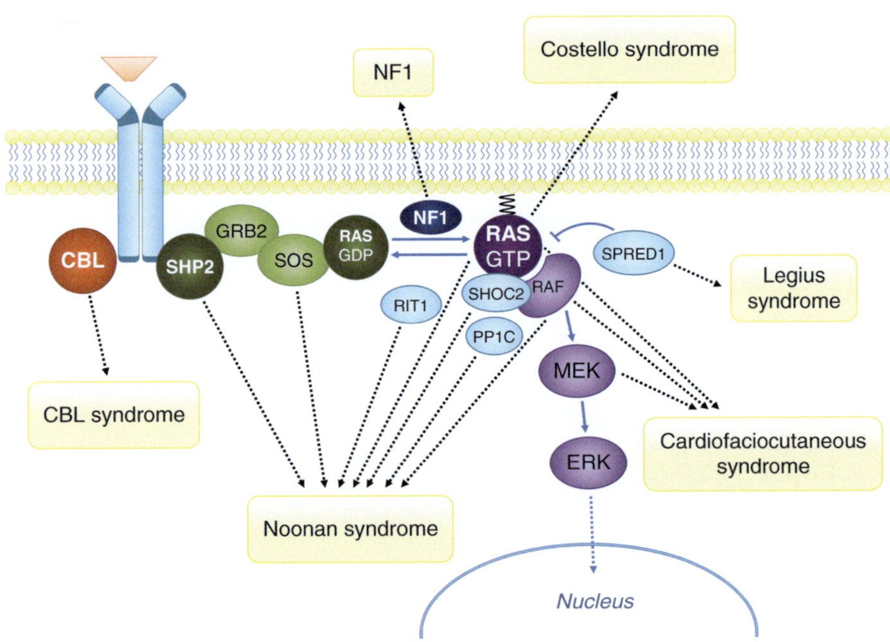

Fig. 17.1 RAS/MAPK pathway and corresponding RASopathies

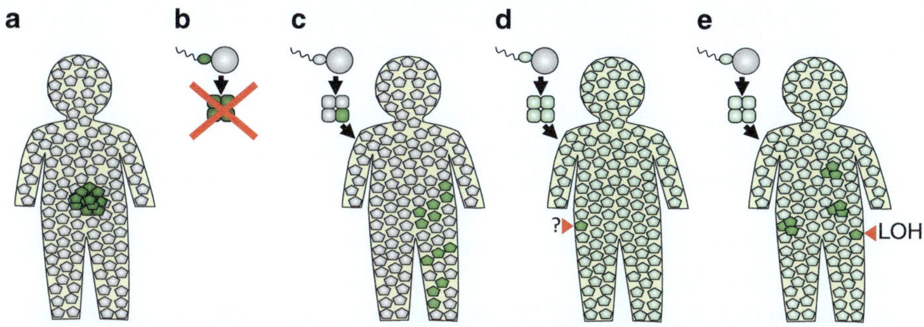

Fig. 17.2 Various consequences of RAS/MAPK pathway dysregulation: (**a**), Oncogenic mutation in a sporadic tumor: a strongly activating (oncogenic) mutation (green color) occurs as a somatic event in a cell and—together with other genetic events—gives rise to proliferation and tumor formation. (**b**), Oncogenic mutation in the germline: strongly activating mutations may arise in germ cells (more likely in sperm), but after fertilization perturbed embryonic development will lead to prenatal lethality in most cases. (**c**), Mosaic RASopathy due to postzygotic ocurrence of an oncogenic mutation: If the same mutation as in (**a**) and (**b**) emerges as a postzygotic mutational event in the embryo, it may be able to survive in the mosaic state and lead to specific lesions in regions affected by the mutation. (**d**), Mildly activating mutation in Noonan syndrome: a mildly activating mutation (light green color) is tolerated in the germline, but the generalized dysregulation of RAS/MAPK signalling leads to characteristic developmental anomalies. The switch from mild to strong activation (arrowhead, green color) by a single genetic event is unlikely and oncogenesis usually requires independent mutational events. (**e**), Inactivating NF1 mutations in neurofibromatosis: The defect of one allele is present in the germline and leads to a mild generalized overactivation of RAS/MAPK signaling that gives rise to mild Noonan syndrome-like features (haploinsufficiency). The switch to severe RAS/MAPK pathway dysregulation may occur with a single secondary genetic event of loss of heterozygosity at the NF1 locus (arrowhead). This is likely to occur at multiple sites during lifetime and, if it is sufficient to lead to tumor formation from certain cells, numerous tumors of that kind will occur

implications for human health. Germline, mosaic, and somatic aberrations in the genes of RAS/MAPK pathway are associated with developmental syndromes, congenital disorders, and cancers, respectively (Fig. 17.2). Herein, we review the cancer risk and spectrum associated with disorders related to germline or mosaic RAS/MAPK pathway disturbances as well as examine practical surveillance guidelines and therapeutic implications.

17.2 RASopathies and Cancer: General Thoughts

Mutations of various genes leading to dysregulation of the RAS signaling pathway occur in the germline and cause syndromes including neurofibromatosis type 1 (NF1), Noonan syndrome (NS), NS with multiple lentigines (NSML), Costello syndrome (CS), cardio-facio-cutaneous syndrome (CFCS), NF1-NS, Legius syndrome, and NS-like disorder with or without juvenile myelomonocytic leukemia (NSLL or CBL syndrome). Although certain clinical characteristics distinguish one syndrome from another, due to a common mechanism of RAS/MAPK pathway dysfunction, many affected individuals exhibit overlapping NS-like phenotypic features such as dysmorphic craniofacial features, congenital heart defects, short stature, skin abnormalities, and variable intellectual disability [5]. It is considered that the expression of NS-like abnormalities mainly reflects the degree of systemic dysregulation of the RAS/MAPK pathway in the developing embryo and child. In fact, the genetic relatedness of these clinically overlapping conditions was postulated long prior to identifying their related genetic basis. Collectively, these syndromes are called the RASopathies, defined by the combination of a germline defect of a RAS signaling component and NS-like features.

It is important to recognize that, in the case of activating mutations of RAS pathway genes, the mutation spectrum observed in the germline differs substantially from the mutation spectrum observed in cancer. This difference can be explained by the notion that in the case of germline mutations biochemically "strong" cancer-associated defects have a higher chance of being embryonic lethal, while in somatic (cancer) cells, "strong" mutations represent key steps during cancerogenesis. The prenatal selection against germline mutations with strong activating effects on the RAS/MAPK pathway is supported by the observation that prenatal testing of *PTPN11* (and other genes) in fetuses with severe abnormalities (such as hydrops fetalis) may detect mutations that are otherwise typically found as somatic mutations in cancer ([6]; and unpublished findings from our lab). Consistently, rare live-born children with "strong" activating mutations usually harbor de novo mutations and tend to have severe developmental defects and a high risk of developing cancer. The occurrence and viability of "strong" mutations in the germline may also depend on the biologic function of the mutated gene [7]. For example, mutations of residues 12 or 13 of HRAS (leading to CS) is observed more frequently in the germline than identical mutations of KRAS. Another chance for prenatal survival of severely dysregulating "oncogenic" RAS/MAPK pathway mutations is in a postzygotic mosaic state which leads to mosaic RASopathies discussed later in this chapter.

In contrast, biochemically "mild" (hypomorphic) mutations are tolerated more commonly as a germline defect without leading to embryonic death. Due to their milder effect, these mutations are rarely seen as somatic cancer-related lesions. The cancer risk of individuals with "mild" mutations is only moderately elevated. From the cancer risk perspective, these "mild" defects represent examples of rare moderate cancer risk alleles (such rare moderate disease risk alleles, unless they have a systemic phenotype, are largely unknown because they typically escape standard gene discovery approaches) [8]. These mutations may also occur as familial mutations, depending on the degree of physical and intellectual impairment and their effects on fertility.

In the case of predominantly loss-of-function germline mutations in negative regulators of the RAS/MAPK pathway (e.g., NF1), the systemic dysregulation of the pathway caused by the defect of one allele (haploinsufficiency) may have settled disadvantageous effects on the developing embryo that lead to mild NS-like manifestations. These genes act in a recessive manner on the cellular level and loss or mutation of the second allele in somatic cells is the key step for tumor development. This explains the observation that the tumor risk can be high in patients with syndromes caused by this mechanism despite the fact that the primary lesions are well tolerated during embryogenesis. Of note, mutations can be both, activating for some biological properties and inactivating for others. Hence, the differentiation is not always clear cut.

While in this theoretical model, the degree of systemic RAS/MAPK dysregulation determines the expression of NS-like developmental anomalies, the tumor risk for a certain entity is not solely depending on the oncogenic potential of the underlying germline event but also on the probability of occurrence of additional genetic hit(s) that are sufficient to confer the transformation in a sensitive cell. For example, in individuals with NF1 the risk of developing neurofibroma is substantially higher than the risk of developing malignant peripheral nerve sheet tumors because the latter requires a more complex pattern of somatic defects. The tumor types that develop in individuals with RASopathies are biologically highly plausible. For example, chromosome 11 band p15 rearrangements are a common event in sporadic embryonal rhabdomyosarcoma which is also associated with somatic defects of *HRAS* (also located on chromosome 11p15). In CS, *HRAS* mutations are present in all cells, including mesenchymal cells with the potential to transform into rhabdomyosarcoma cells. Additional acquired rearrangements of 11p15 in this premalignant tissue contributes to the high rhabdomyosarcoma risk in individuals with CS [9]. With these general thoughts in mind we now briefly review various RASopathies focusing on the cancer risk and spectrum associated with each condition.

17.3 Cancer and Noonan Syndrome

The most common neurodevelopmental syndrome associated with an aberrant RAS/MAPK pathway is NS. Approximately 1 in 1000–2000 newborns are affected. Individuals with NS have distinctive craniofacial dysmorphism including broad forehead, hypertelorism, ptosis, down-slanting palpebral fissures, and low-set posteriorly rotated ears. As noted above, many of these craniofacial features are also observed in other RASopathies and give clue to the presence of a RAS/MAPK pathway anomaly. In addition, in NS congenital cardiac defects, reduced growth, bleeding diathesis, and neurocognitive delay may be present. Disease causative mutations have been identified in *PTPN11* (50%), *SOS1* (13%), *RAF1* (5%), *RIT1* (5%), *KRAS*, *NRAS*, *BRAF*, *MAP 2K1*, *RRAS*, *MRAS*, *RASA2*, *SOS2*, and *LZTR1*. Mutations of *SHOC2* und *PPP1CB* cause NS-like disorders with loose anagen hair. Affected individuals show cardiac anomalies (NS spectrum, semilunar valve dysplasias), characteristic hair, diffuse hyperpigmentation, mild mental retardation, short stature, and a recognizable facial phenotype.

As noted above, the RAS pathway mutations observed in patients with NS differ from the variations typically driving tumorigenesis. As far as this has been studied functionally, NS-associated mutations have been shown to confer less severely dysregulating effects on signaling compared to oncogenic mutations in the respective genes [10, 11]. Consequently, the cancer risk among individuals with NS is not strongly increased and cancer is a rare complication encountered in affected families. As expected, a moderate increase in cancer risk can be confirmed epidemiologically—a recent study observed 8 cases of childhood cancer among 632 patients, while 1 neoplasm was expected when comparing it to the healthy population (Standardized Incidence Ratio: 8.1 [3.5–16.0]) [8]. Tumors that occur in individuals with NS include embryonal rhabdomyosarcoma, neuroblastoma, and astrocytoma, among others. Interestingly, several cases of dysembryoplastic neuroepithelial tumor (DNET) have been reported suggesting that DNET is a rare complication in NS [8]. Moreover, several NS patients with acute lymphoblastic leukemia have been reported. Most patients had a hyperdiploid karyotype [12] providing evidence for a non-random association between ALL and NS. A non-malignant tumor manifestation in NS is multiple giant cell lesions predominantly affecting the jaw bones. These tumors may also occur in other RASopathies [13].

Infants with NS and specific mutations of *PTPN11* (or rarely *KRAS*) are at increased risk of developing a polyclonal myeloproliferative disease that resembles juvenile myelomonocytic leukemia (JMML). Although myeloproliferative disease in children with NS can resolve without treatment, malignant transformation can occur [14–16]. Taken together, the cancer risk is only slightly increased in individuals with NS.

Individuals with NSML have clinical features most akin to NS but these patients display a high penetrance for multiple lentigines and hypertrophic cardiomyopathy. The disorder was previously called LEOPARD syndrome as an acronym for lentigines, electrocardiogram abnormalities, ocular hypertelorism, pulmonary stenosis, abnormal genitalia, retardation of growth, and deafness. The disorder is caused by specific mutations in *PTPN11* (particularly p.T468M, p.Y279C) and rarely in other genes. Rare cases of childhood cancer have been reported, suggesting that the risk is slightly elevated [8]. Recent evidence suggested that neurofibroma-like nerve-sheath tumors and hypertrophic neuropathy is associated with NSML in adulthood [17, 18]. Like in NS, the cancer risk is not strongly increased.

17.4 Cancer and Cardio-Facio-Cutaneous Syndrome

CFCS is a more rare disorder caused by germline mutations of the RAS/MAPK pathway. CFCS patients have macrocephaly, broad forehead, bitemporal narrowing, hypoplastic supraorbital ridges, sparse or missing eyebrows, down-slanting palpebral fissures, ocular abnormalities (strabismus, nystagmus, myopia, ptosis, hyperopia, and astigmatism), short nose with low nasal bridge and anteverted nares, high-arched palate, and low-set posteriorly rotated ears. As indicated by the name, CFCS patients may display more severe ectodermal abnormalities including sparse, curly, thin or thick, woolly and occasionally brittle hair, hyperkeratosis, keratosis pilaris, hemangioma, ichthyosis, and nevi. Moreover, approximately 75% of individuals with CFCS have cardiac defects that include pulmonic stenosis, atrial and ventricular septal defect, hypertrophic cardiomyopathy, and heart valve anomalies [19]. Musculoskeletal and neurologic abnormalities are also frequently encountered in CFCS patients. The degree of intellectual impairment is usually much more severe than in NS. Finally, during infancy, CFCS patients may experience failure to thrive, gastrointestinal reflux, vomiting, oral aversion, and constipation. Mutations in *BRAF*, *MEK1*, *MEK2*, and *KRAS* are responsible for the syndrome. Like in NS, cancer is a rare complication in patients with CFCS. Leukemia, lymphoma, hepatoblastoma, and rhabdomyosarcoma have been reported in rare cases [20]. No risk figure is available, but it seems that cancer risk in CFCS does not exceed the risk that has been reported for NS.

17.5 Cancer and Costello Syndrome

Besides NF1, CS is the RASopathy with the highest cancer risk. First symptoms of the disorder may be observed even during pregnancy. In utero, there may be polyhydramnios secondary to poor swallowing, fetal overgrowth with macrocephaly, and cardiac arrhythmia [5, 19, 21, 22]. Prematurity and generalized edema are not uncommon [21, 23]. During neonatal period, patients usually display feeding difficulties and may show gastro-esophageal reflux secondary to pyloric stenosis and secondary failure to thrive [22, 24]. Likewise, hypotonia, irritability, and hypersensitivity of sound and touch, shyness, and sleep disturbances have been noted in CS infants [25]. The craniofacial features of CS include macrocephaly with a prominent forehead, epicanthal folds, down-slanting palpebral fissures, short nose with depressed nasal bridge and a broad base, low-set posteriorly rotated ears with thick helices and lobes, full cheeks, and large mouth and lips. Dermatologic manifestations consist of soft loose skin, excessive wrinkling, redundancy of the skin of the hands and feet with deep palmar and plantar creases. Hypertrophic cardiomyopathy is also present in CS patients as well as valve anomalies, septal defects, and arrhythmia. CS is caused by de novo germline mutations in *HRAS* [26–28]. The typical CS-associated *HRAS* mutations are located at codons 12 or 13 which are also mutated in solid tumors. Notably, however, the more common CS-associated substitutions (e.g., p.G12S) are less common in cancer.

The fact that CS-associated germline *HRAS* mutations resemble those found as somatic events in tumors is considered to explain the high risk for benign and malignant tumors such as cutaneous papillomas, embryonal rhabdomyosarcoma, transitional cell carcinoma of the bladder, and neuroblastoma in CS. Cancer occurs in 15% of patients by age 20 years [29, 30] justifying cancer surveillance.

17.6 Cancer and CBL Syndrome

The condition NSLL or CBL syndrome (CBLS) is caused by germline mutations of *CBL* and many patients typically display craniofacial and other anomalies reminiscent of NS [31–33]. However, the NS-like phenotype is not always clinically obvious. A particular complication in CBLS is a vasculopathy of medium-sized arteries. As discussed further below, CBLS patients appear to have a high risk of developing

JMML. CBLS-related JMML is a clonal condition and characterized by loss of heterozygosity in hematopoietic cells. Despite the fact that CBLS-related JMML is a clonal disease, some individuals demonstrate spontaneous regression with a benign course.

17.7 Cancer and RASopathies That Lack a NS-Like Appearance

Capillary malformation arteriovenous malformation syndrome (CM-AVM) is another RAS/MAPK pathway disease. Here, multifocal capillary malformations which may be associated with arteriovenous malformations and fistulas. The vascular lesions may be located in many tissues including skin, muscle, bone, heart, and brain. Inactivating mutations in the *RASA1* gene cause CM-AVM. *RASA1* encodes for a RAS-GAP, and the CM-AVM associated mutation results in decreased hydrolysis of RAS-GTP and increased RAS/MAPK signaling [34]. Interestingly, capillary and vascular malformations do also occur as rare cutaneous anomalies in NS and related disorders.

Synaptic RAS GTPase-activating protein 1 (SYNGAP1) is in humans encoded by the *SYNGAP1* gene. SYNGAP1 is a RAS GTPase-activating protein that is critical for the development of cognition and proper synapse function. The protein is expressed exclusively in the brain and mutations in humans can cause intellectual disability or epilepsy. Specifically, Hamdan et al. identified de novo truncating mutations in *SYNGAP1* in approximately 3% of patients with nonsyndromic mental retardation [35]. Patients do not have NS features likely due to expression of *SYNGAP1* limited to the brain. There are no data indicating that individuals with these two conditions have an increased cancer risk.

17.8 Cancer and Mosaic RASopathies

The presence of two genetically distinct populations of cells within an individual derived from a postzygotic mutation is termed mosaicism. In the 1930s it was recognized that some individuals developed NF1 features such as café-au-lait spots, freckling, and neurofibromas limited to a segment of the body. Termed segmental NF1, it would later be established that in most cases, the disorder represented a form of mosaicism of the disease [36]. Subsequently, we have come to learn that there is a broad range of symptoms and disorders involving mosaicism for RASopathy-associated mutations. Indeed, patients with classic features of CS have been recognized who have both normal and mutation-harboring cells within one tissue type demonstrating mosaicism [37, 38]. These are examples for mosaicism of typical mutations associated with a typical—albeit sometimes milder or regionally expressed phenotype.

The term "mosaic RASopathies" has been introduced to describe mosaicism for "oncogenic" RAS/MAPK pathway mutations that are usually embryonically lethal when occurring in the germline, but may survive in the mosaic state. The conditions belonging to the group of mosaic RASopathies are neurocutaneous disorders that usually lack NS-like features, because the percentage of mutated cells in the body is too small to cause manifestations that are seen with a systemic (generalized) RAS/ MAPK pathway overactivation. The majority of mosaic RASopathies belong to the group of systematized or isolated congenital nevi. The great variability of mosaic disorders is related not only to the genotype but also to the localization and distribution of mutated cells in the body.

Keratinocytic epidermal nevi and sebaceous nevus as well as their systematized forms, epidermal nevus syndrome, and Schimmelpenning syndrome, respectively, are caused by mosaic *RAS* mutations with *HRAS* being the most commonly affected *RAS* gene and the p.G13R substitution representing the predominant mutation [39, 40]. The mutations can typically be found in affected but not in unaffected tissue and are usually absent from blood cells [40]. Congenital melanocytic nevi and systematized variant named neurocutaneous melanocytosis typically have oncogenic missense mutations in *NRAS* as mosaic in affected tissue. More recent studies have associated oculoectodermal syndrome with specific *KRAS* mosaic mutations [41], extracranial arteriovenous-malformations with *MAP2K1* (*MEK1*) mutations [42], and *KRAS* mutations in arteriovenous-malformations of the brain [43].

For epidermal nevi there is probably a small risk for malignant transformation. Melanoma occurs in roughly 1–2% of patients with congenital melanocytic nevi and those patients with larger nevi have a higher risk for malignant transformation [44, 45].

The wide-ranging phenotype of the mosaic RASopathies may be explained by the timing of the mutation, the type of the mutation, the particular lineage and the viability of the cells bearing the mutation, as well as by the body region involved [36]. However, there are other yet to be elucidated factors that may be important for a mosaic presentation of RASopathies. A report of a young patient with NSML where the left trunk and arm lacked lentigines that were present on other parts of the body. Fibroblasts from normal appearing skin as well as skin with lentigines showed the *PTPN11* mutation, suggesting an unknown mechanism of "silencing" of the mutation in the normal skin [46].

17.9 Cancer Surveillance for Individuals with RASopathies

Individuals affected by a RASopathy often have multi-system involvement and comprehensive care is often necessary. However, only a subset of patients, specifically those with NF1 (not discussed in detail here), CS, and CBL syndrome, have a clinically relevant (i.e., >5%) increase in cancer risk, and for individuals with these conditions, cancer surveillance is recommended. In patients with CS < 10 years of age, physical exam, and abdominal-pelvic ultrasound are recommended—to screen for rhabdomyosarcoma and neuroblastoma—every 3–4 months. After 10 years of age an annual urinalysis should be completed as a screening tool to detect bladder cancer [29, 30]. CBL syndrome patients have a high but not precisely defined JMML risk during early childhood. Therefore, from 0 to 5 years of age, physical exam (with assessment of spleen) and complete blood count with white blood cell differential every 3–6 months has been recommended [30].

Some patients with mosaic RASopathies, such as patients with multiple/large congenital melanocytic naevi with involvement of the CNS, may also have a clinically relevant increase in cancer risk [47]. Patients affected by a mosaic RASopathy should be monitored clinically on a regular basis. The melanoma risk in patients with large and/or multiple congenital melanocytic nevi justifies screening with MRI of the CNS starting within the first year of life [47] and close clinical monitoring. In addition to what is recommended in the literature [47], annual brain MRIs may be justified due to the significant risk of cerebral melanoma in patients with CNS involvement.

If cancer occurs in patients with RASopathies, there is no evidence that standard therapies are not effective. Nevertheless, due to the likely involvement of the RAS signaling pathway in these cancer patients, the use of targeted therapies (such as MEK inhibitors) may be discussed and considered, especially in the absence of effective standard protocols.

17.10 Conclusion

Germline RAS pathway mutations lead to an increased cancer risk. For most RASopathies, the elevated cancer risk is mild and does not warrant cancer surveillance. Exceptions include NF1, CS, and CBL syndrome. Patients with specific *PTPN11* or *KRAS* mutations may benefit from surveillance (3-monthly blood counts and clinical monitoring during the first 5 years of life) due to their risk of developing a JMML-like myeloproliferation. Depending on the timing and cell type expression of the mutant allele mosaic mutations putatively lead to variable phenotypes. The risk of melanoma observed in patients with congenital melanocytic nevi justifies MRI of the brain and regular physical exams. The wide range of disorders associated with RAS/MAPK pathway dysfunction highlights the critical role of the pathway in man. Excitingly, novel therapies based on inhibition of the RAS pathway are being developed for these disorders.

References

1. Cox AD, Der CJ. Ras history: the saga continues. Small GTPases. 2010;1(1):2–27.
2. Harvey JJ. An unidentified virus which causes the rapid production of tumours in mice. Nature. 1964;204:1104–5.
3. Kirsten WH, Mayer LA. Morphologic responses to a murine erythroblastosis virus. J Natl Cancer Inst. 1967;39(2):311–35.
4. Wennerberg K, Rossman KL, Der CJ. The Ras superfamily at a glance. J Cell Sci. 2005;118(Pt 5):843–6.
5. Rauen KA. The RASopathies. Annu Rev Genomics Hum Genet. 2013;14:355–69.
6. Lee KA, Williams B, Roza K, Ferguson H, David K, Eddleman K, et al. PTPN11 analysis for the prenatal diagnosis of Noonan syndrome in fetuses with abnormal ultrasound findings. Clin Genet. 2009;75(2):190–4.

7. Nussinov R, Tsai CJ, Jang H. Oncogenic Ras isoforms signaling specificity at the membrane. Cancer Res. 2018;78(3):593–602.
8. Kratz CP, Franke L, Peters H, Kohlschmidt N, Kazmierczak B, Finckh U, et al. Cancer spectrum and frequency among children with Noonan, Costello, and cardio-facio-cutaneous syndromes. Br J Cancer. 2015;112(8):1392–7.
9. Kratz CP, Steinemann D, Niemeyer CM, Schlegelberger B, Koscielniak E, Kontny U, et al. Uniparental disomy at chromosome 11p15.5 followed by HRAS mutations in embryonal rhabdomyosarcoma: lessons from Costello syndrome. Hum Mol Genet. 2007;16(4):374–9.
10. Schubbert S, Zenker M, Rowe SL, Boll S, Klein C, Bollag G, et al. Germline KRAS mutations cause Noonan syndrome. Nat Genet. 2006;38(3):331–6.
11. Mohi MG, Williams IR, Dearolf CR, Chan G, Kutok JL, Cohen S, et al. Prognostic, therapeutic, and mechanistic implications of a mouse model of leukemia evoked by Shp2 (PTPN11) mutations. Cancer Cell. 2005;7(2):179–91.
12. Cave H, Caye A, Strullu M, Aladjidi N, Vignal C, Ferster A, et al. Acute lymphoblastic leukemia in the context of RASopathies. Eur J Med Genet. 2016;59(3):173–8.
13. Neumann TE, Allanson J, Kavamura I, Kerr B, Neri G, Noonan J, et al. Multiple giant cell lesions in patients with Noonan syndrome and cardio-facio-cutaneous syndrome. Eur J Hum Genet. 2009;17(4):420–5.
14. Tartaglia M, Niemeyer CM, Fragale A, Song X, Buechner J, Jung A, et al. Somatic mutations in PTPN11 in juvenile myelomonocytic leukemia, myelodysplastic syndromes and acute myeloid leukemia. Nat Genet. 2003;34(2):148–50.
15. Loh ML, Vattikuti S, Schubbert S, Reynolds MG, Carlson E, Lieuw KH, et al. Mutations in PTPN11 implicate the SHP-2 phosphatase in leukemogenesis. Blood. 2004;103(6):2325–31.
16. Bader-Meunier B, Tchernia G, Mielot F, Fontaine JL, Thomas C, Lyonnet S, et al. Occurrence of myeloproliferative disorder in patients with Noonan syndrome. J Pediatr. 1997;130(6):885–9.
17. Conboy E, Dhamija R, Wang M, Xie J, Dyck PJ, Bridges AG, et al. Paraspinal neurofibromas and hypertrophic neuropathy in Noonan syndrome with multiple lentigines. J Med Genet. 2016;53(2):123–6.
18. Maridet C, Sole G, Morice-Picard F, Taieb A. Hypertrophic neuropathy in Noonan syndrome with multiple lentigines. Am J Med Genet A. 2016;170(6):1570–2.
19. Bezniakow N, Gos M, Obersztyn E. The RASopathies as an example of RAS/MAPK pathway disturbances – clinical presentation and molecular pathogenesis of selected syndromes. Dev Period Med. 2014;18(3):285–96.
20. Kratz CP, Rapisuwon S, Reed H, Hasle H, Rosenberg PS. Cancer in Noonan, Costello, cardiofaciocutaneous and LEOPARD syndromes. Am J Med Genet C Semin Med Genet. 2011;157C(2):83–9.
21. Smith LP, Podraza J, Proud VK. Polyhydramnios, fetal overgrowth, and macrocephaly: prenatal ultrasound findings of Costello syndrome. Am J Med Genet A. 2009;149A(4):779–84.
22. Umans S, Decock P, Fryns JP. Costello syndrome: the natural history of a true postnatal growth retardation syndrome. Genet Couns. 1995;6(2):121–5.
23. Piccione M, Piro E, Pomponi MG, Matina F, Pietrobono R, Candela E, et al. A premature infant with Costello syndrome due to a rare G13C HRAS mutation. Am J Med Genet A. 2009;149A(3):487–9.
24. Okamoto N, Chiyo H, Imai K, Otani K, Futagi Y. A Japanese patient with the Costello syndrome. Hum Genet. 1994;93(5):605–6.
25. Kawame H, Matsui M, Kurosawa K, Matsuo M, Masuno M, Ohashi H, et al. Further delineation of the behavioral and neurologic features in Costello syndrome. Am J Med Genet A. 2003;118A(1):8–14.
26. Aoki Y, Niihori T, Kawame H, Kurosawa K, Ohashi H, Tanaka Y, et al. Germline mutations in HRAS proto-oncogene cause Costello syndrome. Nat Genet. 2005;37(10):1038–40.
27. Kerr B, Delrue MA, Sigaudy S, Perveen R, Marche M, Burgelin I, et al. Genotype-phenotype correlation in Costello syndrome: HRAS mutation analysis in 43 cases. J Med Genet. 2006;43(5):401–5.

28. Gripp KW, Lin AE, Stabley DL, Nicholson L, Scott CI Jr, Doyle D, et al. HRAS mutation analysis in Costello syndrome: genotype and phenotype correlation. Am J Med Genet A. 2006;140(1):1–7.
29. Gripp KW. Tumor predisposition in Costello syndrome. Am J Med Genet C Semin Med Genet. 2005;137C(1):72–7.
30. Villani A, Greer MC, Kalish JM, Nakagawara A, Nathanson KL, Pajtler KW, et al. Recommendations for cancer surveillance in individuals with RASopathies and other rare genetic conditions with increased cancer risk. Clin Cancer Res. 2017;23(12):e83–90.
31. Niemeyer CM, Kang MW, Shin DH, Furlan I, Erlacher M, Bunin NJ, et al. Germline CBL mutations cause developmental abnormalities and predispose to juvenile myelomonocytic leukemia. Nat Genet. 2010;42(9):794–800.
32. Perez B, Mechinaud F, Galambrun C, Ben Romdhane N, Isidor B, Philip N, et al. Germline mutations of the CBL gene define a new genetic syndrome with predisposition to juvenile myelomonocytic leukaemia. J Med Genet. 2010;47(10):686–91.
33. Martinelli S, De Luca A, Stellacci E, Rossi C, Checquolo S, Lepri F, et al. Heterozygous germline mutations in the CBL tumor-suppressor gene cause a Noonan syndrome-like phenotype. Am J Hum Genet. 2010;87(2):250–7.
34. Eerola I, Boon LM, Mulliken JB, Burrows PE, Dompmartin A, Watanabe S, et al. Capillary malformation-arteriovenous malformation, a new clinical and genetic disorder caused by RASA1 mutations. Am J Hum Genet. 2003;73(6):1240–9.
35. Hamdan FF, Gauthier J, Spiegelman D, Noreau A, Yang Y, Pellerin S, et al. Mutations in SYNGAP1 in autosomal nonsyndromic mental retardation. N Engl J Med. 2009;360(6):599–605.
36. Tinschert S, Naumann I, Stegmann E, Buske A, Kaufmann D, Thiel G, et al. Segmental neurofibromatosis is caused by somatic mutation of the neurofibromatosis type 1 (NF1) gene. Eur J Hum Genet. 2000;8(6):455–9.
37. Gripp KW, Stabley DL, Nicholson L, Hoffman JD, Sol-Church K. Somatic mosaicism for an HRAS mutation causes Costello syndrome. Am J Med Genet A. 2006;140(20):2163–9.
38. Girisha KM, Lewis LE, Phadke SR, Kutsche K. Costello syndrome with severe cutis laxa and mosaic HRAS G12S mutation. Am J Med Genet A. 2010;152A(11):2861–4.
39. Hafner C, Toll A, Gantner S, Mauerer A, Lurkin I, Acquadro F, et al. Keratinocytic epidermal nevi are associated with mosaic RAS mutations. J Med Genet. 2012;49(4):249–53.
40. Groesser L, Herschberger E, Ruetten A, Ruivenkamp C, Lopriore E, Zutt M, et al. Postzygotic HRAS and KRAS mutations cause nevus sebaceous and Schimmelpenning syndrome. Nat Genet. 2012;44(7):783–7.
41. Peacock JD, Dykema KJ, Toriello HV, Mooney MR, Scholten DJ 2nd, Winn ME, et al. Oculoectodermal syndrome is a mosaic RASopathy associated with KRAS alterations. Am J Med Genet A. 2015;167(7):1429–35.
42. Couto JA, Huang AY, Konczyk DJ, Goss JA, Fishman SJ, Mulliken JB, et al. Somatic MAP 2K1 mutations are associated with extracranial arteriovenous malformation. Am J Hum Genet. 2017;100(3):546–54.
43. Nikolaev SI, Vetiska S, Bonilla X, Boudreau E, Jauhiainen S, Rezai Jahromi B, et al. Somatic activating KRAS mutations in arteriovenous malformations of the brain. N Engl J Med. 2018;378(3):250–61.
44. Krengel S, Hauschild A, Schafer T. Melanoma risk in congenital melanocytic naevi: a systematic review. Br J Dermatol. 2006;155(1):1–8.
45. Kinsler VA, Thomas AC, Ishida M, Bulstrode NW, Loughlin S, Hing S, et al. Multiple congenital melanocytic nevi and neurocutaneous melanosis are caused by postzygotic mutations in codon 61 of NRAS. J Invest Dermatol. 2013;133(9):2229–36.
46. Hafner C, Groesser L. Mosaic RASopathies. Cell Cycle. 2013;12(1):43–50.
47. Kinsler VA, O'Hare P, Bulstrode N, Calonje JE, Chong WK, Hargrave D, et al. Melanoma in congenital melanocytic naevi. Br J Dermatol. 2017;176(5):1131–43.

Therapeutic Approaches for NF1 18

Bruce R. Korf

Contents

18.1 Introduction

NF1 is a multifaceted disorder that affects multiple body systems. The condition is progressive over a person's lifetime and the specific manifestations in an individual are unpredictable. Until recently, treatment was limited to surveillance for

B. R. Korf (✉)
Department of Genetics, University of Alabama at Birmingham, Birmingham, AL, USA
e-mail: bkorf@uabmc.edu

G. Tadini et al. (eds.), *Multidisciplinary Approach to Neurofibromatosis Type 1*,
https://doi.org/10.1007/978-3-319-92450-2_18

complications and interventions such as surgery for removal of tumors or chemotherapy or radiation for treatment of malignancies. Insights into pathogenesis have resulted in identification of potential targets for pharmacological therapy, however, and there are currently clinical trials for many different manifestations of NF1. This chapter will consider the therapy of NF1 from three perspectives. First, we will consider some general therapeutic approaches, including surgical, traditional cancer therapy, and more recent targeted drug treatments. Second, we will explore some specific complications of NF1 and look at the current landscape for treatment of these problems. Third, we will explore the status of preclinical drug development and clinical trials, as well as prospects for treatment based on targeting the gene itself or its protein product. We will not address issues of surveillance or counseling in NF1; although these are part of the overall treatment regimen, they are covered elsewhere in this book and have been the subject of recent published practice resources [1, 2]. Rather, our focus will be on treatments to improve outcomes for specific NF1 manifestations.

18.2 Approaches to Treatment of NF1

NF1 can be an insidiously progressive disorder, with a gradual growth of tumors and slow appearance of new lesions over a lifetime. The mainstay of management to date has been surveillance for treatable complications, and then symptomatic treatments, such as surgery or, in some instances, medication. We will consider some general principles of surgical and medical therapy in this section.

18.2.1 Surgical Treatment in NF1

Surgery is currently the most common approach to treatment of tumors or skeletal disorders associated with NF1. Surgical management of tumors may be useful in diagnosis (e.g., distinguishing a benign from a malignant lesion), cosmesis, and relief of signs and symptoms due to mass effect. The key questions that must be faced in deciding on surgery are (1) what specific goals can be achieved through surgery; (2) what are the risks and benefits of surgery; and (3) when is it most appropriate to intervene surgically? Complete surgical resection of large, complex plexiform neurofibromas is usually not possible, so treatment goals must be clearly defined before embarking on a potentially morbid procedure [3, 4]. For example, a plexiform neurofibroma that cannot be fully resected might still be debulked to relieve symptoms of airway or spinal cord compression. Risks such as damage to major nerves, bleeding, and further disfigurement or scarring need to be considered. Also, plexiform neurofibromas may grow back after surgery, particularly in young children in whom the plexiform neurofibroma may still be actively growing. Often a staged approach is necessary and requires a dialog between the surgeon and patient/family to decide on the best course. Surgical treatment in NF1 often presents challenges that are different from surgical treatment in non-NF patients, and may be best done by a surgeon and medical team with experience in management of NF1.

18.2.2 Chemotherapy in NF1

The fact that tumors are the most common manifestations of NF1 raises the possibility of chemotherapeutic approaches to treatment. Standard cancer chemotherapies mostly work through cytotoxicity, usually targeting rapidly growing cells for relatively selective destruction. Such chemotherapeutic approaches tend to be ineffective in treatment of neurofibromas, however. Neurofibromas are benign tumors that grow very slowly—over months to years rather than days to weeks as is typical for malignancies. Cytotoxic chemotherapies therefore do not result in shrinkage of neurofibromas or prevent their continued growth. Moreover, the toxicities of these drugs prohibit their use over a lifetime, as may be necessary given the chronic nature of neurofibroma growth. The same can be said for radiation treatment, with the added caveat that exposure to radiation might stimulate the development of malignancies or vascular dysplasias [5]. Both chemotherapy and radiation therapy may have roles in the treatment of malignant tumors associated with NF1, as will be outlined below.

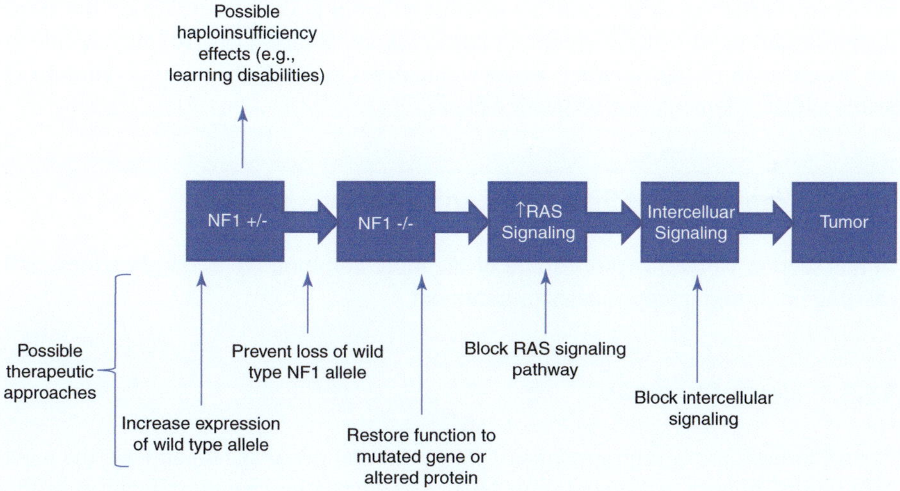

Fig. 18.1 Chain of events leading to tumor such as neurofibroma, with potential therapeutic interventions

18.2.3 Drug Treatment in NF1

As the pathogenetic mechanisms underlying the various manifestations come to light (Fig. 18.1), opportunities arise to develop new approaches to treatment aimed at underlying biochemical mechanisms. This offers the possibility of therapies that target the basic cellular defects, maximizing efficacy and minimizing side effects. Because of the central role of the RAS signaling pathway in NF1, small molecule inhibitors of this pathway have been the main focus of preclinical development and clinical trials [6]. Hyperactive RAS may not account for all aspects of the NF1 phenotype, however. For example, intercellular signaling is also thought to play a role in neurofibroma development [7, 8]. Some targeted therapeutic approaches have already been tested, and it is likely that others will emerge in the coming years. Drug treatments are a new therapeutic area for NF1 and continue to benefit from basic cell biological study and preclinical assessments of candidate therapeutics in animal models, especially mouse [9] and, more recently, pig models [10].

18.2.4 Alternative Therapies for NF1

Given the challenges in treating a progressive disorder such as NF1, it is no surprise that there is widespread interest in use of "alternative therapies" for affected individuals. Although claims have been made for efficacy of specific dietary supplements or approaches [11], these have not been verified in systematic clinical studies. Various nutritional supplements or over-the-counter substances have been tried, generally without convincing tests of efficacy. These include food substances such as turmeric, as well as bee propolis [12], a substance produced by honey bees. There has been conflicting evidence as to whether vitamin D deficiency, which has been demonstrated in NF1 affected individuals in several studies [13–16], plays a role in the progression of the disorder. Recent guidelines support checking of vitamin D levels and supplementation as needed [1, 2].

18.3 Treatment of Specific Manifestations of NF1

In this section we will explore some of the more common NF1 complications, and existing or emerging approaches to treatment.

18.3.1 Neurofibromas

Neurofibromas are benign growths of the peripheral nerve sheath and are the most common of tumors associated with NF1. Although a precise classification of the various types of neurofibromas has been elusive [17], for the purposes of this discussion we will consider three major forms: discrete, solitary tumors that may occur on the skin or anywhere in the body; plexiform neurofibromas, which are longitudinal growths of nerves that may include multiple nerve branches; and spinal neurofibromas, which occur in the paraspinal nerves and may invade the spinal canal, potentially causing cord compression.

The mainstay of treatment for discrete neurofibromas is physical removal, usually by surgery. Surgery is the only approach for removal of internal discrete neurofibromas, though most do not require removal unless they are symptomatic, for example, pressing on a surrounding structure, or causing pain. Some internal solitary neurofibromas—sometimes called "nodular neurofibromas"—are capable of growth and causing pain. These may evolve into malignant peripheral nerve sheath tumors, and some have signs of malignant potential, referred to as "atypical neurofibromatous neoplasms of uncertain biologic potential [18]." Nodular neurofibromas are monitored by imaging and those thought at risk of malignant change may be evaluated by fluoro-deoxyglucose positron emission tomography (PET) [19, 20]. The ultimate diagnosis of potential malignancy requires tissue analysis from biopsy or resection.

The neurofibromas most commonly subjected to treatment are those on the skin, referred to as "cutaneous neurofibromas." Cutaneous neurofibromas do not have malignant potential, but they can be disfiguring or cause discomfort by itching or rubbing on clothing [21, 22]. Some individuals have only a few, though they be unhappy with their appearance. Others are completely covered with more than could ever be counted. In the former case, surgery may be unnecessary or reserved for a specific bothersome tumor. In the latter, it may be impossible to remove all the tumors, but specific tumors may be targeted because of appearance or discomfort; some individuals with large numbers of tumors elect to have many removed in a single procedure. The standard approach to removal of cutaneous neurofibromas is surgical, usually done by a dermatologist or plastic surgeon. Although there is no formal study, the likelihood of regrowth is probably related to how much, if any, tumor is left behind; further, if there is a large number of tumors, others may grow nearby a resected lesion. Aside from the trauma of minor surgery, and potential complications such as infection or bleeding, the procedure is straightforward, and may leave a scar. Alternative approaches include use of the laser or electrodessication ([23–27]. These approaches can be used to remove large numbers of tumors in a single session. Short-term outcomes have been reported to be good, but there are no formal data on the frequency of scarring and long-term benefits.

The treatment of plexiform neurofibromas can be very challenging. Surgery has long been the only option but is limited by the infiltrative nature of plexiform neurofibromas, making it difficult or impossible to completely remove the tumor and risking damage to surrounding tissues. Surgery for plexiform neurofibromas is therefore usually limited to debulking to relieve symptoms of pressure or cosmetic restoration. Regrowth of tumors is common, often necessitating multiple procedures over a period of years.

Chemotherapy has not been effective for these slow-growing tumors, and radiation is both ineffective and may risk future malignant change. Knowledge of the underlying mechanisms of tumorigenesis has, however, opened the door to targeted therapies. It is now known that hyperactivity of RAS-GTP is a major contributor to neurofibroma growth, so inhibitors of components of the RAS signaling pathway have been tested in preclinical models and clinical trials. Early trials with a farnesyltransferase inhibitor, which inhibits binding of Ras to the cell membrane, and pirfenidone, a fibroblast growth inhibitor, did not show clinically significant activity [28, 29]. Some tumor shrinkage was reported in a clinical trial with pegylated interferon [30]. A trial with the RAF inhibitor sorafenib revealed that the drug was not tolerated due to pain [31]. A single case report of response to imatinib [32] led to a subsequent clinical trial that showed 20% or more reduction in plexiform neurofibroma volume in six of 36 participants [33]. A clinical trial with sirolimus, an mTOR inhibitor tested because of evidence of mTOR hyperactivity in neurofibromas, showed insufficient activity to justify clinical use [34, 35]. In contrast, the MEK inhibitor selumetinib has shown significant ability to reduce the volume of plexiform neurofibromas—in one clinical trial 71% of participants experienced a 20% or greater decrease in tumor volume [36], verified in a subsequent phase II study [37]. Selumetinib has been granted FDA approval for treatment of inoperable plexiform neurofibromas in children age 2-18 years. Additional studies are ongoing with selumetinib and other MEK inhibitors in the hope of verifying this activity and determining the long-term tolerability and durability of treatment, and studies of additional drugs, either alone or in combination, are also ongoing.

18.3.2 Gliomas

The most common gliomas seen in association with NF1 are optic pathway tumors, which occur in 15% of children with NF1 [38]. These tend to occur in the early years of life, usually before 6 years of age, and often are asymptomatic. Rare instances of spontaneous regression have been reported [39]. Associated symptoms can include proptosis, interference with eye movements, and loss of visual acuity for intraorbital lesions, and loss of vision, constriction of visual fields, and neuroendocrine disturbance for chiasmatic lesions. Asymptomatic lesions are usually followed clinically and radiographically, and not treated. Progressive, symptomatic tumors are most often treated with chemotherapy, commonly with combinations of vinblastine and carboplatin [40]. Clinical trials are underway with other chemotherapies or targeted therapeutics, such as mTOR inhibitors and MEK inhibitors (see Table 18.1 below). Other gliomas are usually treated similarly to gliomas in the general population, including the use of surgery, radiation, and chemotherapy.

18.3.3 Malignancies

Details about the treatment of malignant tumors, particularly malignant peripheral nerve sheath tumors (MPNST), but also other sarcomas, leukemias, and gastrointestinal stromal cell tumors, are beyond the scope of this chapter. Overall, the success in treating MPNST has not been encouraging, with poor survival for individuals with metastatic tumors [41, 42]. The best "treatment" at present is therefore vigilance for the occurrence of signs and symptoms, such as pain, progressive growth, or change in texture of a lesion from soft to hard, and prompt surgical resection if

Table 18.1 List of clinical trials conducted by NF Clinical Trials Consortium

Medication	Disorder	Indication	ClinicalTrials.gov
Sirolimus	NF1	PN	NCT00634270
Lovastatin	NF1	LD	NCT00853580
Everolimus	NF1	LGG	NCT01158651
Everolimus + bevacizumab[a]	NF1	MPNST	NCT01661283
Bevacizumab	NF2	VS	NCT01767792
Cabozantinib	NF1	PN	NCT02101736
PD-0325901 (MEKi)	NF1	PN	NCT02096471
Bone morphogenetic protein 2	NF1	TD	NCT02718131
Binimetinib (MEKi)	NF1	PN	NCT03231306
MEK162 (MEKi)[b]	NF1	LGG	NCT03231306
Selumetinib+sirolimus[a]	NF1	MPNST	NCT02285439

Abbreviations: *MEKi* MEK inhibitor, *PN* Plexiform neurofibroma, *LD* Learning disabilities; *LGG* low grade glioma; *MPNST* Malignant peripheral nerve sheath tumor; *VS* Vestibular schwannoma, *TD* Tibial dysplasia

[a]Conducted in collaboration with Sarcoma Alliance for Research (SARC)

[b]Conducted in collaboration with Pacific Pediatric Neuro-Oncology Consortium

possible. Clinical trials have been undertaken with a variety of targeted therapies, for example, with mTOR or MEK inhibitors, so far without major success.

18.3.4 Skeletal Dysplasias

Skeletal dysplasias associated with NF1 include long bone dysplasia (most commonly tibial), non-ossifying fibromas, and scoliosis. Specific orthopedic procedures are beyond the scope of this chapter, though in general early detection and prompt orthopedic management are recommended before complications such as fracture and pseudoarthrosis occur [43]. A clinical trial assessing the effectiveness of bone morphogenetic protein 2 in healing of tibial dysplasia was attempted, but was closed due to slow accural (see Table 18.1 below).

18.3.5 Neurocognitive Problems

Learning disabilities, as well as problems including attention deficit disorder, hypotonia, social immaturity, and delayed language development are very commonly seen in children with NF1, who have and may have effects that are lifelong [44, 45]. Early detection and intervention are important to avoid long-term problems with school performance and adverse effects on socioeconomic status. Children with NF1 who have attention deficit disorder can be treated with medications, such as stimulant medications, with similar benefits as in the general population [46]. Clinical trials with statins, based on preclinical evidence of efficacy in a mouse model system, have not demonstrated benefit in persons with NF1 [47–49].

18.4 The Future of NF1 Treatment

18.4.1 Preclinical Drug Development and Clinical Trials

Most of the focus for preclinical drug development has been in repurposing of drugs developed for other reasons, mostly treatment of cancer. The fact that NF1 involves hyperactivation of the RAS signaling pathway, which is also involved in many common cancers, has led to development of drugs that target various components of the pathway. There is also evidence that the tumor microenvironment is important to support growth of tumors such as neurofibromas, offering another avenue for possible drug action [8, 50, 51]. Most of the preclinical studies have been done in mouse models, which usually have a germline *Nf1* mutation together with the other allele in a conditional knockout under the control of tissue-specific *cre* recombinase [9]. In this way, specific complications such as neurofibromas, optic gliomas, or tibial dysplasias have been modeled and can be used to test potential therapies.

Clinical trials involve test of a treatment according to a protocol with defined outcome measures. Some of these may be double blinded, placebo-controlled trials, whereas others are open-labeled studies. The Response Evaluation in Neurofibromatosis and Schwannomatosis (REiNS) Consortium has been working to define evaluation criteria for various aspects of the different forms of neurofibromatosis [52]. An up-to-date directory of active clinical trials is available at www.clinicaltrials.gov. Clinical trials have been done by individual investigators, collaborations, or by the Neurofibromatosis Clinical Trials Consortium [53]. The latter is funded by the Congressionally Directed Medical Research Program of the Department of Defense and currently includes 13 primary sites and 10 affiliated sites. A list of previous or current clinical trials is provided in Table 18.1.

18.4.2 Novel Therapeutic Approaches

As noted above, the focus of preclinical drug testing and clinical trials has so far been on small molecule inhibitors of RAS signaling or intercellular signaling. In principle, it might be possible to target the *NF1* gene or gene product more directly. Most *NF1* pathogenic variants lead to lack of expression of a gene product, e.g., through gene deletion, stop mutation, frameshift, *etc.,* [54]. A subset of missense variants might be compatible with protein production, and possibly could be treated with small molecules that prevent degradation of the altered protein ("correctors") or improve function of a dysfunctional protein ("enhancers"). This approach has been successful in treatment of some *CFTR* pathogenic variants in cystic fibrosis [55]. Variants that lead to lack of protein expression might be targeted at the mRNA level; this can include use of drugs such as aminoglycoside derivatives to read through stop mutations [56] or modulation of splicing pharmacologically or with antisense oligonucleotides to skip exons with mutations or restore normal processing to variants that alter RNA splicing [57, 58]. Ribozyme-mediated RNA editing might also be considered.

Progress in genome editing using the CRISPR-Cas9 system has generated interest as a possible therapeutic approach. In principle it should be possible to use this system to edit a pathogenic variant out of the DNA and replace it with the wild type sequence. Although there are major ethical, as well as technical issues regarding germ line genome editing, it might be a consideration for somatic cell gene editing. The major challenge to overcome, however, is targeting such therapeutic editing to all the target cells, for example, Schwann cells.

18.5 Conclusion

Management of NF1 has, to date, been focused mostly on surveillance and symptomatic treatment, usually surgical for neurofibromas, and cytotoxic treatments for malignancies. Insights into pathogenesis of various manifestations along with preclinical models and infrastructure to perform clinical trials offer hope that more targeted and proactive approaches to treatment may be on the horizon, with one drug now appoved for clinical use.

References

1. Miller DT, Freedenberg D, Schorry E, Ullrich NJ, Viskochil D, Korf BR, Council on Genetics and American College of Medical Genetics and Genomics. Health supervision for children with neurofibromatosis type 1. Pediatrics. 2019;143:e20190660.
2. Stewart DR, Korf BR, Nathanson KL, Stevenson DA, Yohay K. Care of adults with neurofibromatosis type 1: a clinical practice resource of the American College of Medical Genetics and Genomics (ACMG). Genet Med. 2018;20:671–82.
3. Canavese F, Krajbich JI. Resection of plexiform neurofibromas in children with neurofibromatosis type 1. J Pediatr Orthop. 2011;31:303–11.
4. Needle MN, Cnaan A, Dattilo J, Chatten J, Phillips PC, Shochat S, Sutton LN, Vaughan SN, Zackai EH, Zhao H, Molloy PT. Prognostic signs in the surgical management of plexiform neurofibroma: the Children's Hospital of Philadelphia experience, 1974-1994. J Pediatr. 1997;131:678–82.
5. Ullrich NJ, Robertson R, Kinnamon DD, Scott RM, Kieran MW, Turner CD, Chi SN, Goumnerova L, Proctor M, Tarbell NJ, Marcus KJ, Pomeroy SL. Moyamoya following cranial irradiation for primary brain tumors in children. Neurology. 2007;68:932–8.
6. Gutmann DH, Ferner RE, Listernick RH, Korf BR, Wolters PL, Johnson KJ. Neurofibromatosis type 1. Nat Rev Dis Primers. 2017;3:17004.
7. Fletcher JS, Wu J, Jessen WJ, Pundavela J, Miller JA, Dombi E, Kim MO, Rizvi TA, Chetal K, Salomonis N, Ratner N. Cxcr3-expressing leukocytes are necessary for neurofibroma formation in mice. JCI Insight. 2019;4:e98601.
8. Yang FC, Staser K, Clapp DW. The plexiform neurofibroma microenvironment. Cancer Microenviron. 2012;5:307–10.
9. Brossier NM, Carroll SL. Genetically engineered mouse models shed new light on the pathogenesis of neurofibromatosis type I-related neoplasms of the peripheral nervous system. Brain Res Bull. 2012;88:58–71.
10. White KA, Swier VJ, Cain JT, Kohlmeyer JL, Meyerholz DK, Tanas MR, Uthoff J, Hammond E, Li H, Rohret FA, Goeken A, Chan CH, Leidinger MR, Umesalma S, Wallace MR, Dodd RD, Panzer K, Tang AH, Darbro BW, Moutal A, Cai S, Li W, Bellampalli SS, Khanna R, Rogers CS, Sieren JC, Quelle DE, Weimer JM. A porcine model of neurofibromatosis type 1 that mimics the human disease. JCI Insight. 2018;3:e120402.

11. Esposito T, Schettino C, Polverino P, Allocca S, Adelfi L, D'amico A, Capaldo G, Varriale B, Di Salle A, Peluso G, Sorrentino G, Lus G, Sampaolo S, Di Iorio G, Melone MAB. Synergistic interplay between curcumin and polyphenol-rich foods in the mediterranean diet: therapeutic prospects for neurofibromatosis 1 patients. Nutrients. 2017;9:783.
12. Demestre M, Messerli SM, Celli N, Shahhossini M, Kluwe L, Mautner V, Maruta H. CAPE (caffeic acid phenethyl ester)-based propolis extract (Bio 30) suppresses the growth of human neurofibromatosis (NF) tumor xenografts in mice. Phytother Res. 2009;23:226–30.
13. Kluwe L, Hagel C, Friedrich RE, Schnabel C, Schon G, Mautner V. Vitamin D receptor expression and serum 25(OH)D concentration inversely associates with burden of neurofibromas. Eur J Cancer Prev. 2019;28:220–4.
14. Schnabel C, Dahm S, Streichert T, Thierfelder W, Kluwe L, Mautner VF. Differences of 25-hydroxyvitamin D3 concentrations in children and adults with neurofibromatosis type 1. Clin Biochem. 2014;47:560–3.
15. Schnabel C, Jett K, Friedman JM, Frieling I, Kruse HP, Mautner V. Effect of vitamin D3 treatment on bone density in neurofibromatosis 1 patients: a retrospective clinical study. Joint Bone Spine. 2013;80:315–9.
16. Souza Mario Bueno L, Rosset C, Aguiar E, Pereira Fde S, Izetti Ribeiro P, Scalco R, Matzenbacher Bittar C, Brinckmann Oliveira Netto C, Gischkow Rucatti G, Chies JA, Camey SA, Ashton-Prolla P. Vitamin D status and VDR genotype in NF1 patients: a case-control study from Southern Brazil. Int J Endocrinol. 2015;2015:402838.
17. Ortonne N, Wolkenstein P, Blakeley JO, Korf B, Plotkin SR, Riccardi VM, Miller DC, HUSON S, Peltonen J, Rosenberg A, Carroll SL, Verma SK, Mautner V, Upadhyaya M, Stemmer-Rachamimov A. Cutaneous neurofibromas: current clinical and pathologic issues. Neurology. 2018;91:S5–S13.
18. Miettinen MM, Antonescu CR, Fletcher CDM, Kim A, Lazar AJ, Quezado MM, Reilly KM, Stemmer-Rachamimov A, Stewart DR, Viskochil D, Widemann B, Perry A. Histopathologic evaluation of atypical neurofibromatous tumors and their transformation into malignant peripheral nerve sheath tumor in patients with neurofibromatosis 1-a consensus overview. Hum Pathol. 2017;67:1–10.
19. Chirindel A, Chaudhry M, Blakeley JO, Wahl R. 18F-FDG PET/CT qualitative and quantitative evaluation in neurofibromatosis type 1 patients for detection of malignant transformation: comparison of early to delayed imaging with and without liver activity normalization. J Nucl Med. 2015;56:379–85.
20. Ferner R, Lucas J, O'doherty M, Hughes R, Smith M, Cronin B, Bingham J. Evaluation of 18fluorodeoxyglucose positron emission tomography (18FDG PET) in the detection of malignant peripheral nerve sheath tumours arising from within plexiform neurofibromas in neurofibromatosis 1. J Neurol Neurosurg Psychiatry. 2000;68:353–7.
21. Armand ML, Taieb C, Bourgeois A, Bourlier M, Bennani M, Bodemer C, Wolkenstein P. Burden of adult neurofibromatosis 1: development and validation of a burden assessment tool. Orphanet J Rare Dis. 2019;14:94.
22. Cannon A, Chen MJ, Li P, Boyd KP, Theos A, Redden DT, Korf B. Cutaneous neurofibromas in neurofibromatosis type I: a quantitative natural history study. Orphanet J Rare Dis. 2018;13:31.
23. Chiang YZ, Al-Niaimi F, Ferguson J, August PJ, Madan V. Carbon dioxide laser treatment of cutaneous neurofibromas. Dermatol Ther (Heidelb). 2012;2:7.
24. Kim HJ, Lee KG, Yi SM, Kim JH, Kim IH. Successful treatment of multiple cutaneous neurofibromas using a combination of shave excision and laser photothermocoagulation with a 1,444-nm neodymium-doped yttrium aluminum garnet laser. Dermatol Surg. 2012;38: 960–3.
25. Kriechbaumer LK, Susani M, Kircher SG, Distelmaier K, Happak W. Comparative study of CO- and Er:YAG laser ablation of multiple cutaneous neurofibromas in von Recklinghausen's disease. Lasers Med Sci. 2013;5:5.
26. Kriechbaumer LK, Susani M, Kircher SG, Happak W. Vaporization of cutaneous neurofibromas with an erbium: yttrium-aluminum-garnet laser: a comparative histologic evaluation. Plast Reconstr Surg. 2012;129:602e–4e.

27. Lutterodt CG, Mohan A, Kirkpatrick N. The use of electrodessication in the treatment of cutaneous neurofibromatosis: a retrospective patient satisfaction outcome assessment. J Plast Reconstr Aesthet Surg. 2016;69:765–9.
28. Widemann BC, Babovic-Vuksanovic D, Dombi E, Wolters PL, Goldman S, Martin S, Goodwin A, Goodspeed W, Kieran MW, Cohen B, Blaney SM, King A, Solomon J, Patronas N, Balis FM, Fox E, Steinberg SM, Packe RJ. Phase II trial of pirfenidone in children and young adults with neurofibromatosis type 1 and progressive plexiform neurofibromas. Pediatr Blood Cancer. 2014;22:25041. https://doi.org/10.1002/pbc.25041.
29. Widemann BC, Dombi E, Gillespie A, Wolters PL, Belasco J, Goldman S, Korf BR, Solomon J, Martin S, Salzer W, Fox E, Patronas N, Kieran MW, Perentesis JP, Reddy A, Wright JJ, Kim A, Steinberg SM, Balis FM. Phase 2 randomized, flexible crossover, double-blinded, placebo-controlled trial of the farnesyltransferase inhibitor tipifarnib in children and young adults with neurofibromatosis type 1 and progressive plexiform neurofibromas. Neuro-Oncology. 2014;16:707–18.
30. Jakacki RI, Dombi E, Steinberg SM, Goldman S, Kieran MW, Ullrich NJ, Pollack IF, Goodwin A, Manley PE, Fangusaro J, Allen R, Widemann BC. Phase II trial of pegylated interferon alfa-2b in young patients with neurofibromatosis type 1 and unresectable plexiform neurofibromas. Neuro-Oncology. 2017;19:289–97.
31. Kim A, Dombi E, Tepas K, Fox E, Martin S, Wolters P, Balis FM, Jayaprakash N, Turkbey B, Muradyan N, Choyke PL, Reddy A, Korf B, Widemann BC. Phase I trial and pharmacokinetic study of sorafenib in children with neurofibromatosis type I and plexiform neurofibromas. Pediatr Blood Cancer. 2013;60:396–401.
32. Yang FC, Ingram DA, Chen S, ZHU Y, Yuan J, Li X, Yang X, Knowles S, Horn W, Li Y, Zhang S, Yang Y, Vakili ST, Yu M, Burns D, Robertson K, Hutchins G, Parada LF, Clapp DW. Nf1-dependent tumors require a microenvironment containing Nf1+/–– and c-kit-dependent bone marrow. Cell. 2008;135:437–48.
33. Robertson KA, Nalepa G, Yang FC, Bowers DC, Ho CY, Hutchins GD, Croop JM, Vik TA, Denne SC, Parada LF, Hingtgen CM, Walsh LE, Yu M, Pradhan KR, Edwards-Brown MK, Cohen MD, Fletcher JW, Travers JB, Staser KW, Lee MW, Sherman MR, Davis CJ, Miller LC, Ingram DA, Clapp DW. Imatinib mesylate for plexiform neurofibromas in patients with neurofibromatosis type 1: a phase 2 trial. Lancet Oncol. 2012;13:1218–24.
34. Weiss B, Widemann BC, Wolters P, Dombi E, VINKS A, CANTOR A, Perentesis J, Schorry E, Ullrich N, Gutmann DH, Tonsgard J, Viskochil D, Korf B, Packer RJ, Fisher MJ. Sirolimus for progressive neurofibromatosis type 1-associated plexiform neurofibromas: a neurofibromatosis clinical trials consortium phase II study. Neuro-Oncology. 2015;17:596–603.
35. Weiss B, Widemann BC, Wolters P, Dombi E, Vinks AA, Cantor A, Korf B, Perentesis J, Gutmann DH, Schorry E, Packer R, Fisher MJ. Sirolimus for non-progressive NF1-associated plexiform neurofibromas: an NF clinical trials consortium phase II study. Pediatr Blood Cancer. 2014;61:982–6.
36. Dombi E, Baldwin A, Marcus LJ, Fisher MJ, Weiss B, Kim A, Whitcomb P, Martin S, Aschbacher-Smith LE, Rizvi TA, Wu J, Ershler R, Wolters P, Therrien J, Glod J, Belasco JB, Schorry E, Brofferio A, Starosta AJ, Gillespie A, Doyle AL, Ratner N, Widemann BC. Activity of selumetinib in neurofibromatosis type 1-related plexiform neurofibromas. N Engl J Med. 2016;375:2550–60.
37. Gross AM, Wolters PL, Dombi E, Baldwin A, Whitcomb P, Fisher MJ, Weiss B, Kim A, Bornhorst M, Shah AC, Martin S, Roderick MC, et al. Selumetinib in children with inoperable plexiform neurofibromas. New Engl J Med. 2020;382:1430–42.
38. Campen CJ, Gutmann DH. Optic pathway gliomas in neurofibromatosis type 1. J Child Neurol. 2018;33:73–81.
39. Rozen WM, Joseph S, Lo PA. Spontaneous regression of low-grade gliomas in pediatric patients without neurofibromatosis. Pediatr Neurosurg. 2008;44:324–8.
40. Avery RA, Fisher MJ, Liu GT. Optic pathway gliomas. J Neuroophthalmol. 2011;31:269–78.
41. Evans DGR, Baser ME, Mcgaughran J, Sharif S, Howard E, Moran A. Malignant peripheral nerve sheath tumours in neurofibromatosis 1. J Med Genet. 2002;39:311–4.
42. Reilly KM, Kim A, Blakely J, Ferner RE, Gutmann DH, Legius E, Miettinen MM, Randall RL, RATNER N, Jumbe NL, Bakker A, Viskochil D, Widemann BC, Stewart DR. Neurofibromatosis

type 1-associated MPNST state of the science: outlining a research agenda for the future. J Natl Cancer Inst. 2017;109:djx124.
43. Stevenson DA, Little D, Armstrong L, Crawford AH, Eastwood D, Friedman JM, Greggi T, Gutierrez G, Hunter-Schaedle K, Kendler DL, Kolanczyk M, Monsell F, Oetgen M, Richards BS, Schindeler A, Schorry EK, Wilkes D, Viskochil DH, Yang FC, Elefteriou F. Approaches to treating NF1 tibial pseudarthrosis: consensus from the Children's Tumor Foundation NF1 bone abnormalities consortium. J Pediatr Orthop. 2013;33:269–75.
44. Vaucheret Paz E, Lopez Ballent A, Puga C, Garcia Basalo MJ, Baliarda F, Ekonen C, Ilari R, Agosta G. Cognitive profile and disorders affecting higher brain functions in paediatric patients with neurofibromatosis type 1. Neurologia. 2017;34:353–9.
45. Vogel AC, Gutmann DH, Morris SM. Neurodevelopmental disorders in children with neurofibromatosis type 1. Dev Med Child Neurol. 2017;59:1112–6.
46. Lion-François L, Gueyffier F, Mercier C, Gérard D, Herbillon V, Kemlin I, Rodriguez D, Ginhoux T, Peyric E, Coutinho V, Bréant V. The effect of methylphenidate on neurofibromatosis type 1: a randomised, double-blind, placebo-controlled, crossover trial. Orphanet J Rare Dis. 2014;9:142.
47. Bearden CE, Hellemann GS, Rosser T, Montojo C, Jonas R, Enrique N, Pacheco L, Hussain SA, Wu JY, Ho JS, Mcgough JJ, Sugar CA, Silva AJ. A randomized placebo-controlled lovastatin trial for neurobehavioral function in neurofibromatosis I. Ann Clin Transl Neurol. 2016;3:266–79.
48. Payne JM, Barton B, Ullrich NJ, Cantor A, Hearps SJ, Cutter G, Rosser T, Walsh KS, Gioia GA, Wolters PL, Tonsgard J, Schorry E, Viskochil D, Klesse L, Fisher M, Gutmann DH, Silva AJ, Hunter SJ, Rey-Casserly C, Cantor NL, Byars AW, Stavinoha PL, Ackerson JD, Armstrong CL, Isenberg J, O'neil SH, Packer RJ, KORF B, Acosta MT, North KN. Randomized placebo-controlled study of lovastatin in children with neurofibromatosis type 1. Neurology. 2016;87:2575–84.
49. Van der Vaart T, Plasschaert E, Rietman AB, Renard M, Oostenbrink R, Vogels A, De Wit MC, Descheemaeker MJ, Vergouwe Y, Catsman-Berrevoets CE, Legius E, Elgersma Y, Moll HA. Simvastatin for cognitive deficits and behavioural problems in patients with neurofibromatosis type 1 (NF1-SIMCODA): a randomised, placebo-controlled trial. Lancet Neurol. 2013;12:1076–83.
50. Fletcher JS, Springer MG, Choi K, Jousma E, Rizvi TA, Dombi E, Kim MO, Wu J, Ratner N. STAT3 inhibition reduces macrophage number and tumor growth in neurofibroma. Oncogene. 2019;38:2876–84.
51. Staser K, Yang FC, Clapp DW. Pathogenesis of plexiform neurofibroma: tumor-stromal/hematopoietic interactions in tumor progression. Annu Rev Pathol. 2012;7:469–95.
52. Plotkin SR, Blakeley JO, Dombi E, Fisher MJ, Hanemann CO, Walsh KS, Wolters PL, Widemann BC. Achieving consensus for clinical trials: the REiNS International Collaboration. Neurology. 2013;81:S1–5.
53. Gutmann DH, Blakeley JO, Korf BR, Packer RJ. Optimizing biologically targeted clinical trials for neurofibromatosis. Expert Opin Investig Drugs. 2013;22:443–62.
54. Wimmer K, Yao S, Claes K, Kehrer-Sawatzki H, Tinschert S, De Raedt T, Legius E, Callens T, Beiglböck H, Maertens O, Messiaen L. Spectrum of single- and multiexon NF1 copy number changes in a cohort of 1,100 unselected NF1 patients. Genes Chromosomes Cancer. 2006;45:265–76.
55. Burgener EB, Moss RB. Cystic fibrosis transmembrane conductance regulator modulators: precision medicine in cystic fibrosis. Curr Opin Pediatr. 2018;30:372–7.
56. Keeling KM, Wang D, Conard SE, Bedwell DM. Suppression of premature termination codons as a therapeutic approach. Crit Rev Biochem Mol Biol. 2012;47:444–63.
57. Castellanos E, Rosas I, Solanes A, Bielsa I, Lazaro C, Carrato C, Hostalot C, Prades P, Roca-Ribas F, Blanco I, Serra E, Hugtip-Ico-Imppc NFMC. In vitro antisense therapeutics for a deep intronic mutation causing Neurofibromatosis type 2. Eur J Hum Genet. 2013;21:769–73.
58. Pros E, Fernández-Rodríguez J, Benito L, Ravella A, Capellá G, Blanco I, Serra E, Lázaro C. Modulation of aberrant NF1 pre-mRNA splicing by kinetin treatment. Eur J Hum Genet. 2010;18:614–7.

Medical Follow-Up in Neurofibromatosis Type 1

19

Christina Bergqvist and Pierre Wolkenstein

Contents

C. Bergqvist
Department of Dermatology, American University of Beirut Medical Center, Beirut, Lebanon

P. Wolkenstein (✉)
French Referral Centers for Neurofibromatoses and for Toxic Bullous Dermatoses, Créteil Cedex, France

Division Cancers Immunity Transplantation Infections, Henri-Mondor Hospital, APHP, Créteil Cedex, France

EA-7379, EpiDermE, University Paris Est Créteil, Créteil Cedex, France

Faculty of Medicine, University Paris Est Créteil, Créteil Cedex, France

G. Tadini et al. (eds.), *Multidisciplinary Approach to Neurofibromatosis Type 1*,
https://doi.org/10.1007/978-3-319-92450-2_19

Neurofibromatosis type 1 (NF1) is a multisystem genetic disorder that is primarily associated with cutaneous, neurologic, and orthopedic manifestations; some of which are progressive and result in substantial morbidity or mortality. Indeed, NF1 is associated with an increased risk of malignancy and a life expectancy of about 10–15 years shorter than the general population [1]. The mainstay of management of patients with NF1 is a longitudinal care with age specific monitoring of disease manifestations, aiming at the early detection and symptomatic treatment of complications as they arise. The multi-organ involvement of neurofibromatosis frequently entails care from a variability of medical subspecialists and surgical specialists. Active partnership and an active engagement between multiple health care providers using a multidisciplinary approach optimizes the management and monitoring of this rare disease.

Lifetime monitoring is recommended as soon as the diagnosis of NF1 is suspected. Early recognition of NF1 allows for appropriate surveillance. Once the diagnosis is considered, referral should be made to any physician conversant with the diagnosis of NF1, including dermatologists, geneticists, neurologists, or pediatricians. This team should examine the child for diagnostic criteria, identify potential complications, deliver anticipatory guidance, and refer to specialists when needed.

In the absence of complications, clinical evaluation should take place on a yearly basis for both children and adults with NF1, as annual examinations allow for early detection of complications, decreasing morbidity and improving quality of life. Clinical evaluation seems to be more useful in detecting complications than are routine screening investigations in asymptomatic patients [2].

Children and adults with subcutaneous neurofibromas (termed high-risk phenotype as they have a higher risk of developing malignant peripheral nerve sheath tumors (MPNSTs) [3]) should be followed up by a NF1 specialist annually. Otherwise, NF1 patients without the high-risk phenotype or complications should visit the NF1 specialist every 2–3 years, with the rest of the visits taking place with a primary care physician, dermatologist, or pediatrician [4].

Table 19.1 summarizes the essential evaluations to be undertaken in the medical follow-up of patients with NF1.

19.1 Confirming the Diagnosis

To date, NF1 is diagnosed primarily on clinical grounds. Although the diagnosis relies mainly on the basis of the National Institutes of Health (NIH) diagnostic criteria [5], most experts in the NF1 community believe that the diagnostic criteria should include molecular testing. Generally, NF1 can be diagnosed by physical examination and by evaluating the patient's family history. However, the age at

Table 19.1 Medical follow-up of individuals with neurofibromatosis 1

Medical follow-up of individuals with neurofibromatosis 1	
At the time of diagnosis	*Confirming the diagnosis*
	– on the basis of NIH diagnostic criteria
	– perform physical examination
	– evaluate family history
	– genetic testing for select cases (does not meet diagnostic criteria or unusual phenotype)
	– define phenotype and NF1 score
	Screening family members
	– All first-degree relatives
	– complete physical examination
	– slit-lamp examination
	– genetic testing in questionable cases
	Announcing the diagnosis
	– well-planned, dedicated, face-to-face consultation
	– review clinical manifestations, variability, natural history, prognosis, risk of complications, and the warning signs
	– offer consultation with a well-trained psychologist or a specialist in genetic counseling
	– inform about the location of neurofibromatosis clinics
	– provide available NF1 resources such as books, pamphlets, reliable website addresses, and support groups
	Genetic counseling
	– Prenatal and pre-implantation genetic testing
Infancy and early childhood	– Clinical examination on a yearly basis
	– Yearly ophthalmologic evaluation
	– Yearly blood pressure monitoring
	– Yearly measurements of weight, height, and head circumference
	– Examine skin for CALMs, plexiform neurofibromas, skinfold freckling
	– Evaluate for skeletal changes including scoliosis, vertebral changes, and limb abnormalities
	– Check for proptosis, a rapidly increasing head size, and focal neurologic signs
	– Check neurodevelopmental progress
	– Evaluation of learning, speech, language, and motor abilities
	– Evaluation of family's psychological support

(continued)

Table 19.1 (continued)

Late childhood and adolescence	– Clinical examination on a yearly basis
	– Yearly ophthalmologic evaluation up until the age of 8 years (then yearly or every 2 years depending on country's guidelines)
	– Yearly blood pressure monitoring
	– Yearly measurements of weight, height, and head circumference
	– Examine skin for neurofibromas, plexiform neurofibromas
	– Assess for persistent, substantial, or difficult to control pain or a rapid increase in the size of an existing plexiform neurofibroma or alteration in its consistency from soft to hard. If present, order an MRI to evaluate for possible malignant transformation into a MPNST
	– Complete neurologic examination to check for deep plexiform neurofibromas
	– Evaluate for signs of early puberty. If present, order MRI of the brain and orbits to investigate for an OPG
	– Evaluate learning disabilities and attention-deficit hyperactivity disorder
	– Evaluate school progress
	– Evaluate the patient's social adjustment
	– Evaluate the physical and psychological impacts of the disease and refer to psychologist or psychiatrist for further evaluation and therapy if needed
Adulthood	– Yearly blood pressure monitoring
	– Assess the degree of cosmetic disfigurement caused by skin tumors and refer to surgery or CO2 laser
	– Evaluation of literacy and numeracy problems
	– Evaluation of social difficulties
	– Evaluate the physical and psychological impacts of the disease and refer to psychologist or psychiatrist for further evaluation and therapy if needed
	– Discuss the effect of pregnancy on NF1
	– Discuss prenatal diagnosis and refer the patient to a geneticist
	– Cancer screening guidelines similar to that of the general population
	– Consider regular mammography-based or MRI-based screening starting at the age of 30 years

which these diagnostic findings develop is variable, with some patients exhibiting a late onset and others never developing certain signs and symptoms. Definitive diagnosis may therefore be delayed by years. Studies have shown that NIH diagnostic criteria help reaching a diagnosis of NF1 in the majority of children at the age of 5 years, but are insufficient for reaching a diagnosis at an earlier age [6]. Indeed, only 50% of children with sporadic NF1 younger than 2 years have been reported to fulfil only 1 NIH criterion, leading to delayed diagnosis [6].

Genetic testing can thus be helpful in confirming the diagnosis for children who do not meet diagnostic criteria or those who present with an unusual phenotype. A positive genetic test shortens the period of diagnostic uncertainty and early recognition of NF1 allows for appropriate surveillance and helps provide the parents with the appropriate genetic counseling regarding any future planned pregnancy.

Patients with Legius syndrome and constitutional mismatch repair-deficiency syndrome may present with both café-au-lait macules (CALMs) and axillary freckling, and patients with Noonan syndrome may present with CALMs. Thus, children who present with CALMs as the sole clinical feature with no family history of NF1 might need genetic testing to confirm a diagnosis of NF1. In a study of 71 patients <20 years of age with six or more CALMs and no non-pigmentary criterion, 66.2% were discovered to have NF1, 8.5% had Legius syndrome, and 25.3% harbored no disease causing variant [7].

In adults, the clinical presentation may be incomplete in some rare forms, necessitating genetic analysis for the confirmation of the diagnosis. Patients with limited and localized clinical features and no family history of NF1 may possibly have segmental NF1 [4].

Mutations associated with NF1 disrupt the function of the *NF1* gene [8]. Molecular diagnosis of NF1 is challenging due to the large size of the tumor suppressor gene *NF1* and the lack of mutation hotspots [8]. A huge number of different pathogenic *NF1* mutations have been reported. Molecular testing with high sensitivity is clinically available and around 95% of *NF1* gene mutations can already be identified using various molecular analysis methods (multistep approach including a cDNA, DNA Sanger sequencing, and copy number alteration study) [8]. Hence a negative test using those methods cannot completely exclude the diagnosis, and patients with segmental NF1 and mosaicism can also test negative.

A new targeted next-generation sequencing of *NF1* and *SPRED1* using a multiplex PCR approach was developed and its high sensitivity was recently validated in a cohort study whereby 98.5% of all targeted bases were covered by at least 20X and 96% by at least 100X [9].

Generally speaking, a positive *NF1* mutation test does not predict the severity or complications of the disorder. For patients with intragenic *NF1* mutations which represent over 90% of all NF1 cases, no straightforward genotype–phenotype correlations have been identified [10] with two exceptions: a 3-bp in-frame deletion (c.2970-2972 delAAT) in exon 17 of the *NF1* gene and a missense mutations involving codon 1809; these have been associated with a milder phenotype and the absence of cutaneous neurofibromas.

In 5–10% of patients, NF1 results from microdeletions that encompass the entire *NF1* gene and a variable number of flanking genes. These large *NF1* locus deletions have been associated with a more severe phenotype including developing neurofibromas at an earlier age, having a lower mean IQ, abnormal facial features, and an elevated risk for MPNST [11].

19.2 Screening Family Members

When the diagnosis of NF1 is made in a child, a detailed family history should be obtained. All first-degree relatives should be evaluated with a complete examination of the skin looking for the characteristic NF1 signs; as well as a slit-lamp examination to look for Lisch nodules, which are found in 90% of adults with NF1. Genetic testing can be performed to confirm the diagnosis in questionable cases using targeted testing for the mutation identified in the proband rather than a comprehensive mutation analysis of the entire gene.

19.3 Genetic Counseling

NF1 is an autosomal dominant genetic disorder that is fully penetrant (without skipped generations or asymptomatic carriers). If one of the parents has the disease, the risk of having a child with NF1 is 50% but is roughly 5% for a parent with segmental disease [12]. Prenatal and pre-implantation genetic testing can be offered when the causative *NF1* mutation has been identified in the parent, but as mentioned above it generally does not predict the disease severity.

19.4 Announcing the Diagnosis

The announcement of a genetic disorder such as NF1 is a crucial event in the lives of both the parents and the child as it is often traumatic, eliciting strong emotions such as the anxiety of an unknown disease in non-familial forms, guilt in familial forms, and for all, fear of the prognosis and the possible complications [4].

The announcement of the diagnosis should be a well-planned, dedicated, face-to-face consultation which needs experience and unlimited time. It should be adapted to family history, depending on whether the newly detected disease is familial or sporadic. The parents should be offered a consultation with a well-trained psychologist or a specialist in genetic counseling for a more in-depth discussion of clinical findings and future reproductive options. An important step in the announcement is discussing the possibility of the extension of the diagnosis to other members of the family. The clinical manifestations, variability, natural history, prognosis, risk of complications, and the warning signs that should prompt rapid medical consultation must be reviewed. All these consultations should also address the current scientific progress with the latest therapeutic and supportive care possibilities, including their efficacy, complications, and adverse effects. Parents should be informed about the neurofibromatosis clinics in their region for further guidance, therapy, and consultation. Parents should also be provided with available NF1 resources such as books, pamphlets, reliable website addresses, and support groups.

19.5 Dermatological Evaluation

The medical follow-up of patients with NF1 relies on a multidisciplinary team within which the dermatologist plays an important role, including in the diagnosis. Indeed, the seven diagnostic criteria of the NIH include three cutaneous manifestations (café-au-lait macules, freckling on flexural areas, and cutaneous neurofibromas) [5]; however, the age at which these diagnostic findings develop is variable, with some patients exhibiting a late onset and others never developing certain symptoms. Definitive diagnosis may therefore be delayed by years. As mentioned above, the NIH diagnostic criteria are insufficient for reaching a diagnosis at an early age [6]; hence, other cutaneous lesions found in this age group can be identified by dermatologists to help with the diagnosis.

The dermatological exam consists of examining the skin carefully for the specific NF1 skin lesions which usually appear in the following order: café-au-lait macules (CALMs); plexiform neurofibromas; axillary and/or inguinal lentigines; subcutaneous neurofibromas; and cutaneous neurofibromas.

19.6 Dermatological Examination in Infancy and Childhood

The dermatological examination of a newborn can help in confirming the diagnosis, as the initial clinical manifestation of NF1 are CALMs which are usually present at birth or appear in infancy. CALMs may increase in number and size in early childhood. Around 80% of patients with NF1 will have more than five CALMs by 1 year of age, and the physician should be aware that their absence does not exclude the diagnosis of NF1. They tend to darken with sun exposure and fade with age or become obscured by numerous neurofibromas. CALMs have no malignant potential and the family should be reassured that CALMs have no functional significance. Sun protection and camouflage advice can be offered to patients who are bothered by the pigmentation [13]. The smooth borders of the CALMs associated with NF1 have been likened to the coast of California and tend to have a poor response using Q-switched or picosecond lasers [14]. There is not enough evidence to warrant the routine use of laser treatment for CALMs [13]. Hypopigmented macules and nevus anemicus are other associated features observed in patients with NF1 of this age group [4].

Plexiform neurofibromas are also congenital and externally visible plexiform neurofibromas are present in around 25% of individuals with NF1 [15]. However, only in 10% to 15% of neonates, will a plexiform neurofibroma be recognized [15]. These lesions consist of a subtle enlargement of soft tissue or a patch of hyperpigmentation with or without hypertrichosis. Substantial increase in growth usually occurs during the first decade of life and adolescence [4]. These tumors can invade surrounding structures, leading to considerable pain and bone destruction. Plexiform neurofibroma of the face may be potentially devastating and associated with considerable disfigurement, necessitating surgical excision. These tumors have a risk of malignant transformation. Twenty to forty percent of adult patients have internal tumors that cannot always be detected on clinical examination and whole-body magnetic resonance imaging (MRI) is used in some centers to evaluate the tumor burden and growth [16]. Although plexiform neurofibromas may remain asymptomatic, they can lead to significant morbidities such as pain, neurological deficit, disfigurement, risk of progression to MPNST, and the potential for life-threatening hemorrhage and infection during surgery.

The management of these complex lesions is unclear. Radiotherapy is contraindicated in benign tumors because of the risk of malignant degeneration. Excision of benign plexiform neurofibromas is often very challenging due to impingement of the tumor on contiguous nerves and structures and its inherent extensive vascularity might lead to life-threatening hemorrhage in particular with facial plexiform neurofibromas [13]. Hence, expert advice should be sought from experienced plastic surgeons and those experienced with soft tissue tumor resection. No specific medical treatment exists so far. Several treatments are being tested in clinical trials and volumetric MRI along with whole-body MRI allows a precise evaluation of tumor response to new therapy [17]. The farnesyltransferase inhibitor tipifarnib, the mammalian target of rapamycin inhibitor sirolimus, and the fibroblast inhibitor pirfenidone were not proven to have enough benefit to support their use. Both imatinib and pegylated interferon have been shown to lead to a reduction in the size of plexiform neurofibromas in a limited number of patients [4]. Selumetinib, an oral selective mitogen-activated protein kinase inhibitor, has shown promising results in a phase 1 study whereby children with neurofibromatosis type 1 and inoperable plexiform neurofibromas benefited from long-term dose-adjusted administration of selumetinib without excess toxic effects [18]. So far, patients with NF1 can benefit from these treatments only within clinical trials.

Skinfold freckling is usually the second feature noticed in children with NF1 and is found in 85% of NF1 individuals [13, 4]. It is typically detected between the ages of 3 and 5 years. It can appear in any area where skinfolds are in apposition, including the axilla, inguinal area, base of the neck, upper eyelid, and under the breasts in women. Parents should be reassured that CALMs and freckling only have a cosmetic significance.

Juvenile xanthogranulomas (JXG) are benign yellowish papules and multiple JXG lesions are highly prevalent in children younger than 2 years with NF1. They are transient and generally spontaneously disappear before a child reaches 5 years, and they do not require treatment unless they are located in the eye, where they can lead to hyphema [19].

Its presence has been considered an alarming sign for juvenile myelomonocytic leukemia (JMML). However, the relationship among JXG, NF1, and JMML has generated lots of confusion; especially that in two retrospective series of JXG in patients with NF1, an increased incidence of JMML was not found [20, 15]. Other studies have shown that patients with NF1 and multiple JXG lesions have a 20–30 fold higher risk of developing JMML than those without JXG lesions but nevertheless, this condition remains extremely rare [21]. And hence, there is no evidence to recommend approaching children with NF1 and JXG differently from those who have NF1 alone, and there is not sufficient information to recommend routine screening for JMML in patients with NF1.

However, physicians should be aware of the presenting signs and symptoms of JMML. Clinical examination must, therefore, be thorough and directed: if NF1 patients develop hepatosplenomegaly, lymphadenopathy, or pallor, they should directly be assessed for JMML and complete blood counts should then be obtained.

As mentioned earlier, 50% of children with sporadic NF1 younger than 2 years have been reported to fulfil only 1 NIH criterion, leading to delayed diagnosis. Both JXG and nevus anemicus have been diagnosed in most children with NF1 aged younger than 2 years and were found in 80% of patients with insufficient criteria for diagnosis at that time. Hence, JXG and nevus anemicus appear helpful in improving the early diagnosis of NF1 in young children and infants.

19.7 Dermatological Examination in Late Childhood and Adolescence

From there on, during each visit of patients in late childhood and adolescence, the skin should be examined for new neurofibromas, the progression of existing ones, and whether they are causing pruritus, pain, bleeding, interference with function, or disfigurement. A consultation with a specialist should be offered to patients if surgery is required to improve appearance or function. A thorough skin evaluation of plexiform neurofibromas and a complete neurologic examination to check whether they are encroaching on deeper structures should be done. Some centers recommend that whole-body MRI be performed between 16 and 18 years of age to assess the neurofibroma load and to evaluate the size and extent of individual tumors [16].

19.8 Neurofibromas

Neurofibromas are benign peripheral nerve sheath tumors and are the cardinal feature of NF1. There are different subtypes: cutaneous, subcutaneous, spinal nerve root, and nodular or diffuse plexiform tumors.

Cutaneous (or dermal) neurofibromas are found in the vast majority of patients with NF1 and usually develop in late adolescence, but can occasionally appear in younger children [22]. They are soft flesh-colored or purplish nodules that become pedunculated as they grow. The number of neurofibromas varies between patients and within families [23, 22]. Although these skin tumors are benign, they can cause significant discomfort including transient stinging and itching, pain, bleeding, catching on clothing, and cosmetic problems. Pruritus does not usually respond to antihistamines and the use of mast cell stabilizers is unclear [24]; patients should be advised to avoid excessive heat and to use emollients [13]. Management of dermal neurofibromas includes referral to surgeons who are familiar with the excision of neurofibromas and plastic surgeons should be considered for neurofibromas on the face and neck, although patients should be informed of the risks of delayed wound healing and thickened scars. Laser ablation for small lesions on the face and neck may be helpful [13, 25]. Electrodessication is another useful tool as it enables the treatment of hundreds of neurofibromas in a single operation under general anesthesia, with low complication rates and high levels of clinical and patient-reported outcomes [26]. Patient should also be offered advice on camouflage make-up and psychological support.

Subcutaneous neurofibromas are firm discrete palpable lesions, they may be tender to touch and can cause tingling along the affected nerve or even neurological deficits. Malignant change can rarely occur [27]. If removal is considered, NF1 specialists or soft tissue tumor or peripheral nerve surgeons should be consulted as removal can lead to neurological deficit [13].

Spinal neurofibromas are usually asymptomatic but may become symptomatic by causing nerve root or spinal cord compression. Neurofibromas located in the upper cervical region are prone to lead to spinal cord compression especially at the second cervical nerve root which is susceptible to repeated low-grade trauma as it exits from the neural foramen [28]. Fortunately, the neurological signs and symptoms are frequently mild and spinal cord compression can be present even in the absence of neurological signs and symptoms. Surgical intervention should be undertaken on the grounds of progressive neurological symptoms and risk of permanent deficit.

19.9 Malignant Peripheral Nerve Sheath Tumors

MPNSTs are a subtype of sarcoma with an assumed Schwann cell origin. The cumulative lifetime risk of developing MPNST in NF1 is approximately 8–13% and occurs mostly in individuals aged 20–35 years [29, 30]. These tumors usually arise in preexisting plexiform neurofibromas or subcutaneous NF. They are difficult to identify, have the ability to metastasize, and entail a poor prognosis [29, 30]. MPNST displays clinical heterogeneity: some high-grade tumors metastasize widely and have a poor prognosis, whereas low-grade MPNST treated appropriately can be associated with long-term survival [29].

The symptoms of MPNST are similar to the benign symptomatic plexiform neurofibromas, and NF1 patients should be informed to consult the neurofibromatosis clinics urgently if they develop any of these symptoms within their plexiform neurofibroma: Persistent, substantial, or difficult to control pain, new neurological deficit or sphincter anomaly, a rapid increase in the size of an existing plexiform neurofibroma or alteration in its consistency from soft to hard [29]. Clinicians should also keep in mind that symptoms may arise from internal plexiform neurofibroma. Risk factors for MPNST include previous treatment with radiotherapy, a large internal neurofibroma burden or numerous subdermal neurofibromas, atypical neurofibromas, neurofibromatous neuropathy, optic pathway glioma, a personal or family history of MPNST, and microdeletions of the NF1 locus [29]. Patients with symptomatic plexiform neurofibromas or those with one of the above risk factors require careful clinical monitoring, and further studies are needed to evaluate the usefulness of regular screening with MRI and fluorodeoxyglucose (FDG)-PET/CT. Nonetheless, it is crucial to educate patients on how to recognize important symptoms and to seek specialist advice promptly.

The diagnosis of MPNSTs is not always easy, as NF1 patients may have many tumors and as mentioned above, symptoms of malignant tumors overlap with those of benign plexiform neurofibromas. MRI can help define the location and the size of the lesion but cannot always distinguish between malignant disease and benign tumors. The most sensitive and specific noninvasive indicator of malignant potential is [18F]2-fluoro-2-dexoy-D-glucose positron emission tomography computed tomography (FDG PET CT) using visual assessment and semiquantitative assessments with a cut-off SUV [31]. Indeed, FDG PET CT has the potential to predict the grade of tumor, as a significant difference in mean delayed SUVmax between benign and malignant lesions was detected in one study [32]. For patients with tumors with an SUVmax in the overlapping range between benign and malignant, they can be further assessed using another tracer [11C] methionine (MET) to evaluate the malignant potential [33]. MET is an amino acid that reflects cell proliferation more strongly than FDG and therefore has a better ability to reflect malignant change as compared to FDG. The heterogeneous nature of some MPNST makes it likely for blind biopsy to miss the area of malignant change in a tumor with mixed features [29]. It is thus recommended to use MRI-guided or FDG PET CT-guided biopsy.

Once the diagnosis of MPNST is suspected, patients should be evaluated and managed by a multidisciplinary team including surgeons, radiologists, neurologists, pathologists, oncologists, and radiation oncologists to efficiently apply a strategy for biopsy and treatment. Complete surgical resection of MPNST with tumor-free margins is the best treatment option for patients with malignant peripheral nerve sheath tumors [34]. Radiotherapy offers local control and could delay the onset of recurrence but does not affect long-term survival [29]. Neoadjuvant chemotherapy with an anthracycline such as doxorubicin and ifosfamide can be used to downstage tumors and facilitate surgical removal; however, this practice has not been adopted widely [29]. Adjuvant chemotherapy using the combination of an anthracycline and ifosfamide also remains controversial. Single-agent anthracycline is often used as front-line therapy for palliative care in patients with metastatic disease [29]. Newer therapies are currently in clinical trials. PET CT can help in assessing treatment response and in distinguishing tumor recurrence from the secondary effects arising from radiotherapy [35].

19.10 Other Dermatological Manifestations

Glomus tumors have also been associated with NF1 with an estimated prevalence of 5% in adult patients with NF1, they are usually multiple and recurring and should be differentiated from symptomatic subcutaneous neurofibromas [36, 37]. Around 30% of patients with glomus tumors have NF1 [36, 37]. Surgical exploration should be considered if the diagnosis is suspected, as excision relieves the symptoms.

Benign cherry angiomas have also been described in patients with neurofibromatosis [38].

19.11 Defining a "High-Risk" Subpopulation

In order to provide optimal care for patients with NF1, it is useful to define a "high-risk" subpopulation that is most likely to develop MPNST and to require close monitoring. Indeed, early identification of patients with this phenotype would allow for adapted surveillance. The major risk factor for the development of MPNST is the presence of many subcutaneous neurofibromas, often associated with peripheral neuropathy and the presence of at least one internal neurofibroma [3].

A clinical score for predicting internal neurofibromas in adults was developed and validated. Four variables were independently associated with internal neurofibromas: at least two subcutaneous neurofibromas, age ≤ 30, absence of cutaneous neurofibromas, and fewer than six café-au-lait macules [39].

Although MRI is not systematically recommended, NF-1 score directs physicians as to which patient warrants a radiological assessment. Faced with a patient with a high NF-1 score value, the French guidelines recommend screening for internal neurofibromas by imaging (preferably by MRI) at NF1 diagnosis if the NF1 score is high [4]. If no internal neurofibromas are detected, then there is no need to repeat imaging. Whether systematic imaging to evaluate for MPNST is recommended in patients with a high NF1 score remains to be investigated.

19.12 Defining a "Complex NF1"

Neurofibromatosis type 1 presents with a heterogeneous clinical picture with some affected individuals having uncomplicated NF1 but others developing rare "complex" manifestations which may affect any system of the human body [40]. NF1 is considered "complex" whenever it includes one of the following:

- Extensive plexiform neurofibromas
- Spinal cord compression arising from cervical plexiform neurofibromas
- Neurofibromatous neuropathy
- Atypical neurofibromas and malignant peripheral nerve sheath tumor
- Optic pathway glioma
- Brain and spine glioma
- Refractory epilepsy due to structural lesion
- Multiple sclerosis
- Complex neurovascular disease
- Pseudarthrosis of the long bones
- Sphenoid wing dysplasia
- Atypical NF1 phenotypes
- Genetic counseling for segmental NF1

Patients with uncomplicated NF1 require a clinical setup focused on diagnosis, genetic counseling, education, monitoring of blood pressure, bone health, and neurofibromas. However, patients with complex NF1 are in an even more particular need of a specialized setting composed of a multidisciplinary team of caregivers familiar with the diagnosis and management of rare and unusual complications of NF1, as well as the development of new treatments. This classification is a flexible one, as patients with uncomplicated NF1 may develop one of the above complications and become a complex NF1, and conversely, patients with complex NF1 may have resolution of their complex manifestation and become a non-complex NF1 [40].

19.13 Ophthalmology Evaluation

Pigmented iris hamartomas, or Lisch nodules, start developing around the age of 3 years and are found in about 90% of NF1 patients who are 20 years of age and older and almost 100% by the age of 30 years [6]. Lisch nodules are among the criteria for NF1 diagnosis (two or more nodules). They are asymptomatic 1–2 mm yellow brown dome shaped papules of the iris, varying depending on the color of the iris and the age of the patient. They are best visualized using careful slit-lamp examination of the non-dilated iris.

The choroid is one of the most commonly affected structures by NF1. The choroidal abnormalities are detected by near-infrared reflectance and appear as bright patchy nodules. They have been recognized as being a highly specific finding for NF1 [41]. Since they sometimes precede the appearance of Lisch nodules, they can facilitate the diagnosis.

A unique, generally single, isolated, and unilateral abnormality of a small second- or third-order retinal venule, which takes on a corkscrew-like tortuosity, can also be detected in a third of cases using direct ophthalmoscopy [42].

Congenital and acquired glaucoma, idiopathic congenital ptosis, and neurofibromas that impinge on the eyelid are other recognized complications of NF1 [43].

19.14 Optic Pathway Gliomas

All children diagnosed with NF1 should have a regular and formal pediatric ophthalmological examination to assess for signs of optic glioma and to follow their progression closely. The evaluation should begin when NF1 is first suspected and be repeated at regular intervals or when symptoms develop.

Optic pathway gliomas (OPG) are frequent benign tumors associated with NF1. They are present in 15% to 20% of children with NF1 and constitute the most common central nervous system (CNS) tumor in patients with NF1 [44, 45]. These tumors usually appear early, in children younger than 6 years, with a median age of clinical presentation at 4.2 years [44, 45]. Although symptomatic tumors have been identified in older individuals, the risk of having a symptomatic optic glioma is greatest in children under 7 years; older individuals rarely develop tumors that necessitates medical intervention.

Histologically these gliomas are juvenile pilocytic astrocytomas, they are slow growing with a low potential of malignancy. They frequently develop within the optic pathway, optic nerve, optic chiasma, and postchiasmatic radiations, but may also be present in the brainstem. OPG in NF1 are subdivided according to their anatomical location: the prechiasmatic tracts of the optic nerves, the chiasmatic–hypothalamic region, and the posterior optic pathways [46]. Although their natural history is often indolent, they are locally invasive and compressive and clinical consequences of these tumors are caused by their space-occupying characteristics and can become symptomatic in a good proportion of patients with NF1 [44, 45]. Indeed, optic pathway gliomas in patients with NF1 can lead to the rapid onset of proptosis associated with moderate-to-severe visual loss in the affected eye; or to abnormal ophthalmological examinations without any visual symptoms. Precocious puberty is another possible complication if the optic pathway tumor impinges on the optic chiasm [47, 48] and more rarely hypothalamus [49]. One factor related to decreased visual acuity seems to be gender; with girls with optic pathway gliomas being 5–10-times more likely to have visual loss requiring treatment [50]. Presentation before the age of 2 years or after the age of 10 years and rapidly progressive proptosis, were also found to be associated with poor visual outcome [51].

19.15 Screening for Optic Pathway Gliomas

The most useful screening tool is measurement of visual acuity; nystagmus, squint, and impaired color vision are usually all associated with visual acuity loss when due to OPG in NF1 [49]. Toddlers and young children do not complain of visual loss until it is very pronounced and sometimes only when they have visual loss bilaterally. Parents should be counseled about the possible hints for visual impairment such as bumping into objects and failure to pick up small toys [13]. Since infants and young children seldom complain of visual loss despite its severity, regular ophthalmological examinations are critical in children with NF1. In the USA, a NF1 Optic Pathway Glioma task force proposed in 1997 a set of guidelines which were reviewed in 2007 for the diagnosis and management of NF1-associated OPG [52]. They recommended that all children with NF1 younger than 8 years should undergo an annual ophthalmological examination performed by an ophthalmologist or neuro-ophthalmologist familiar with young children with NF1. The exam should include measurement of visual acuity, confrontation visual field testing, color vision evaluation, and assessment of pupils, eyelids, ocular motility, irises, and fundi, with formal computerized or kinetic evaluation of visual fields as an adjunctive test if the patient is reliable. Visual evaluation is challenging in young children and those with cognitive deficits. Recognition of visual acuity can be evaluated at a developmental age of 3 years, color vision at 5 years, and visual fields at the age of 8 years [13]. Ophthalmological signs of optic pathway glioma involve optic nerve atrophy, an afferent pupillary defect, strabismus, papilledema, or color vision defects [49].

Children 8 years of age and older have a significantly lower risk for developing OPG making the data insufficient to recommend the optimal interval at which ophthalmological examinations should be performed and at up to what age before its discontinuation [51]. However, the task force recommended that children in this age group should receive complete ophthalmologic examinations every 2 years up until 18 years of age. Finally, no specialized ophthalmological follow-up is necessary for adults with NF1 except for routine eye care. In the UK, published guidelines recommend yearly ophthalmological screening of all children until 8 years of age, reduced to every 2 years until 18 years of age [49]. Published French guidelines recommend that all children diagnosed with NF1 should be subject to specific pediatric ophthalmological follow-up every 6 months, at least up until the age of 18 years [53].

Due to the variable and unpredictable evolution of OPG tumors, management and neuroimaging for these tumors have been the subject of controversy. Although the natural history of OPG is not completely understood, they are indolent for the vast majority in patients with NF1 [45, 44]. However, OPG have the dreadful ability to disturb vision and hypothalamic function in a small proportion of patients and some specialists advocate an initial screening MRI when the diagnosis of NF1 is made to detect the presence of an optic glioma. A routine neuroimaging screening of asymptomatic children with NF1 would be useful if early detection of OPG will allow vision preservation. Few studies have assessed the usefulness of brain or orbital MRI screening in young children with NF1.

A longitudinal study of 227 children with NF1 failed to detect any OPG in which early detection changed the clinical outcome [44]. Half of the identified OPG never lead to any symptoms, nor did they grow; and the vast majority of symptomatic OPG did not necessitate treatment. Only three of the 26 children with OPG had tumor progression following their discovery, out of which only two required treatment. However, both of these children had abnormal ophthalmological findings on examination and would have been detected even if screening neuroimaging had not been done. Furthermore, OPG can develop in young children with NF1 soon after normal neuroimaging, indicating that normal neuroimaging findings in an infant or young child with NF1 is not a guarantee that the optic nerves and chiasm will remain intact [54–56]. Based on these pieces of evidence, the National Neurofibromatosis Foundation Optic Pathway Task Force recommended against routine screening neuroimaging of children with neurofibromatosis type 1 [52].

The outcome of systematic screening for optic glioma using both MRI and ophthalmic examinations yearly in young children was assessed in a clinical study of 84 children younger than 6 years with NF1, whereby 13 children (15% of patients) were found to have OPG [48]. The authors compared the group of children with OPG discovered by screening to those referred during the same period with already discovered OPG. Three "screened" children were treated with chemotherapy (due to progressive enlarging chiasmal lesions on subsequent MRI and or ophthalmic examination) and had preservation of vision. In contrast, the 13 children with OPG diagnosed outside of screening guidelines included five children with substantial visual loss. The authors thus suggested that routine surveillance for OPG could improve outcomes. However this was not a randomized study, and other authors responded to the article claiming that one of the three "screened" patients who needed chemotherapy was not treated until he had specific ophthalmologic signs, which would have been identified by an ophthalmologic exam and that four of the five patients in the "unscreened" had orbital tumors with distinctly different biologic properties that are more aggressive than their chiasmal counterparts [57].

Despite expert opinions recommending against the use of screening MRI for OPGs in children with NF1, substantial variability across institutions exists. A subsequent study of 826 children with NF1 who had systematic MRI evaluation at one center demonstrated that screening could improve and preserve visual outcome in young children with OPG [58]. OPGs were identified on brain or orbital MRI in a total of 18% of patients (149 patients), and in 15% of out these patients (22 patients) radiologic or clinical progression of OPG was detected and required chemotherapy. Out of these 22 patients, 12 children were treated with chemotherapy based on both abnormal MRI findings and ophthalmologic findings, and ten children were treated with chemotherapy based on high-risk MRI findings, without any abnormalities on ophthalmologic examination. These high-risk MRI findings consisted of chiasmatic or postchiasmatic involvement, bilateral involvement, marked tumor progression, or tumor extending beyond the optic tracts. Results showed that children with OPGs with visual anomalies prior to therapy were more likely to experience a visual decline (10/12) when compared to children treated based on imaging progression of OPGs alone (2/10) ($p < 0.012$). Since none of the children with progressive OPG who were identified solely with MRI developed vision loss, the authors concluded that screening MRIs in patients with NF1could help in detecting aggressive lesions earlier and initiate treatment in order to preserve visual outcomes.

In 2001, members of the NF France network established recommendations for the management of NF1. The authors considered that MRI for early detection of OPG in young children was a controversial issue due to the difficulty of achieving complete and reliable ophthalmologic examinations in children under 6 years of age and in children with cognitive impairment. Accordingly, they recommended systematic MRI in all newly diagnosed NF1 children under 6 years of age and/or in children with cognitive impairment (along with annual systematic ophthalmologic assessment in all NF1 children) [59]. However, in 2015, the NF France network reviewed the medical records of 306 children who were screened systematically by ophthalmologic and MRI examinations in order to determine the outcome of this screening on the therapeutic management of children with OPG. Forty-five patients had confirmed OPG (14.7%) and the majority (80%) of these patients were asymptomatic at the time of diagnosis. Progression was observed in 16 patients (35%) out of which 87% patient were managed conservatively and six children (13%) were treated with chemotherapy due to worsening visual function. All of these children had severe or mild visual impairment at the end of follow-up. The authors concluded that there was no convincing benefit of systematic MRI screening in NF1 children under 6 years old as it had no impact on therapeutic management of OPG patients since treatment was initiated only when visual acuity was decreased, and although OPG were diagnosed earlier, treatment with chemotherapy did not improve the final visual outcome. Furthermore, the majority of NF1 children who acquired OPGs did not necessitate treatment and only children who developed progressive visual deterioration required treatment. Hence, the authors concluded that the main indication for neuroimaging should be determined by yearly clinical and ophthalmological assessments. In 2016, the National Diagnosis and Treatment Protocol (NDTP) for Neurofibromatosis 1 recommended against the systematic imaging of the optic and cerebral pathways by MRI, maintaining that MRI at diagnosis in young children without symptoms was controversial, and that it should be undertaken only if an OPG is suspected [4].

Since most of the patients with incidentally discovered OPG on MRI will not experience any progression or could regress spontaneously, a potentially negative outcome of brain and orbital MRI screening is unwarranted parental anxiety and high costs associated with frequent imaging. Another drawback to screening is that clinical or radiological changes and real tumor progression were not found to be correlated. Serial alterations in visual function do not reliably identify tumor progression and conversely, radiological evidence of tumor progression does not reliably correlate with alterations of visual function [60].

The natural history of OPG is variable and unpredictable in NF1 children. In order to provide optimal care for children with NF1-associated OPG, studies have tried to define a "high-risk" population that is most likely to progress and require treatment. Some studies have suggested that the anatomic location of the OPG is an important indicator for tumor progression and need for therapy post-chiasmal involvement of OPG has been found to be associated with visual acuity loss [55]; however, this finding was not confirmed by other studies [61, 62]. Isolated prechiasmatic tumors have been found to be more indolent and more likely to regress than chiasmatic and postchiasmatic OPGs [63]. Further studies will help elucidate whether neuroimaging surveillance could be altered based on OPG location.

19.16 Management of Optic Pathway Gliomas

Once a child with NF1 develops visual symptoms or physical signs (proptosis, decreased visual acuity, or precocious puberty) or an ophthalmological abnormality is detected, MRI of the brain and orbits to investigate for an OPG is the appropriate imaging modality. There is no role for the use of visual evoked potentials in the diagnosis or follow-up of children with OPG [49].

There is little consensus regarding the surveillance of children with known OPG. The frequency of ophthalmologic examination and neuroimaging varies between 3 months and 24 months depending on the degree of visual impairment and associated symptoms, the site of the tumor, and evidence of progression [49]. National Neurofibromatosis Foundation Optic Pathway Task Force recommends ophthalmological and MRI studies every 3 months for the first year, with subsequent gradual lengthening of test intervals over the next 2–3 years [49]. Determining retinal nerve fiber thickness potentially has a role in the sensitive detection of loss of visual acuity in children with optic gliomas [64], and diffusion-weighted and dynamic contrast-enhanced imaging may be a helpful biomarker for establishing which tumors will behave aggressively and require treatment [65]. Larger prospective longitudinal studies are needed to confirm those findings.

Treatment is only necessary in the small percentage of patients who develop symptomatic tumors with clinically significant growth and progressive visual loss. Optimal management of OPGs is controversial and opinions differ regarding the timing and suitability of treatment for OPG. The NF1 Optic Pathway Task Force recommends that a two-line reduction in visual acuity, using standardized visual assessment tools such as the Snellen chart, combined with progressive changes on MRI is the principle deciding factor [49].

The first-line treatment for most patients with symptomatic OPG is chemotherapy with carboplatin and vincristine [66, 67]. It leads to radiological tumor regression and stabilization or improvement in vision in many children. Other chemotherapy combinations have been used successfully; however, further randomized control trials are needed to compare them to one another [4]. However, very few children have a normal visual acuity after treatment [49]. Furthermore, visual acuity data after chemotherapy is difficult to obtain, especially that NF1 patients are lumped together with patients with sporadic OPG, and large studies focus more on MRI outcome and as mentioned already radiographic outcomes do not necessarily correlate with visual outcomes [35]. In a multicenter retrospective study of neurofibromatosis type 1-associated optic pathway glioma treated with chemotherapy visual acuity improved in 32% of patients, remained stable in 40%, and declined 28% at completion of chemotherapy [68].

Radiotherapy treatment of OPG is not recommended for children with NF1 due to the increased likelihood of developing secondary malignancies, either gliomas or MPNST [69]; as well as developing neurovascular, endocrine, and neuropsychological problems [70, 49]. Surgery has a very limited indication in the treatment of optic pathway gliomas as it can lead to permanent neurological damage [49]. However, one can resort to surgery to treat corneal exposure or large proptosis for cosmetic reasons as well as to remove large orbital tumors with no useful vision [49]. Surgical decompression of hypothalamic or chiasmal gliomas is occasionally required especially in the context of third ventricular compression with secondary hydrocephalus [49].

19.17 Orthopedic Evaluation

19.17.1 Growth and Development

Macrocephaly affects most individuals with NF1 [71]. However, a child with an acute acceleration in head growth should be evaluated for hydrocephalus secondary to aqueductal stenosis or intracranial tumors.

All children with NF1 should have yearly measurements of weight and height plotted on standard growth charts. Short stature is found in a third of patients with NF1 and is not associated with disease severity. During childhood height-growth velocity is normal for both genders and children with NF1 grow normally until puberty after which the growth spurt is slightly reduced, attaining a mean adult height close to the 25th percentile for the general population. There are specific growth charts made especially for children with NF1 [71].

Older children should be assessed for abnormal growth acceleration or early development of secondary sexual characteristics as they may be associated with an optic glioma involving the chiasm [49]. Delayed puberty has also been frequently reported in NF1 and is seen in 20–30% of adolescents with NF1 [53].

19.17.2 Scoliosis

Scoliosis usually affects the lower cervical and upper thoracic spine and is either dystrophic or non-dystrophic with the latter being more common in patients with

NF1 [22]. Dystrophic scoliosis results from primary bone dysplasia and is usually recognizable in early childhood; it creates a sharply angulated curve that involves several vertebral bodies [72]. Scoliosis can also be due to the presence of paraspinal neurofibromas, which lead to vertebral erosion.

Scoliosis can affect 10–26% of patients with NF1. Therefore, patients with NF1 need yearly assessment of the spine during childhood and early adolescence. Patients with clinical evidence of scoliosis should have appropriate imaging and be referred to an orthopedist.

Once scoliosis is detected, unpredictability in progression makes it difficult to determine the prognosis and close monitoring is necessary. Excessive snoring and disturbed sleep can signal respiratory impairment and regular pulmonary function tests are indicated for patients with severe scoliosis. Dystrophic scoliosis usually requires corrective surgery with fusion of the abnormal vertebral bodies. This should usually be performed by surgeons familiar with NF1 as the inherent bone properties of these patients make manipulation and instrumentation challenging. Surgical intervention is usually achieved at a younger age and at smaller angles than in patients with non-dystrophic scoliosis. Expectant management or bracing to prevent progression is the usual treatment of most children with non-dystrophic scoliosis [4].

19.17.3 Osteopenia or Osteoporosis

Individuals with NF1 have an increased incidence of bone mineralization disorders (osteopenia in 48% and osteoporosis in 25% of patients with NF1). Both children and adults have a greater risk of fracture. A large registry-based study of NF1 showed that patients with NF1 had increased age-dependent fracture risk in non-dysplastic bones compared to healthy controls, with roughly fivefold increase in fracture risk in adults older than 40 years, and a threefold increase in children younger than 16 years [73]. This might be related to low vitamin D levels or deregulated osteoclast function and prophylactic measures such as lifestyle modifications should be indicated in these patients.

Clinicians should therefore be cautious about the possibility of osteoporosis and have a low threshold for performing dual-energy X-ray absorptiometry (DXA) scans. Identifying osteoporosis early in patients with NF1 allows for more timely and optimal management to prevent significant morbidity related to increased fracture risk.

Low concentrations of vitamin D have been found in patients with NF1. In a retrospective study vitamin D supplementation improved the bone mineral density significantly in adult NF1 patients [74].

19.17.4 Tibial Dysplasia

Congenital tibial dysplasia is characterized by congenital anterolateral bowing of the lower leg on plain radiographs. The presence of bowing in an infant requires prompt radiographic assessment and referral to an orthopedic surgeon familiar with the management of NFl-related orthopedic problems in children. Bowing of long bones leads to visible deformity and fragile bone that is susceptible to fracture [73]. Prevention of fracture is crucial in affected patients and bracing is recommended to prevent bone fracture.

Repeated fractures with failure to heal can lead to development of pseudarthrosis (failure of primary union of the separate bone ends can create a false joint) and sometimes limb amputation is the only option left. Prompt referral to a skilled pediatric orthopedic surgeon is warranted to start appropriate treatment and prevent this bad outcome.

19.17.5 Sphenoid Wing Dysplasia

The sphenoid bones consist of multiple ossification centers that fuse to become the important elements of the orbits. Around 5% of patients with NF1 have sphenoid wing dysplasia, and it is often unilateral. Sometimes, thinning or absence of the sphenoid wing is secondary to the existence of an associated orbital plexiform neurofibroma. The deformity can lead to proptosis, and around half of patients with NF1 with sphenoid wing dysplasia will manifest ipsilateral temporal-orbital plexiform neurofibroma [22]. Patients with sphenoid wing dysplasia can also develop pulsating exophthalmus without visual loss, and absence of sphenoid wing can lead to herniation of the temporal lobe into the orbit [43]. Surgical correction is occasionally indicated for cosmetic purposes but should be carried out by cranio-facial teams familiar with the surgical management of NF1 individuals.

19.17.6 Nonossifying Fibromas

Nonossifying fibromas of the long bones, mostly the distal femur and proximal tibia, might occur infrequently in adolescence or adulthood and may lead to fracture. It has been suggested to obtain screening radiograph of both knees in early adolescence as a routine study to deliver early appropriate intervention [75]. However, at present there is not enough evidence to support routine screening.

19.17.7 Cardiovascular Evaluation

Patients with NF1 can develop a variety of cardiovascular manifestations.

Vasculopathy is a common finding in NF1 patients and can affect any arterial vessel, leading to cerebrovascular events, renal artery stenosis, or peripheral vascular insufficiency. One of the potentially serious manifestation of NF1 is cerebrovascular disease which presents as stenosis or occlusion of the internal carotid, middle cerebral and anterior cerebral arteries, moyamoya disease, and aneurysm formation. Although cerebrovascular disease is commonly mentioned as a cause of early death in NF1, this was not found in large NF1 study in the USA [76].

Congenital heart disease, especially pulmonary stenosis, is observed in patients with NF1 [77]. A thorough physical examination of the heart should be performed and if any murmur is found, the child should be referred to a pediatric cardiologist [77].

Hypertension is a common finding in adults with NF1 and may first appear during childhood, and it is significantly associated with mortality [77]. Although essential hypertension is the most common cause of hypertension in NF1, it can also result from renovascular disease, paragangliomas, pheochromocytoma, and coarctation of the aorta. Blood pressure should thus be evaluated at least annually in patients with NF1, and evaluation of renovascular causes should be initiated in children with NF1 and hypertension. Renovascular hypertension is less likely in older NF1 patients but this possibility should still be entertained if an upper abdominal bruit is heard or if the hypertension is severe or refractory to treatment. Appropriate imaging studies such as CT angiography of the renal arteries or arteriography must be performed in NF1 patients with hypertension; laboratory evaluations should include serum creatinine and electrolytes, plasma renin, and urinalysis. These vascular malformations may recur after revascularization and long-term monitoring is therefore required in affected patients [4].

Clinicians should consider evaluation for paragangliomas and pheochromocytoma in all NF1 patients with symptoms of catecholamine excess (sweating, palpitations, headache) and classically labile hypertension and/or hypertension refractory to standard treatment [4]. It usually presents in adult NF1 patients with a mean age at presentation of 42 years of age [78]. The diagnosis of pheochromocytoma and paraganglioma is based on the plasma and/or urinary free metanephrine levels and abdominal imaging. Any increase in metanephrine levels should prompt referral for imaging with MRI or CT scans exploring the adrenal areas. F-DOPA PET may be useful for detecting extra-abdominal paragangliomas, when available, but functional imaging using 123I-tagged metaiodobenzylguanidine may also prove to be useful [78]. Treatment involves alpha and beta blockade before surgery.

Although pheochromocytomas are rare in individuals with NF1, one series demonstrated frequent simultaneous occurrence of gastrointestinal stromal tumors (GIST) and pheochromocytoma in one series, advocating that patients should be screened first for pheochromocytoma before undergoing surgical procedures for a GIST as an undiagnosed pheochromocytoma could be a potential life-threatening cardiovascular complication during surgery [79]. Moreover, physicians should be on the lookout for any sign or symptoms of a carcinoid tumor as an association has been identified in NF1 patients between the presence of pheochromocytomas and carcinoid tumors.

19.18 Neurological Evaluation

Neurofibromatosis can have an important impact on the central nervous system. The most common neurological complication is mild cognitive impairment [80]. Epilepsy, cerebrovascular disease, and multiple sclerosis occur with increased frequency in NF1 and necessitate referral to a specialist for management.

Neurological complications develop from tumors of the central and peripheral nervous system as well as malformations which include aqueduct stenosis [22]. Sphenoid wing dysplasia can be complicated by temporal lobe herniation into the orbit with resulting pulsating exophthalmos [22]. Severe scoliosis can lead to spine deformities with resulting cord compression and respiratory insufficiency [22]. Neurofibromas can lead to neurological sequalae due to peripheral nerve, spinal nerve root, and cord compression.

Children with NF1 should be monitored for developmental progress and should undergo neurological and psychological screening evaluations early in life (as early as possible and definitely before school), followed by more elaborate testing when appropriate [81]. Neurological examination should be performed during the annual assessment and a developmental history should be obtained. Any unexplained neurological signs and symptoms should prompt a referral to a neurologist. Morning vomiting, headaches on waking, and altered consciousness are indicative of increased intracranial pressure and should be dealt with urgently. Patients with NF1 who develop acute or progressive sensory disturbance, motor deficit, incoordination, or sphincter disturbance should consult urgently to rule out intracranial lesion or spinal cord compression. Parents should be asked about progress at school along with enquiries about the child's distractibility and ability to focus on an activity, sleep patterns, social interaction, and fine and gross motor skills.

Neuroimaging such as brain MRI should only be performed to evaluate specific neurologic deficits, and should not be part of a routine diagnostic evaluation.

19.18.1 Cognitive Impairment

Neurocognitive impairment is among the most common manifestations of NF1, with an average IQ in the low average range (88–94), behavioral problems, and specific learning difficulties [80]. These learning difficulties include visuospatial and visuomotor impairments, language disorders, and fine and gross motor impairments. Attention-deficit hyperactivity disorder, behavioral abnormalities, autism spectrum disorders, and psychosocial problems are also features encountered in patients with NF1 [82].

Any delay in psychomotor and/or language development should lead the clinician to refer the child for early management by an appropriate professional. Recognizing learning and behavioral disabilities in children early is important to facilitate intervention in a timely fashion. Children with NF1-associated cognitive impairment might benefit from an individually tailored learning support and multidisciplinary approach, in which educational psychologists, pediatric neuropsychologists, speech therapists, physical therapists, and occupational therapists join forces to enhance the child's abilities and optimize their academic and social progress. Close communication between teachers, pediatricians, occupational therapists, and educational psychologists contributes to the optimal assessment of the child with NF1 with the appropriate remedial support. Attention-deficit disorder can be well managed with methylphenidate, and cognitive behavioral therapy can be helpful [83]. Adult individuals with NF1 have literacy and numeracy problems as well as social difficulties [84].

A preclinical trial using a mouse model of NF1 with learning deficits demonstrated that the deficits in neuronal plasticity as well as the spatial and attention impairments are due to increased RAS/ERK (rat sarcoma viral oncogene homolog/extracellular signal-regulated kinase) signaling. Subsequently, treatment with 3-hydroxy-3-methylglutaryl coenzyme A (HMG-COA) reductase inhibitors reversed these deficits in those mice [85]. In the first randomized, controlled 12-week trial of statins in 62 children aged 8–16 years with NF1, simvastatin did not improve cognitive function [86]. A following study with a longer duration of treatment (12 months) likewise did not demonstrate an improvement in cognitive function [87]. A phase-I study of lovastatin in 24 children with NF1 and learning disabilities showed improvements in verbal and nonverbal memory and visual attention and efficiency [88]; however, the phase-II trial did not reveal benefits after 16 weeks of treatment with lovastatin on cognitive functioning [89]. At present, there is not enough evidence to justify the use of statins in the treatment of cognitive impairment in NF1 individuals. An ongoing clinical trial is currently assessing the use of lamotrigine on cognition in NF1 (NCT02256124).

19.19 Epilepsy

Compared to the general population, seizures are more common in individuals with NF1. It occurs in 4–13% of NF1 patients and could possibly be due to an underlying cortical dysgenesis or intracranial structural lesions [90, 91]. The onset of epilepsy has been reported to range from infancy to late middle age [90]. It is often mild and not correlated with the severity of the disease [90]. All seizure types are encountered but focal seizures are predominant [90]. Focal seizures may be due to an intracranial neoplasm [91]. Thus, the onset of seizures should lead to systematic neuroimaging searching for a lesion of the central nervous system (tumors, aqueduct stenosis, vasculopathy). Patients with epilepsy associated with intracranial structural lesions should therefore undergo appropriate evaluation to assess whether surgical excision is possible as it can be a potential cure.

Management of NF1-related epilepsy is similar to that in the general population, and outcomes of epilepsy associated with NF1 seem to be better than other neurocutaneous disorders [90, 91]. Levetiracetam may cause worsening of behavior in patients with cognitive impairment [92]. In almost 30% of cases, epilepsy is resistant to treatment and associated with severe mental retardation [90].

19.20 Oncologic Evaluation

Malignancies are the leading cause of death in NF1 [1, 4]. Many malignancies occur more commonly in individuals with NF1 patients as compared to the general population, often occurring at an earlier age and with variable prognoses. There is up to a fivefold increase in cancer incidence in the NF1 population and the lifetime cancer risk for patients with NF1 was estimated to be 59.6% in a Finnish cancer registry study [93]. The most common malignancies associated with NF1 are intracranial gliomas and MPNST. CNS tumors occur in approximately 20% of patients with NF1 and are usually detected in early childhood [1].

A study on NF1 patients in England showed an increased relative risk (4.3) of cancer development for all cancers, and risks were significantly high for cancer of the esophagus (3.3), stomach (2.8), colon (2.0), liver (3.8), lung (3.0), bone (19.6), thyroid (4.9), malignant melanoma (3.6), non-Hodgkin's lymphoma (3.3), chronic myeloid leukemia (6.7), female breast (2.3), and ovary (3.7) [94]. Other studies have shown up to a fivefold increase in the risk for breast cancer in patients with NF1, mainly occurring in women younger than 50 years, with mortality rates higher than those for women with breast cancer in the general population [4]. Based on the increased risk of early-onset breast cancer in female patients with NF1, annual breast screening with mammography should begin at the age of 30 years [95]. Screening with breast MRI could also be considered. As of age 50 years, breast cancer risk in women with NF1 may not significantly differ from that of women in the general population; therefore, breast MRI screening in individuals with NF1 may be stopped at the age of 50 years. Risk-reducing mastectomy is not recommended in patients with NF1 as there are no data regarding their benefit; but it may be considered based on family history. Treatment of NF1-associated breast cancer is similar to that of breast cancer in the general population.

Patients with NF1 are also at an increased risk of developing gastrointestinal stromal tumors (GIST). In patients with NF1, GIST tend to occur at an earlier age, are often multiple, and frequently occur in the small intestine [96]. These do not harbor the mutations in *KIT* and *PDGFRA*, which are typically associated with sporadic GIST. These tumors are therefore poorly responsive to the tyrosine kinase inhibitor imatinib, although sunitinib, another tyrosine kinase receptor inhibitor, could be useful in metastatic disease.

Carcinoid tumors are neuroendocrine tumors that originate from endocrine cells within the gastrointestinal tract and have also been reported in patients with NF1 [97]. As mentioned previously, an association has been identified in NF1 patients between the presence of pheochromocytomas and carcinoid tumors [98].

Children with NF1 are predisposed to the development of juvenile myelomonocytic leukemia and juvenile chronic myelogenous leukemia, as well as acute lymphocytic leukemia, and non-Hodgkin lymphoma. Treatment does not differ from that for individuals without NF1.

Rhabdomyosarcomas are non-neurogenic sarcomas and are more frequently found in children with NF1 than in the general population. It tends to occur at an early age and often arises in a genitourinary site that presents clinically as palpable masses. Management is usually surgical resection when possible, with radiation therapy and adjuvant chemotherapy reserved for select patients.

Given the higher risk of neoplasia in NF1 patients, thorough clinical examination should be performed regularly, at each visit, with referral to appropriate specialists and oncologists when needed.

Patients with NF1 should follow the same screening guidelines as those for the general population [4]. However, since in the setting of NF1 breast cancer occurs in women younger than 50 years, it has been suggested that women with NF1 should undergo regular mammography-based screening starting at the age of 30 years; however, large prospective studies are needed in order to construct formal recommendations for this special population.

19.21 Pain Evaluation

With a prevalence of 7%, pain is a very common reason for consultation [4]. The physical manifestations of NF1 such as nodular neurofibromas (subcutaneous or internal), plexiform neurofibromas, and skeletal deformations can all cause chronic pain. At each visit, patients should be asked, particularly in adolescence, about any change in pain associated with a preexisting plexiform neurofibroma to evaluate for a possible malignant transformation into a MPNST. More frequent pain leads to functional disability, and higher pain interference in daily activities is associated with poorer overall QOL [99, 100]. Pain control in patients with NF1 follows the pain management guidelines whereby drugs from different steps of the "pain ladder" should be prescribed after assessing the severity of nociceptive pain. Antidepressants or antiepileptic agents are the preferred agents for neuropathic pain. Complementary nonpharmacological therapy, such as physiotherapy, occupational therapy, and functional rehabilitation, should also be offered to patients.

19.22 Quality of Life Evaluation

The quality of life (QOL) of NF1 patients is often impaired, even if the disease is very mild or the affected area is very small [4].

In children and adolescents with NF1, studies consistently report a decreased QOL as compared to population norms, with parent-reported ratings lower than child self-report. Factors attributed to poorer QOL in children are: greater disease severity, orthopedic manifestations, learning disabilities, and plexiform neurofibromas. Pain interferes with daily functioning in the majority of NF1 patients, which in turn is associated with poorer QOL. Cognitive impairments in patients with NF1 are also associated with poorer QOL.

In adults with NF1, studies have also reported a decreased QOL relative to population norms. Body image is an important link between disease visibility and psychological well-being and higher self-perceived disease visibility is related to decreased QOL. More severe complications of NF1, older age, worse headache, worse health, and poorer health are all associated with poorer QOL. Furthermore, depressive symptoms are frequently found in patients with NF1 and strongly impact the overall QOL.

INF1-QOL is another reliable validated and disease specific questionnaire that correlates moderately well with disease severity as it covers a wide range of themes representative of NF1 manifestations. Its main advantage relies in the fact that is quick and simple to complete [4].

Disease acceptance and self-esteem preservation vary considerably between individuals. Making assumptions about the psychological impact of NF1 on a particular patient is difficult, and QOL evaluations should therefore be systematic and regularly repeated.

19.23 Evaluation of Physical and Psychological Impact

Assessing the physical and psychological impacts of the disease on patients with NF1 is important and helps improve their management and referral to specialist teams. This evaluation can be performed using scales that are not specific for NF1.

The Riccardi's severity index is used to determine the severity of NF1 according to the degree of cutaneous involvement and disabling complications. Ablon's visibility index can be used to grade the cosmetic disfigurement of NF1.

The doctor–patient relationship is of paramount in assessing the physical and psychological impact. Self-assessment scales such as the Skindex, SF-36 (Short Form 36 health survey), Children's Dermatology Life Quality Index (CDLQI) and DISABKIDS, and PedsQL™ Neurofibromatosis Module are useful tools.

19.24 Psychological Support

Psychological support can be offered to patients and their families at diagnosis as well as throughout the management of patients with NF1. The chronic pain, esthetic complications of the disease, the cognitive impairment and learning disabilities, pregnancy planning, and the complex and unpredictable nature of neurofibromatosis may all lead to psychological distress (anxiety, social isolation, decreased self-esteem) with a negative impact on relationships and functionality. As patients are often unwilling to raise these issues, the physician should evaluate systematically the need for psychological support for patients and their families and offer it if required.

19.25 Social Support

Social support should be offered to patients and their families, along with assistance and guidance through the various fields of social intervention: coping with disability, dealing with social deprivation, obtaining social security rights, workforce integration, home support, school placement, among others. The social support should take into account the medical, psychological, and environmental impacts on individuals with NF1, to ensure the best possible outcome. This social management implicates multidisciplinary teams, third parties, and external partners.

In summary, given the complexity of this disorder, the management of children and adults with NF1 requires the access to the full complement of health care providers. Coordination among the multiple specialties is crucial. Lifetime monitoring is recommended as soon as the diagnosis of NF1 is suspected; however, the modalities and frequency of disease surveillance should be carefully weighed against the risk of eliciting unnecessary parental and patient anxiety.

Given the heterogeneity in the clinical picture, management of NF1 differs greatly depending on whether patients belong to the uncomplicated group or complex group. Patients who lack the serious complications can be followed up regularly by their local clinicians in partnership with lay organizations in a clinical setup focused on diagnosis, genetic counseling, education, monitoring of blood pressure, bone health, and neurofibromas. Conversely, patients with complex NF1 need to be followed closely within a specialized referral center by a multidisciplinary team of caregivers familiar with the diagnosis and management of rare and unusual complications of NF1, as well as with the development of new treatments. Further studies should hopefully help elucidate optimal strategies for disease surveillance. Furthermore, new insights into the molecular pathogenesis of NF1 and the development of accurate preclinical models of NF1-associated malignant disease in genetically engineered mice have set the stage to conceive rational biologically informed, molecular-targeted drugs.

References

1. Duong TA, Sbidian E, Valeyrie-Allanore L, Vialette C, Ferkal S, Hadj-Rabia S, et al. Mortality associated with neurofibromatosis 1: a cohort study of 1895 patients in 1980-2006 in France. Orphanet J Rare Dis. 2011;6:18. https://doi.org/10.1186/1750-1172-6-18.
2. Wolkenstein P, Freche B, Zeller J, Revuz J. Usefulness of screening investigations in neurofibromatosis type 1. A study of 152 patients. Arch Dermatol. 1996;132(11):1333–6.
3. Sbidian E, Bastuji-Garin S, Valeyrie-Allanore L, Ferkal S, Lefaucheur JP, Drouet A, et al. At-risk phenotype of neurofibromatose-1 patients: a multicentre case-control study. Orphanet J Rare Dis. 2011;6:51. https://doi.org/10.1186/1750-1172-6-51.
4. Bergqvist C, Servy A, Valeyrie-Allanore L, Ferkal S, Combemale P, Wolkenstein P, et al. Neurofibromatosis 1 French national guidelines based on an extensive literature review since 1966. Orphanet J Rare Dis. 2020;15(1):37. https://doi.org/10.1186/s13023-020-1310-3.
5. Neurofibromatosis. Conference statement. National Institutes of Health Consensus Development Conference. Arch Neurol. 1988;45(5):575–8.
6. DeBella K, Szudek J, Friedman JM. Use of the national institutes of health criteria for diagnosis of neurofibromatosis 1 in children. Pediatrics. 2000;105(3 Pt 1):608–14.
7. Evans DG, Bowers N, Burkitt-Wright E, Miles E, Garg S, Scott-Kitching V, et al. Comprehensive RNA analysis of the NF1 gene in classically affected NF1 affected individuals meeting NIH criteria has high sensitivity and mutation negative testing is reassuring in isolated cases with pigmentary features only. EBioMedicine. 2016;7:212–20. https://doi.org/10.1016/j.ebiom.2016.04.005.
8. Sabbagh A, Pasmant E, Imbard A, Luscan A, Soares M, Blanche H, et al. NF1 molecular characterization and neurofibromatosis type I genotype-phenotype correlation: the French experience. Hum Mutat. 2013;34(11):1510–8. https://doi.org/10.1002/humu.22392.
9. Pasmant E, Parfait B, Luscan A, Goussard P, Briand-Suleau A, Laurendeau I, et al. Neurofibromatosis type 1 molecular diagnosis: what can NGS do for you when you have a

large gene with loss of function mutations? Eur J Hum Genet. 2015;23(5):596–601. https://doi.org/10.1038/ejhg.2014.145.
10. Pasmant E, Vidaud M, Vidaud D, Wolkenstein P. Neurofibromatosis type 1: from genotype to phenotype. J Med Genet. 2012;49(8):483–9. https://doi.org/10.1136/jmedgenet-2012-100978.
11. De Raedt T, Brems H, Wolkenstein P, Vidaud D, Pilotti S, Perrone F, et al. Elevated risk for MPNST in NF1 microdeletion patients. Am J Hum Genet. 2003;72(5):1288–92.
12. Ruggieri M, Huson SM. The clinical and diagnostic implications of mosaicism in the neurofibromatoses. Neurology. 2001;56(11):1433–43.
13. Ferner RE, Huson SM, Thomas N, Moss C, Willshaw H, Evans DG, et al. Guidelines for the diagnosis and management of individuals with neurofibromatosis 1. J Med Genet. 2007;44(2):81–8. https://doi.org/10.1136/jmg.2006.045906.
14. Belkin DA, Neckman JP, Jeon H, Friedman P, Geronemus RG. Response to laser treatment of café au lait macules based on morphologic features. JAMA Dermatol. 2017;153(11):1158–61. https://doi.org/10.1001/jamadermatol.2017.2807.
15. Huson SM, Compston DA, Clark P, Harper PS. A genetic study of von Recklinghausen neurofibromatosis in south East Wales. I. Prevalence, fitness, mutation rate, and effect of parental transmission on severity. J Med Genet. 1989;26(11):704–11.
16. Mautner V-F, Asuagbor FA, Dombi E, Fünsterer C, Kluwe L, Wenzel R, et al. Assessment of benign tumor burden by whole-body MRI in patients with neurofibromatosis 1. Neuro-Oncology. 2008;10(4):593–8. https://doi.org/10.1215/15228517-2008-011.
17. Dombi E, Solomon J, Gillespie AJ, Fox E, Balis FM, Patronas N, et al. NF1 plexiform neurofibroma growth rate by volumetric MRI: relationship to age and body weight. Neurology. 2007;68(9):643–7. https://doi.org/10.1212/01.wnl.0000250332.89420.e6.
18. Dombi E, Baldwin A, Marcus LJ, Fisher MJ, Weiss B, Kim A, et al. Activity of selumetinib in neurofibromatosis type 1-related plexiform neurofibromas. N Engl J Med. 2016;375(26):2550–60. https://doi.org/10.1056/NEJMoa1605943.
19. Fenot M, Stalder J-F, Barbarot S. Juvenile xanthogranulomas are highly prevalent but transient in young children with neurofibromatosis type 1. J Am Acad Dermatol. 2014;71(2):389–90. https://doi.org/10.1016/j.jaad.2014.02.049.
20. Cambiaghi S, Restano L, Caputo R. Juvenile xanthogranuloma associated with neurofibromatosis 1: 14 patients without evidence of hematologic malignancies. Pediatr Dermatol. 2004;21(2):97–101. https://doi.org/10.1111/j.0736-8046.2004.21201.x.
21. Burgdorf WH, Zelger B. JXG, NF1, and JMML: alphabet soup or a clinical issue? Pediatr Dermatol. 2004;21(2):174–6. https://doi.org/10.1111/j.0736-8046.2004.21219.x.
22. Korf BR. Diagnostic outcome in children with multiple cafe au lait spots. Pediatrics. 1992;90(6):924–7.
23. Korf BR. Plexiform neurofibromas. Am J Med Genet. 1999;89(1):31–7.
24. Riccardi VM. Mast-cell stabilization to decrease neurofibroma growth. Preliminary experience with ketotifen. Arch Dermatol. 1987;123(8):1011–6.
25. Moreno JC, Mathoret C, Lantieri L, Zeller J, Revuz J, Wolkenstein P. Carbon dioxide laser for removal of multiple cutaneous neurofibromas. Br J Dermatol. 2001;144(5):1096–8.
26. Lutterodt CG, Mohan A, Kirkpatrick N. The use of electrodessication in the treatment of cutaneous neurofibromatosis: a retrospective patient satisfaction outcome assessment. J Plast Reconstr Aesthet Surg. 2016;69(6):765–9. https://doi.org/10.1016/j.bjps.2016.03.024.
27. Tucker T, Wolkenstein P, Revuz J, Zeller J, Friedman JM. Association between benign and malignant peripheral nerve sheath tumors in NF1. Neurology. 2005;65(2):205–11. https://doi.org/10.1212/01.wnl.0000168830.79997.13.
28. Leonard JR, Ferner RE, Thomas N, Gutmann DH. Cervical cord compression from plexiform neurofibromas in neurofibromatosis 1. J Neurol Neurosurg Psychiatry. 2007;78(12):1404–6. https://doi.org/10.1136/jnnp.2007.121509.
29. Ferner RE, Gutmann DH. International consensus statement on malignant peripheral nerve sheath tumors in neurofibromatosis. Cancer Res. 2002;62(5):1573–7.
30. Ducatman BS, Scheithauer BW, Piepgras DG, Reiman HM, Ilstrup DM. Malignant peripheral nerve sheath tumors. A clinicopathologic study of 120 cases. Cancer. 1986;57(10):2006–21.

31. Ferner RE, Golding JF, Smith M, Calonje E, Jan W, Sanjayanathan V, et al. [18F]2-fluoro-2-deoxy-D-glucose positron emission tomography (FDG PET) as a diagnostic tool for neurofibromatosis 1 (NF1) associated malignant peripheral nerve sheath tumours (MPNSTs): a long-term clinical study. Ann Oncol. 2008;19(2):390–4. https://doi.org/10.1093/annonc/mdm450.
32. Warbey VS, Ferner RE, Dunn JT, Calonje E, O'Doherty MJ. [18F]FDG PET/CT in the diagnosis of malignant peripheral nerve sheath tumours in neurofibromatosis type-1. Eur J Nucl Med Mol Imaging. 2009;36(5):751–7. https://doi.org/10.1007/s00259-008-1038-0.
33. Bredella MA, Torriani M, Hornicek F, Ouellette HA, Plamer WE, Williams Z, et al. Value of PET in the assessment of patients with neurofibromatosis type 1. AJR Am J Roentgenol. 2007;189(4):928–35. https://doi.org/10.2214/ajr.07.2060.
34. Dunn GP, Spiliopoulos K, Plotkin SR, Hornicek FJ, Harmon DC, Delaney TF, et al. Role of resection of malignant peripheral nerve sheath tumors in patients with neurofibromatosis type 1. J Neurosurg. 2013;118(1):142–8. https://doi.org/10.3171/2012.9.jns101610.
35. Ferner RE, Gutmann DH. Neurofibromatosis type 1 (NF1): diagnosis and management. Handb Clin Neurol. 2013;115:939–55. https://doi.org/10.1016/b978-0-444-52902-2.00053-9.
36. Kumar MG, Emnett RJ, Bayliss SJ, Gutmann DH. Glomus tumors in individuals with neurofibromatosis type 1. J Am Acad Dermatol. 2014;71(1):44–8. https://doi.org/10.1016/j.jaad.2014.01.913.
37. Harrison B, Moore AM, Calfee R, Sammer DM. The association between glomus tumors and neurofibromatosis. J Hand Surg Am. 2013;38(8):1571–4. https://doi.org/10.1016/j.jhsa.2013.05.025.
38. Wertelecki W, Superneau DW, Forehand LW, Hoff CJ. Angiomas and von Recklinghausen neurofibromatosis. Neurofibromatosis. 1988;1(3):137–45.
39. Sbidian E, Wolkenstein P, Valeyrie-Allanore L, Rodriguez D, Hadj-Rabia S, Ferkal S, et al. NF-1Score: a prediction score for internal neurofibromas in neurofibromatosis-1. J Invest Dermatol. 2010;130(9):2173–8. https://doi.org/10.1038/jid.2010.100.
40. Ferner RE, Huson SM. Management and treatment of "complex neurofibromatosis 1". In: Upadhyaya M, Cooper DN, editors. Neurofibromatosis type 1: molecular and cellular biology. Berlin: Springer; 2012. p. 31–45.
41. Viola F, Villani E, Natacci F, Selicorni A, Melloni G, Vezzola D, et al. Choroidal abnormalities detected by near-infrared reflectance imaging as a new diagnostic criterion for neurofibromatosis 1. Ophthalmology. 2012;119(2):369–75. https://doi.org/10.1016/j.ophtha.2011.07.046.
42. Muci-Mendoza R, Ramella M, Fuenmayor-Rivera D. Corkscrew retinal vessels in neurofibromatosis type 1: report of 12 cases. Br J Ophthalmol. 2002;86(3):282–4.
43. Ferner RE. Neurofibromatosis 1 and neurofibromatosis 2: a twenty first century perspective. Lancet Neurol. 2007;6(4):340–51. https://doi.org/10.1016/s1474-4422(07)70075-3.
44. Listernick R, Charrow J, Greenwald M, Mets M. Natural history of optic pathway tumors in children with neurofibromatosis type 1: a longitudinal study. J Pediatr. 1994;125(1):63–6.
45. Listernick R, Charrow J, Greenwald MJ, Esterly NB. Optic gliomas in children with neurofibromatosis type 1. J Pediatr. 1989;114(5):788–92.
46. Taylor T, Jaspan T, Milano G, Gregson R, Parker T, Ritzmann T, et al. Radiological classification of optic pathway gliomas: experience of a modified functional classification system. Br J Radiol. 2008;81(970):761–6. https://doi.org/10.1259/bjr/65246351.
47. Laue L, Comite F, Hench K, Loriaux DL, Cutler GB Jr, Pescovitz OH. Precocious puberty associated with neurofibromatosis and optic gliomas. Treatment with luteinizing hormone releasing hormone analogue. Am J Dis Child (1960). 1985;139(11):1097–100.
48. Blazo MA, Lewis RA, Chintagumpala MM, Frazier M, McCluggage C, Plon SE. Outcomes of systematic screening for optic pathway tumors in children with neurofibromatosis type 1. Am J Med Genet A. 2004;127a(3):224–9. https://doi.org/10.1002/ajmg.a.20650.
49. Listernick R, Ferner RE, Liu GT, Gutmann DH. Optic pathway gliomas in neurofibromatosis-1: controversies and recommendations. Ann Neurol. 2007;61(3):189–98. https://doi.org/10.1002/ana.21107.

50. Diggs-Andrews KA, Brown JA, Gianino SM, Rubin JB, Wozniak DF, Gutmann DH. Sex is a major determinant of neuronal dysfunction in neurofibromatosis type 1. Ann Neurol. 2014;75(2):309–16. https://doi.org/10.1002/ana.24093.
51. Listernick R, Ferner RE, Piersall L, Sharif S, Gutmann DH, Charrow J. Late-onset optic pathway tumors in children with neurofibromatosis 1. Neurology. 2004;63(10):1944–6.
52. Listernick R, Louis DN, Packer RJ, Gutmann DH. Optic pathway gliomas in children with neurofibromatosis 1: consensus statement from the NF1 optic pathway glioma task force. Ann Neurol. 1997;41(2):143–9. https://doi.org/10.1002/ana.410410204.
53. Centre de référence labellisé neurofibromatoses, Protocole National de Diagnostic et de Soins (PNDS) Neurofibromatose 1. 2016. http://www.orpha.net/data/patho/PNDS/Neurofibromatose_type_1_FR_fr_PNDS.pdf, Last access April 15, 2020.
54. Listernick R, Charrow J, Greenwald M. Emergence of optic pathway gliomas in children with neurofibromatosis type 1 after normal neuroimaging results. J Pediatr. 1992;121(4):584–7.
55. King A, Listernick R, Charrow J, Piersall L, Gutmann DH. Optic pathway gliomas in neurofibromatosis type 1: the effect of presenting symptoms on outcome. Am J Med Genet A. 2003;122a(2):95–9. https://doi.org/10.1002/ajmg.a.20211.
56. Blanchard G, Lafforgue MP, Lion-Francois L, Kemlin I, Rodriguez D, Castelnau P, et al. Systematic MRI in NF1 children under six years of age for the diagnosis of optic pathway gliomas. Study and outcome of a French cohort. Eur J Paediatr Neurol. 2016;20(2):275–81. https://doi.org/10.1016/j.ejpn.2015.12.002.
57. Listernick R, Charrow J. Knowledge without truth: screening for complications of neurofibromatosis type 1 in childhood. Am J Med Genet Part A. 2004;127a(3):221–3. https://doi.org/10.1002/ajmg.a.20654.
58. Millichap JG. MRI Screening for Optic Gliomas in Neurofibromatosis Type 1. Pediatr Neurol Briefs. 2015;29(9):72. https://doi.org/10.15844/pedneurbriefs-29-9-7.
59. Pinson S, Creange A, Barbarot S, Stalder JF, Chaix Y, Rodriguez D, et al. Neurofibromatosis 1: recommendations for management. Annales de dermatologie et de venereologie. 2001;128(4):567–75.
60. Kelly JP, Weiss AH. Detection of tumor progression in optic pathway glioma with and without neurofibromatosis type 1. Neuro-Oncology. 2013;15(11):1560–7. https://doi.org/10.1093/neuonc/not120.
61. Segal L, Darvish-Zargar M, Dilenge ME, Ortenberg J, Polomeno RC. Optic pathway gliomas in patients with neurofibromatosis type 1: follow-up of 44 patients. J AAPOS. 2010;14(2):155–8. https://doi.org/10.1016/j.jaapos.2009.11.020.
62. Opocher E, Kremer LC, Da Dalt L, van de Wetering MD, Viscardi E, Caron HN, et al. Prognostic factors for progression of childhood optic pathway glioma: a systematic review. Eur J Cancer (Oxford, England: 1990). 2006;42(12):1807–16. https://doi.org/10.1016/j.ejca.2006.02.022.
63. Prada CE, Hufnagel RB, Hummel TR, Lovell AM, Hopkin RJ, Saal HM, et al. The Use of Magnetic Resonance Imaging Screening for Optic Pathway Gliomas in Children with Neurofibromatosis Type 1. J Pediatr. 2015;167(4):851–6.e1. https://doi.org/10.1016/j.jpeds.2015.07.001.
64. Avery RA, Liu GT, Fisher MJ, Quinn GE, Belasco JB, Phillips PC, et al. Retinal nerve fiber layer thickness in children with optic pathway gliomas. Am J Ophthalmol. 2011;151(3):542–9.e2. https://doi.org/10.1016/j.ajo.2010.08.046.
65. Jost SC, Ackerman JW, Garbow JR, Manwaring LP, Gutmann DH, McKinstry RC. Diffusion-weighted and dynamic contrast-enhanced imaging as markers of clinical behavior in children with optic pathway glioma. Pediatr Radiol. 2008;38(12):1293–9. https://doi.org/10.1007/s00247-008-1003-x.
66. Packer RJ, Ater J, Allen J, Phillips P, Geyer R, Nicholson HS, et al. Carboplatin and vincristine chemotherapy for children with newly diagnosed progressive low-grade gliomas. J Neurosurg. 1997;86(5):747–54. https://doi.org/10.3171/jns.1997.86.5.0747.
67. Jahraus CD, Tarbell NJ. Optic pathway gliomas. Pediatr Blood Cancer. 2006;46(5):586–96. https://doi.org/10.1002/pbc.20655.

68. Fisher MJ, Loguidice M, Gutmann DH, Listernick R, Ferner RE, Ullrich NJ, et al. Visual outcomes in children with neurofibromatosis type 1-associated optic pathway glioma following chemotherapy: a multicenter retrospective analysis. Neuro-Oncology. 2012;14(6):790–7. https://doi.org/10.1093/neuonc/nos076.
69. Sharif S, Ferner R, Birch JM, Gillespie JE, Gattamaneni HR, Baser ME, et al. Second primary tumors in neurofibromatosis 1 patients treated for optic glioma: substantial risks after radiotherapy. J Clin Oncol. 2006;24(16):2570–5. https://doi.org/10.1200/jco.2005.03.8349.
70. Oh KS, Hung J, Robertson PL, Garton HJ, Muraszko KM, Sandler HM, et al. Outcomes of multidisciplinary management in pediatric low-grade gliomas. Int J Radiat Oncol Biol Phys. 2011;81(4):e481–8. https://doi.org/10.1016/j.ijrobp.2011.01.019.
71. Clementi M, Milani S, Mammi I, Boni S, Monciotti C, Tenconi R. Neurofibromatosis type 1 growth charts. Am J Med Genet. 1999;87(4):317–23.
72. Crawford AH, Herrera-Soto J. Scoliosis associated with neurofibromatosis. Orthop Clin North Am. 2007;38(4):553–62,. vii. https://doi.org/10.1016/j.ocl.2007.03.008.
73. Heerva E, Koffert A, Jokinen E, Kuorilehto T, Peltonen S, Aro HT, et al. A controlled register-based study of 460 neurofibromatosis 1 patients: increased fracture risk in children and adults over 41 years of age. J Bone Miner Res. 2012;27(11):2333–7. https://doi.org/10.1002/jbmr.1685.
74. Schnabel C, Jett K, Friedman JM, Frieling I, Kruse HP, Mautner V. Effect of vitamin D3 treatment on bone density in neurofibromatosis 1 patients: a retrospective clinical study. Joint Bone Spine. 2013;80(3):315–9. https://doi.org/10.1016/j.jbspin.2012.07.010.
75. Colby RS, Saul RA. Is Jaffe-Campanacci syndrome just a manifestation of neurofibromatosis type 1? Am J Med Genet A. 2003;123a(1):60–3. https://doi.org/10.1002/ajmg.a.20490.
76. Rasmussen SA, Yang Q, Friedman JM. Mortality in neurofibromatosis 1: an analysis using U.S. death certificates. Am J Hum Genet. 2001;68(5):1110–8. https://doi.org/10.1086/320121.
77. Friedman JM, Arbiser J, Epstein JA, Gutmann DH, Huot SJ, Lin AE, et al. Cardiovascular disease in neurofibromatosis 1: report of the NF1 cardiovascular task force. Genet Med. 2002;4(3):105–11. https://doi.org/10.1097/00125817-200205000-00002.
78. Pappachan JM, Raskauskiene D, Sriraman R, Edavalath M, Hanna FW. Diagnosis and management of pheochromocytoma: a practical guide to clinicians. Curr Hypertens Rep. 2014;16(7):442. https://doi.org/10.1007/s11906-014-0442-z.
79. Vlenterie M, Flucke U, Hofbauer LC, Timmers HJ, Gastmeier J, Aust DE, et al. Pheochromocytoma and gastrointestinal stromal tumors in patients with neurofibromatosis type I. Am J Med. 2013;126(2):174–80. https://doi.org/10.1016/j.amjmed.2012.07.022.
80. North KN, Riccardi V, Samango-Sprouse C, Ferner R, Moore B, Legius E, et al. Cognitive function and academic performance in neurofibromatosis. 1: consensus statement from the NF1 cognitive disorders task force. Neurology. 1997;48(4):1121–7.
81. Hyman SL, Shores A, North KN. The nature and frequency of cognitive deficits in children with neurofibromatosis type 1. Neurology. 2005;65(7):1037–44. https://doi.org/10.1212/01.wnl.0000179303.72345.ce.
82. Acosta MT, Gioia GA, Silva AJ. Neurofibromatosis type 1: new insights into neurocognitive issues. Curr Neurol Neurosci Rep. 2006;6(2):136–43.
83. Mautner VF, Kluwe L, Thakker SD, Leark RA. Treatment of ADHD in neurofibromatosis type 1. Dev Med Child Neurol. 2002;44(3):164–70.
84. Merker VL, McDannold S, Riklin E, Talaei-Khoei M, Sheridan MR, Jordan JT, et al. Health literacy assessment in adults with neurofibromatosis: electronic and short-form measurement using FCCHL and health LiTT. J Neuro-Oncol. 2017;136:335–42. https://doi.org/10.1007/s11060-017-2657-8.
85. Li W, Cui Y, Kushner SA, Brown RA, Jentsch JD, Frankland PW, et al. The HMG-CoA reductase inhibitor lovastatin reverses the learning and attention deficits in a mouse model of neurofibromatosis type 1. Curr Biol. 2005;15(21):1961–7. https://doi.org/10.1016/j.cub.2005.09.043.
86. Krab LC, de Goede-Bolder A, Aarsen FK, Pluijm SM, Bouman MJ, van der Geest JN, et al. Effect of simvastatin on cognitive functioning in children with neurofibromatosis type 1: a randomized controlled trial. JAMA. 2008;300(3):287–94. https://doi.org/10.1001/jama.300.3.287.

87. van der Vaart T, Plasschaert E, Rietman AB, Renard M, Oostenbrink R, Vogels A, et al. Simvastatin for cognitive deficits and behavioural problems in patients with neurofibromatosis type 1 (NF1-SIMCODA): a randomised, placebo-controlled trial. Lancet Neurol. 2013;12(11):1076–83. https://doi.org/10.1016/s1474-4422(13)70227-8.
88. Acosta MT, Kardel PG, Walsh KS, Rosenbaum KN, Gioia GA, Packer RJ. Lovastatin as treatment for neurocognitive deficits in neurofibromatosis type 1: phase I study. Pediatr Neurol. 2011;45(4):241–5. https://doi.org/10.1016/j.pediatrneurol.2011.06.016.
89. Payne JM, Barton B, Ullrich NJ, Cantor A, Hearps SJ, Cutter G, et al. Randomized placebo-controlled study of lovastatin in children with neurofibromatosis type 1. Neurology. 2016;87(24):2575–84. https://doi.org/10.1212/wnl.0000000000003435.
90. Ferner RE, Jackson MJ. Neurofibromatoses. In: Andermann F, Guerrini R, Shorvon SD, editors. The causes of epilepsy: common and uncommon causes in adults and children. Cambridge: Cambridge University Press; 2011. p. 183–8.
91. Ostendorf AP, Gutmann DH, Weisenberg JL. Epilepsy in individuals with neurofibromatosis type 1. Epilepsia. 2013;54(10):1810–4. https://doi.org/10.1111/epi.12348.
92. Hurtado B, Koepp MJ, Sander JW, Thompson PJ. The impact of levetiracetam on challenging behavior. Epilepsy Behav. 2006;8(3):588–92. https://doi.org/10.1016/j.yebeh.2006.01.003.
93. Uusitalo E, Rantanen M, Kallionpaa RA, Poyhonen M, Leppavirta J, Yla-Outinen H, et al. Distinctive cancer associations in patients with neurofibromatosis type 1. J Clin Oncol. 2016;34(17):1978–86. https://doi.org/10.1200/jco.2015.65.3576.
94. Seminog OO, Goldacre MJ. Risk of benign tumours of nervous system, and of malignant neoplasms, in people with neurofibromatosis: population-based record-linkage study. Br J Cancer. 2013;108(1):193–8. https://doi.org/10.1038/bjc.2012.535.
95. Evans DG. Are we ready for targeted early breast cancer detection strategies in women with NF1 aged 30-49 years? Am J Med Genet A. 2012;158a(12):3054–5. https://doi.org/10.1002/ajmg.a.35585.
96. Salvi PF, Lorenzon L, Caterino S, Antolino L, Antonelli MS, Balducci G. Gastrointestinal stromal tumors associated with neurofibromatosis 1: a single Centre experience and systematic review of the literature including 252 cases. Int J Surg Oncol. 2013;2013:398570. https://doi.org/10.1155/2013/398570.
97. Dayal Y, Tallberg KA, Nunnemacher G, DeLellis RA, Wolfe HJ. Duodenal carcinoids in patients with and without neurofibromatosis. A comparative study. Am J Surg Pathol. 1986;10(5):348–57.
98. Griffiths DF, Williams GT, Williams ED. Duodenal carcinoid tumours, phaeochromocytoma and neurofibromatosis: islet cell tumour, phaeochromocytoma and the von Hippel-Lindau complex: two distinctive neuroendocrine syndromes. Q J Med. 1987;64(245):769–82.
99. Garwood MM, Bernacki JM, Fine KM, Hainsworth KR, Davies WH, Klein-Tasman BP. Physical, cognitive, and psychosocial predictors of functional disability and health-related quality of life in adolescents with neurofibromatosis-1. Pain Res Treat. 2012;2012:975364. https://doi.org/10.1155/2012/975364.
100. Wolters PL, Burns KM, Martin S, Baldwin A, Dombi E, Toledo-Tamula MA, et al. Pain interference in youth with neurofibromatosis type 1 and plexiform neurofibromas and relation to disease severity, social-emotional functioning, and quality of life. Am J Med Genet A. 2015;167a(9):2103–13. https://doi.org/10.1002/ajmg.a.37123.

Brief Notes on Pregnancy, Prenatal Diagnosis, and Preimplantation Procedures in NF1

20

Gianluca Tadini and Donatella Milani

Contents

Few reports in literature have investigated pregnancy in NF1. Some of them remain anecdotal, other are small case series published many years ago regarding only severe cases in which are described a high rate of hypertension, preeclampsia, intrauterine growth restriction, preterm labor, and cesarean delivery in NF1 pregnancies [1, 2]. On the contrary, in 1996 a further study on 105 patients failed to confirm these data and more recent reviews in 2010 and 2017 dedicate to this topic only brief comments [3–5].

Nevertheless, Terry et al. in 2013 decided to fill this gap using a large population-based US national registry (United States National Inpatient Sample, NIS) to investigate pregnancy complications in women with NF1, collecting data from 1988 to

G. Tadini (✉)
Pediatric Dermatology Unit, Fondazione IRCCS Ca' Granda, Ospedale Maggiore Policlinico, Department of Physiopathology and Transplantation, Milan, Italy

Paediatric Highly Intensive Care Unit, Fondazione IRCCS Ca' Granda Ospedale Maggiore Policlinico, Milan, Italy

Center for Inherited Cutaneous Diseases, University of Milan, Milan, Italy
e-mail: gtadinicmce@unimi.it

D. Milani
Pediatric Dermatology Unit, Fondazione IRCCS Ca' Granda, Ospedale Maggiore Policlinico, Department of Physiopathology and Transplantation, Milan, Italy

G. Tadini et al. (eds.), *Multidisciplinary Approach to Neurofibromatosis Type 1*,
https://doi.org/10.1007/978-3-319-92450-2_20

Table 20.1 Odds ratio for outcomes of interest between NF1 patients and healthy controls

	NF1 (%)	Control (%)
Gestational hypertension	3.5	2.3
Preeclampsia	9.7	3.5
IUGR[a]	7.9	1.5
Preterm labor	12.4	6.9
Cesarean delivery	43.3	25.7
Stillbirth	0.9	0.5

[a] *IUGR* Intrauterine growth retardation

2009. During this period, NIS registered 19,750,702 pregnancy-related admissions and 1533 were associated with a diagnosis of NF1 [6].

Using data from this study, fertility seems to be normal in NF1 women and they will experience one or more pregnancies. Usually, higher mortality rate related to the disease does not comprise the reproductive years. NF1 pregnant women at the time of hospital admission were in majority between 20 and 35 years of age, 1 year younger than control population and they came from lower socio-economic group. Furthermore, they had a higher rate of pre-existing hypertension (4.7% vs 1.8%) and renal disease (0.8% vs 0.3%).

The odds ratio for outcomes of interest by at-risk group is presented in Table 20.1.

Moreover, NF1 patients experienced more commonly cerebrovascular events both during pregnancy and in the peripartum period. In contrast, no acute cardiac complications were observed and the in-hospital mortality rate was the same in two groups.

Data from Table 20.1 show clearly the higher rate of gestational hypertension and preeclampsia, IUGR, and preterm labor. Even analyzing NF1 group excluding patients with pre-existing hypertension and vascular renal disorders, the results confirm that higher risk of pregnancy complications is not due to pre-existing conditions.

Cesarean sections (43.3% vs 25.7%) were more frequent in NF1 population, even if the authors recommend being cautious analyzing this data because of the preference for more conservative management in NF1 patients even in the absence of complications.

In summary, we can consider that this large analysis (>1500 patients) identified increased risks for many complications that were unreported in previous literature and claimed for counsel in NF1 affected families planning for spontaneous or assisted conception. Furthermore, this study was unable to obtain information on neonatal course.

Finally, we have to remember that there are at least two well-established phenomena during NF1 pregnancy:

1. The increase in number and size of cutaneous neurofibromas and plexiform lesions during pregnancy
2. The rare presence of plexiform tumors on external genitalia and retroperitoneal and/or pelvic masses may interfere with the course of gestation and/or complicate delivery

20.1 Prenatal and Preimplantation Genetic Diagnosis

Also on this argument medical literature is far to be abundant. First, we have to underline that couples at risk for NF1 recur to the prenatal diagnosis (PD) rarely. PD is possible in NF1 families at risk only when molecular analysis reveals pathogenic variants. Usually, detection of family segregated mutation is performed using chorionic villi sample analysis and less frequently with fetal blood sampling [7, 8].

In a recent study performed in the Netherlands [9] analyzing molecular diagnosis of NF1 in a span of 18 years, about 2000 index cases were analyzed. Among them, 46 (2.4%) prenatal diagnoses were performed in 28 families at risk for NF1. Twenty-nine of forty-six index cases received a diagnosis of heterozygosity for the familial pathogenic mutation: from these data the authors emphasize there is a need for prenatal NF1 testing.

Ultrasound and RMI are also used in selected cases for prenatal diagnostic purposes [10].

Preimplantation genetic diagnosis (PDG) allows testing an embryo generated from in vitro fertilization before uterine transfer for specific mutations. In contrast, preimplantation genetic screening may detect chromosomal aneuploidies.

A recent study [11] on a cohort of 1356 embryos obtained from in vitro fertilizations at risk for NF1, 1322 were available for further studies and 1080 obtained a diagnosis. From these 1080 diagnoses, 483 were unaffected and 577 were affected with NF1. In the unaffected generated cycles, 22 had a confirmed unaffected live birth.

Finally, the association of pregnancy complications seen in NF1 women claims for adequate attention in patients who use assisted reproductive technologies because of the increased risk of multiple pregnancies.

Funding Sources None.

Conflict of Interest None declared.

References

1. Hagymasy L, Toth M, Szucs N, Rigo J Jr. Neurofibromatosis type 1 with pregnancy-associated renovascular hypertension and the syndrome of hemolysis, elevated liver enzymes ad low platelets. Am J Obstet Gynecol. 1998;179:272–4.
2. Agarwal U, Dahiya P, Sangwan K. Recent onset neurofibromatosis complicating eclampsia with maternal death: a case report. Arch Gynecol Obstet. 2003;268:241–2.
3. Dugoff L, Sujansky E. Neurofibromatosis type 1 in pregnancy. Am J Med Genet. 1996;66: 7–10.
4. Jett K, Friedman JM. Clinical and genetic aspects of neurofibromatosis 1. Genet Med. 2010;12:1–11.
5. Friedman JM. Neurofibromatosis 1. In: Adam MP, Ardinger HH, Pagon RA, Wallace SE, Bean LJH, Stephens K, Amemiya A, editors. GeneReviews®. Seattle: University of Washington; 1998. 1993–2018. [updated 2018 Jan 11].
6. Terry AR, Barker FG II, Leffert L, et al. Neurofibromatosis type 1 and pregnancy complications: a population-based study. Am J Obstet Gynecol. 2013;209:46.e1–8.

7. Chetty SP, Shaffer BL, Norton ME. Management of pregnancy in women with genetic disorders: part 2: inborn errors of metabolism, cystic fibrosis, neurofibromatosis type 1, and turner syndrome in pregnancy. Obstet Gynecol Surv. 2011;66(12):765–76.
8. Lin S, Wu J, Zhang Z, Ji Y, Fang Q, Chen B, Luo Y. Prenatal genetic diagnosis for a fetus with atypical neurofibromatosis type 1 microdeletion. Zhonghua Yi Xue Yi Chuan Xue Za Zhi. 2016;33(2):212–5.
9. Van Minkelen R, Van Bever Y, Kromosoeto JNR, Whitagen-Hermans CJ, Nieuwlaat A, Halley DJJ, van den Ouweland AMW. A clinical and genetic overview of 18 years neurofibromatosis type 1 molecular diagnostics in the Netherlands. Clin Genet. 2013;85:318–27.
10. McEwing RL, Joelle R, Mohlo M, Bernard JP, Hillion Y, Ville Y. Prenatal diagnosis of neurofibromatosis type 1: sonographic and MRI findings. Prenat Diagn. 2006;26:1110–4.
11. Merker VL, Murphy TP, Hughes JB, Muzikansky A, Hughes MR, Souter I, Plotkin SR. Outcomes of preimplantation genetic diagnosis in neurofibromatosis type 1. Fertil Steril. 2015;103:761–8.e1.

Proposal of New Diagnostic Criteria

21

Gianluca Tadini, Hilde Brems, and Eric Legius

Content

At the end of this book, we are aware of the fact that, despite NF1 is not a rare disease, there is a tendency to leave this "troublesome diagnosis" only to physicians working on dedicated centers and, notwithstanding a higher consciousness and raised knowledge from pediatricians, early diagnosis is reached in few cases.

As already stated, clear-cut demonstration show that in NF1 patients "new" clinical signs, coming directly from the observation of large series of patients, are available for this purpose.

G. Tadini (✉)
Pediatric Dermatology Unit, Fondazione IRCCS Ca' Granda, Ospedale Maggiore Policlinico, Department of Pathophysiology and Transplantation, Milan, Italy

Paediatric Highly Intensive Care Unit, Fondazione IRCCS Ca' Granda Ospedale Maggiore Policlinico, Milan, Italy

Center for Inherited Cutaneous Diseases, University of Milan, Milan, Italy
e-mail: gtadinicmce@unimi.it

H. Brems
Department of Human Genetics, Catholic University of Leuven, Leuven, Belgium

Department of Human Genetics O&N I, KU Leuven, Leuven, Belgium

E. Legius
Department of Human Genetics, Catholic University of Leuven, Leuven, Belgium

Center for Human Genetics, Universitaire Ziekenhuizen Leuven Center for Human Genetics, Leuven, Belgium

G. Tadini et al. (eds.), *Multidisciplinary Approach to Neurofibromatosis Type 1*,
https://doi.org/10.1007/978-3-319-92450-2_21

Table 21.1 Laboratory, cutaneous, and extra-cutaneous signs to discuss in order to revise the classical diagnostic criteria of NF1

From laboratory	Molecular analysis of the neurofibromatosis 1 gene
From imaging	Unidentified bright objects (UBOs) at MRI
Cutaneous signs	Juvenile xanthogranulomas Anemic nevus (nevus anemicus) Hypochromic macules Hyperpigmentation "Soft-touch" skin Vascular malformations ("blue-red" macules and cherry angiomas)
Extra-cutaneous signs	Choroidal nodules Elevated head circumference and hypertelorism (facies) The peculiar neuropsychological pattern (learning, speech, and behavioral disabilities) Headache and seizures Unidentified bright objects Endocrinological disorders (precocious puberty, short stature, deficient bone mineralization, vitamin D deficiency) Neoplasms (MPNST, CNS tumors) Cancer proneness

A critical revision of the classical grid of diagnostic criteria is now mandatory in order to actualize and mix together the "classical" diagnostic criteria and recent knowledge.

On the contrary, we can't deny that there is a sort of resistance in modifying such a well-established concepts, and for that reasons we propose to integrate and complete the grid and not to abruptly erase more than 30 years of medical history of neurofibromatosis 1.

In the following table, we try to resume all the notions exposed in previous chapters that will be the platform for further discussion about the revision of diagnostic criteria, useful for patients of all ages (Table 21.1).

In conclusion, the established diagnostic criteria may be very specific but, on the contrary, they are not enough sensitive being absent in infancy, leading to at best a delayed diagnosis and to all the clinical and psychological implications they have for the patients and their relatives.

Furthermore, many of the new diagnostic findings are not so specific, being present or associated with overlapping disorders (i.e., Legius syndrome, constitutional mismatch repair syndrome, and other rasopathies), although they could make the diagnostic pathway more sensitive.

After an "embryonic" meeting in Milan in winter 2014 and a first discussion in the Barcelona Neurofibromatoses Meeting in September 2015, the project of revision took place after 2 years under the supervision of Susan Huson, Eric Legius, Ludvine Messiaen, Gareth Evans, Scott Plotkin, and Pierre Wolkenstein in San Francisco in September 2017 at the NF Conference. This group of scientists formed a committee (early 2018) that proposed a first Delphi Process [1] with a target focused on neurofibromatois 1, Legius syndrome, neurofibromatosis 2, schwannomatosis and related mosaicisms with the aim to clarify the wording, to include molecular biology, to add new suggested criteria and to increase specificity and sensitivity.

The first DELPHI [1] Process questionnaire has been evaluated by the experts' groups in May 2018.

In June 2018 was held at Sloan Kettering Institute in New York a 3 days NF Criteria Reform Workshop, composed from experts' groups meeting in any special field, conclusion and recommendations from these experts' groups and a further synthesis of comments and suggestions were reached.

During summer 2018 a dense e-mail exchange and debates raised convergences and divergences and the committee created a second DELPHI Process questionnaire to be evaluated by the experts' group (October 2018) in order to have an acceptable synthesis of 2 years hard work to be proposed at the Global Joint Meeting in Paris in November 2018.

Here we report only the results and the proposed revised NF1 diagnostic criteria.

It must be noted that, contemporaneously, the second group of scientists lead by Gareth Evans and Scott Plotkin discussed the revision of definitions and criteria for NF2/schwannomatoses chapter. The results of this DELPHI process will not be reported here.

The guiding principles of the revision of the diagnostic criteria would:

1. Represent best consensus among NF1 experts
2. Address diagnostic rather than clinical management issues
3. Be broadly representative of medical specialties and national groups
4. Be accessible to generalists as well as NF specialists
5. Recognize advances in genetics over the last 30 years without requiring genetic analysis for diagnosis
6. Be valid in different countries and health care systems

General principles based on feedback from the two rounds of DELPHI Process and following debates are:

1. Keep criteria simple and easy to use for non-experts (NF1 experts do not need criteria for diagnosis)
2. No complicated explanations or "*" referral in the list of criteria
3. No A/B or minor/major criteria
4. Concern about sensitivity for diagnosis in children based on clinical findings, preferring overdiagnosis rather than missing a case (sensitivity > specificity), with the aim to diagnose young children as soon as possible for proper surveillance and clinical care
5. NF1 mutation analysis is not always readily available
6. Proper discussion and illustrations in a dedicated accompanying test with details on potential pitfalls

Table 21.2 Revised and approved new diagnostic criteria for NF1

Need ≥ 2 for diagnosis
Six or more café-au-lait spots • Greater than 5 mm in prepubertal children • Greater than 15 mm in postpubertal children
Bilateral freckles in axilla or groin
Two or more neurofibromas of any type or one plexiform neurofibroma
Two or more iris Lisch nodules **or two or more choroidal abnormalities**
Optic pathway glioma
A distinctive osseous lesion such as: Sphenoid wing dysplasia, **anterolateral bowing of tibia (tibial dysplasia), or pseudoarthrosis of a long bone**
A NF1 heterozygous pathogenic variant
A **parent** with NF1 by the above criteria

In **bold** the changes compared to the previous list of diagnostic criteria for NF1

We must underline that café-au-lait spots criterion remains unchanged as well as the criterion of neurofibromas and plexiform neurofibromas and optic way glioma.

On the contrary, revision of criteria modifies some of the previous or introduces new ones (Table 21.2):

New Criteria

1. *A NF1 heterozygous pathogenic variant*
   Recommendations:
   - Accept this definition as diagnostic criterion but not as "stand-alone criterion"
   - One additional criterion required
   - NF1 heterozygous mutation is used already in clinical practice for diagnostic purposes
   - Ninety-five percent support in DELPHI Process for adding mutation analysis to revised criteria
   - High sensitivity (>90%)
   - Pathogenicity of the single mutation should be determined by the proper criteria established by the professional societies
   - Mosaicism for a pathogenic mutation will be discussed separately in this text (see Chap. 3)
   - Still possible to diagnose NF1 based on clinical criteria with the same sensitivity as before
2. Two or more iris Lisch nodules *or two or more choroidal abnormalities* (see also Chap. 6)
   Recommendations:
   - Choroidal abnormalities (CAs) are defined as bright, patchy nodules investigated by "near infrared"(NIR) technique
   - CAs seem to be a more precocious sign compared to Lisch nodules
   - If Lisch nodules are present, there is no advantage to search for CAs also

- NIR technique assessment for CAs should be limited to cases of diagnostic uncertainty and where OCT scan can be easily obtained in the outpatient clinic (i.e., without sedation/anesthesia, related to the age of pediatric patients)

3. Osseous lesions:

Tibial dysplasia and/or pseudoarthrosis of a long bone is added to the sphenoid wing dysplasia as a new diagnostic criterion.

Modified Criteria

1. Criterion for "freckling" is modified introducing *"bilateral"* as a further characterization, in order to separate clearly the monolateral pattern typical of NF1 mosaic.
2. The last criterion in the new list is modified: *"parent"* substitutes "a 1st degree relative."

In conclusion, we remind that some of the proposed new clinical signs did not reach a unanimous consensus for different reasons among the experts to be introduced as new criteria, such as anemic nevus, UBOs, elevated head circumference, neuropsychological pattern, but in our opinion may help the clinicians for early diagnosis.

Funding Sources None.

Conflict of Interest None declared.

Reference

1. Humphrey-Murto S, Varpio L, Wood TJ, Gonsalves C, Ufholz LA, Mascioli K, Wang C, Foth T. The use of the Delphi and other consensus group methods in medical education research: a review. Acad Med. 2017;92(10):1491–8.

MIX
Papier aus verantwortungsvollen Quellen
Paper from responsible sources
FSC® C105338

If you have any concerns about our products,
you can contact us on
ProductSafety@springernature.com

In case Publisher is established outside the EU,
the EU authorized representative is:
Springer Nature Customer Service Center GmbH
Europaplatz 3, 69115 Heidelberg, Germany

Printed by Libri Plureos GmbH
in Hamburg, Germany